Sociocultural Issues in Psychiatry

Sociocultural Issues in Psychiatry

A Casebook and Curriculum

EDITED BY NHI-HA T. TRINH

AND

JUSTIN A. CHEN

Oxford University Press is a department of the University of Oxford. It furthers
the University's objective of excellence in research, scholarship, and education
by publishing worldwide. Oxford is a registered trade mark of Oxford University
Press in the UK and certain other countries.

Published in the United States of America by Oxford University Press
198 Madison Avenue, New York, NY 10016, United States of America.

Library of Congress Cataloging-in-Publication Data
Names: Trinh, Nhi-Ha, editor. | Chen, Justin A., editor.
Title: Sociocultural issues in psychiatry : a casebook and curriculum /
[edited by] Nhi-Ha T. Trinh, Justin A. Chen.
Description: Oxford ; New York : Oxford University Press, [2019] |
Includes bibliographical references and index.
Identifiers: LCCN 2018028701 | ISBN 9780190849986 (pbk. : alk. paper)
Subjects: | MESH: Community Psychiatry | Ethnopsychology |
Sociological Factors | Models, Psychological | Professional-Patient Relations
Classification: LCC RC455 | NLM WM 31 | DDC 616.89—dc23
LC record available at https://lccn.loc.gov/2018028701

9 8 7 6 5 4 3 2 1

Printed by Webcom, Inc., Canada

CONTENTS

FOREWORD

The American Psychiatric Association (APA) has four strategic priorities: advancing psychiatry, supporting research, educating about mental disorders, and supporting and increasing diversity. While diversity stands as a separate pillar, it is also a common thread across all the priorities, especially education.

Since its inception in 1974, APA's Division of Diversity and Health Equity has primarily focused on developing and educating a culturally competent workforce to meet the needs of minority and underserved populations. As early as 1969, APA's official policies included the "Position Statement on the Delineation of Transcultural Psychiatry as a Specialized Field of Study," and in 2013, APA's Board of Trustees reaffirmed the 1969 policy regarding the importance of cultural teaching with its "Position Statement on Cultural Psychiatry as a Specific Field of Study Relevant to the Assessment and Care of All Patients." Through many policies, strategies, and bylaws, the world's largest psychiatric organization executes its mission of providing cultural education to its 38,000 members.

In their textbook, Drs. Nhi-Ha Trinh and Justin Chen spotlight the importance and challenges of teaching cultural and social issues in medicine today. As the U.S. population continues to become more culturally diverse, "cultural psychiatry" will soon be synonymous with "U.S. psychiatry." Additionally, these ethnographic changes add complexity and numbers to people at the intersection of minority statuses or who have multiple social identities.

This textbook demonstrates that mental health providers can no longer understand culture as a unidimensional construct. Similarly, the latest *Diagnostic and Statistical Manual* (DSM) deepens our understanding of cultural psychiatry. DSM-5 provides greater utility than its predecessors by introducing a focus on cultural concepts of distress.

Today's generation of educators and mental health providers are required to be lifelong learners. They must commit to understanding many evolving areas relevant to cultural psychiatry, including social determinants of mental health, structural competency, cultural humility, minority stress theory, implicit bias, religion and sexuality, and the impact of patient–physician concordance. *Sociocultural Issues in Psychiatry* is timely for the well-prepared psychiatrist of today who is, at the same time, both culturally competent and curious.

Ranna Parekh, MD, MPH
Deputy Medical Director
Director, Diversity and Health Equity
American Psychiatric Association

CONTRIBUTORS

Gowri G. Aragam, MD
Resident, Adult Psychiatry
Adult Psychiatry Residency Training
    Program
Massachusetts General Hospital/
    McLean Hospital (MGH/McLean)
Boston, Massachusetts

Tony B. Benning, MBChB,
MSC, PGDIP, MRCPsych (UK),
FRCPC, PhD
Clinical Instructor in Psychiatry
Department of Medicine, University of
    British Columbia
Consultant Psychiatrist
Maple Ridge Mental Health Center and
    Ridge Meadows Hospital
Vancouver, British Columbia, Canada

Justin A. Chen, MD, MPH
Assistant Professor of Psychiatry
Harvard Medical School
Medical Director, Ambulatory
    Psychiatry Services
Massachusetts General Hospital
Boston, Massachusetts

Chun-Yi Joey Cheung, BS
Research Coordinator
Depression Clinical and Research
    Program
Department of Psychiatry
Massachusetts General Hospital
Boston, Massachusetts

Christine Crawford, MD, MPH
Fellow, Child and Adolescent Psychiatry
Division of Child and Adolescent
    Psychiatry
Department of Psychiatry
Massachusetts General Hospital
Boston, Massachusetts

Andrew Cruz, MD
Resident, Adult Psychiatry
Adult Psychiatry Residency Training
    Program
Massachusetts General Hospital/
    McLean Hospital (MGH/McLean)
Boston, Massachusetts

Jiaying Ding, MDiv
Graduate Student
Harvard Divinity School
Cambridge, Massachusetts

Erin C. Dunn, ScD, MPH
Assistant Professor of Psychiatry
 Harvard Medical School
Psychiatric and Neurodevelopmental
    Genetics Unit
Center for Genomic Medicine
Massachusetts General Hospital
Boston, Massachusetts

Anne Emmerich, MD
Instructor of Psychiatry
Harvard Medical School
Department of Psychiatry
Massachusetts General Hospital
Boston, Massachusetts

Andrea S. Heberlein, PhD
Senior Lecturer
Boston College
Chestnut Hill, Massachusetts

Esther Howe, BA
Program Coordinator
Depression Clinical and Research
    Program
Department of Psychiatry
Massachusetts General Hospital
Boston, Massachusetts

Josepha A. Immanuel, MD
Clinical Faculty
Baylor College of Medicine
Child, Adolescent and Adult
    Psychiatrist
Legacy Community Health
Houston, Texas

David Shumway Jones, MD, PhD
A. Bernard Ackerman Professor of the
    Culture of Medicine
Harvard University
Cambridge, Massachusetts

Maya Nauphal, BA
Research Coordinator
Depression Clinical and Research
    Program
Department of Psychiatry
Massachusetts General Hospital
Boston, Massachusetts

Kristen Nishimi, MPH
PhD Candidate
Department of Social and Behavioral
    Sciences
Harvard T.H. Chan School of
    Public Health
Psychiatric and Neurodevelopmental
    Genetics Unit
Center for Genomic Medicine
Massachusetts General Hospital
Boston, Massachusetts

Siobhan M. O'Neill, MD
Assistant Professor of Psychiatry
    (Part-Time)
Department of Psychiatry
Massachusetts General Hospital
Harvard Medical School
Boston, Massachusetts

Michaela Owusu, MD, MSc
Fellow, Child and Adolescent Psychiatry
Division of Child and Adolescent
    Psychiatry
Department of Psychiatry
Massachusetts General Hospital
Boston, Massachusetts

Christopher M. Palmer, MD
Assistant Professor of Psychiatry
Harvard Medical School
Director, Department of Postgraduate
    and Continuing Education
McLean Hospital
Belmont, Massachusetts

Ranna Parekh, MD, MPH
Deputy Medical Director
Director, Diversity and Health Equity
American Psychiatric Association
Washington, DC

Maria C. Prom, MD
Resident, Adult Psychiatry
Adult Psychiatry Residency Training
    Program
Massachusetts General Hospital/
    McLean Hospital (MGH/McLean)
Boston, Massachusetts

Judith Puckett, MD
Resident, Adult Psychiatry
Adult Psychiatry Residency Training
    Program
Massachusetts General Hospital/
    McLean Hospital (MGH/McLean)
Boston, Massachusetts

Kimberly L. Reynolds, MD
Assistant Professor of Clinical Pediatrics
University of Miami Miller School of
    Medicine
Pediatric Hospitalist
Holtz Children's Hospital at Jackson
    Memorial Medical Center
Miami, Florida

Kira Knight Rodriguez, MD, MS
Association of University Centers on
    Disabilities (AUCD) Diversity Fellow
Mailman Center for Child Development
University of Miami Miller School of
    Medicine
Miami, Florida

Loucresie Rupert, MD
Medical Director of Psychiatry
Winona Health
Adult, Child and Adolescent
    Psychiatrist
Insightful Consultant, LLC
 Winona, Minnesota

Lisa Sangermano, BA
Research Coordinator
Depression Clinical and Research
    Program
Department of Psychiatry
Massachusetts General Hospital
Boston, Massachusetts

Priya Sehgal, MD, MA
Child and Adolescent Psychiatry Fellow
Cambridge Health Alliance/Harvard
    Medical School
Cambridge, Massachusetts

Maya Son, MD
Resident, Adult Psychiatry
Adult Psychiatry Residency Training
    Program
Massachusetts General Hospital/
    McLean Hospital (MGH/McLean)
Boston, Massachusetts

Leslie Tarver, MD, MPH
Resident, Adult Psychiatry
Adult Psychiatry Residency Training
    Program
Massachusetts General Hospital/
    McLean Hospital (MGH/McLean)
Boston, Massachusetts

Julianne Torrence, LICSW
Director
Department of Performance and
    Quality Improvement
Connecticut Junior Republic
Litchfield, Connecticut

Nhi-Ha T. Trinh, MD, MPH
Assistant Professor of Psychiatry
Harvard Medical School
Director, Psychiatry Center for
    Diversity
Director of Multicultural Studies and of
    Clinical Services
Depression Clinical and Research
    Program
Department of Psychiatry
Massachusetts General Hospital
Boston, Massachusetts

Alexander C. Tsai, MD, PhD
Associate Professor of Psychiatry
Harvard Medical School
Department of Psychiatry
Massachusetts General Hospital
Boston, Massachusetts

Introduction to Sociocultural Psychiatry

NHI-HA T. TRINH, CHUN-YI JOEY CHEUNG,
AND JUSTIN A. CHEN ■

Psychiatry must learn from anthropology that culture does considerably more than shape illness as an experience, it shapes the very way we conceive of illness.

—ARTHUR KLEINMAN[1]

From its founding, the United States has been a country composed of people from diverse racial, ethnic, and cultural backgrounds. Furthermore, demographic shifts in the United States have recently accelerated; in the past 20 years, racial and ethnic minorities have increased from 19% to 27% of the U.S. population.[2-4] According to the U.S. Census Bureau, this growth is projected to continue; by 2044 the United States will become a "majority minority" nation, with the largest growth occurring among Hispanic and Asian populations.[2]

Race, ethnicity, and culture may all exert a tremendous impact on medical diagnosis, treatment, and outcomes. This is especially true in psychiatry, given the prominent role that culture plays in patients' interpretation and management of symptoms that fall within the affective, behavioral, and cognitive domains. Although an in-depth understanding of every culture is impossible, familiarity with some basic principles will help minimize cultural clashes and reduce the risk of compromised medical care.

KEY DEFINITIONS

Race is defined as a category of humankind that shares certain distinctive physical traits,[5] such as skin color, facial features, and stature. Most people think of race in biological terms; for more than 300 years, or since the era of white European colonialization of populations of color in the world, race has indeed served as the "premier source of human identity."[6] Anthropologists, sociologists, and many biologists now question the value of these categories and thus the value of race as a helpful biological concept.[7,8] Indeed, DNA studies have debunked race as a biological construct and more of a social construct, as less than 0.1% of all our DNA accounts for physical differences among people associated with racial differences.[8] However, because society has valued these physical differences, the classification of individuals based on physical characteristics has led societies to treat them differently—and unequally.

In contrast, *ethnicity* refers to a particular ethnic affiliation or group,[9] with the term *ethnic* relating to large groups of people classed according to common racial, national, tribal, religious, linguistic, or cultural origin or background ethnic minorities.[10] Thus, ethnic groups also are a social construct and have shared social, cultural, and historical experiences stemming from common national or regional backgrounds.

The term *culture* has multiple meanings. Culture can describe the beliefs, customs, and arts, of a particular society, group, place, or time; culture can be used as a synonym for a particular society that has its own beliefs, ways of life, and art, for example ; finally, culture can refer to a specific way of thinking, behaving, or working that exists in a place or organization.[11] Clearly certain ethnic or racial groups can have their own cultures, but the association is not always one to one; in addition, groups or organizations made up of multiple races or ethnicities can create their own culture, such as, for example, "American culture" or the culture of medicine.

Culture can thus be thought of as the collected body of beliefs, customs, and behaviors that a group of people acquire socially and transmit from one generation to another through symbols and shared meanings. It provides the tools by which members of a given society adapt to their physical environment, to their social environment, and to one another. It organizes groups of ready-made solutions to the problems and challenges that people often face. There are two levels of culture: physical and ideological.

Physical culture—including art, literature, architecture, tools, machines, food, clothing, and means of transportation—can be directly observed through the five senses and/or through items collected in a museum or recorded on film. The physical level of culture yields more easily to change and to adaptation than does the ideological level.

Ideological culture refers to aspects of culture that must be observed indirectly, usually through behaviors, including beliefs and values; reasons for holding some things sacred and others ordinary; the events and characteristics of which a society is proud or ashamed; and the sentiments that underlie patriotism or chauvinism. Religion, philosophy, psychology, literature, and the meanings that people give to symbols are all part of the ideological aspect of culture. Without some understanding of the ideological aspect of culture, it is difficult to understand the meaning of a group purely at the physical level.

One level above culture, *sociocultural* encompasses the combination of the cultural with the social, and hence a broader focus not just on race, ethnicity, or even a cultural group, but all of society and its structures, including, for instance, the institution of medicine, or the historical and political systems of the United States.

In this sociocultural context, a *minority group* is a part of a population differing from others in some characteristics and often subjected to different treatment.[12] Minority groups are differentiated from the social majority, defined as those who hold major positions of social power in a society. The differentiation can be based on one or more observable human characteristics, including ethnicity, race, religion, disability, gender, wealth, health, or sexual orientation, and may be enforced by law. The term is applied to various situations and civilizations within history despite its association with a numerical, statistical minority.[13]

SOCIOCULTURAL CHALLENGES IN CLINICAL PRACTICE

Understanding a patient's sociocultural background will aid in the delivery of high-quality care. However, a little knowledge can also be a dangerous thing. Variability among individuals is inevitable; a particular patient may not fit into a clinician's preconceived notion of his or her culture. Thus, the clinician must probe for clues regarding the patient's background while remaining flexible enough to recognize when a patient's behaviors and clinical presentation do not necessarily match what is expected. The clinician should be aware of his or her own feelings, biases, and preconceptions about other cultures. In addition, clinicians must assess the social context, including the impact of the hospital environment, the attitudes of the medical and ancillary care teams, and the patient's experience within the health care system. Mistrust of the health care system is common and may influence a patient's behavior, level of cooperation, and adherence to treatment.

Furthermore, disparities in health care delivery have been well documented and are influenced by factors such as gender, race, ethnicity, and culture. The 2001 Surgeon General's report "Culture, Race, and Ethnicity" documented the existence of striking disparities for racial, ethnic, and other minorities as compared to white populations in mental health care. In sum, the report found that compared to whites, racial and ethnic minorities have reduced access to mental health services, are less likely to receive needed care, and receive lesser-quality care—if they were to receive mental health care at all. The supplement to the Surgeon General's report suggested multiple reasons for these disparities on various levels—structural, financial, and individual. Rather than operating independently, these factors may intersect, resulting in minorities' failing to receive adequate screening and care for mental health diagnoses and, therefore, presenting for treatment only at later or more severe stages. The Federal Collaborative for Health Disparities Research listed mental health disparities as one of its top research priorities in 2006, underscoring the gravity of the problem.[14]

NEED FOR SOCIOCULTURAL EDUCATION

To meet the needs of the growing minority and underserved populations, clinicians must be educated and well versed in the skills and strategies needed to provide culturally respectful and relevant care for their patients. While the demographic profile of patients is changing rapidly, the demographic profile of mental health professionals is changing more slowly.[15] For instance, a 2013 survey found that a majority of psychologists were white and female (83% and 68.3%). Between 2005 and 2013, the percentage of racial and ethnic minority groups within the psychology workforce grew from 8.9% to 16.4%; this is significantly behind the 39.6% of the overall workforce from racial/ethnic minority backgrounds, and the 25.8% in the general doctoral/professional workforce.[16] Despite these advances, rates of Asian American, Black, and Latino American psychologists have continued to remain low (4.3%, 5.3%, and 5% respectively in 2016).[17] Similarly, in 2013, the racial and ethnic breakdown of U.S. physicians in practice was non-Hispanic white (43.0%), Hispanic or Latino (4.0%), Black or African American (3.7%), Asian (10.9%), and Native American/Alaskan Native (0.3%).[18] For U.S.-trained psychiatrists, the numbers of minorities are even lower than those in the overall U.S. physician workforce.[19,20] For social workers, the situation is slightly less dire; in 2015, 67.3% of social workers were white, 23.3% were Black, and 5.3% were Asian Americans.[21]

In a survey of 689 psychologists, the majority of whom were white, more than 80% reported discussing racial or ethnic differences in at least one cross-racial therapeutic encounter in the previous two years.[22] Yet they also reported that racial or ethnic differences were discussed in less than half of all cross-racial clinical sessions, a finding that is particularly surprising because racial and ethnic identity is central to an individual's experience in the world, similar to sexual or gender identity. Understanding a racial or ethnic minority individual's cultural identity may be crucial to developing a therapeutic alliance and treatment plan. Indeed, with the demographic composition of the United States rapidly evolving, ongoing efforts should be made to increase both the diversity of the physician workforce and the capacity and skill of providers to deliver quality health care for diverse patient populations. Training focused on fostering an attitude of cultural respect will help equip providers for this challenge. Efforts to create and recruit a diverse psychiatric workforce should proceed in tandem with efforts to cultivate a culturally respectful psychiatric workforce.[20]

FROM CULTURAL COMPETENCE TO CULTURAL HUMILITY

Because of this, the term "cultural competence" has become *au courant*, as a clinical solution to bridge the disparities in access and treatment for depression for racial and ethnic minorities specifically, given how central racial and ethnic minority status may inform one's cultural identity. And yet individuals can belong to several cultural groups based on their racial, ethnic, religious, or family backgrounds.[11] Thus cultural competency can be defined as "a set of congruent behaviors, attitudes, and policies that come together in a system, agency or among professionals and enable that system, agency or those professions to work effectively in cross-cultural situations."[23]

Cultural competency encompasses systems as well as individual therapeutic encounters. Betancourt and colleagues[24] define three levels for cultural competence interventions: organizational (leadership/workforce), structural (processes of care), and clinical (provider–patient encounter). They note that at the clinical level, training has often focused on a categorical approach that involves ascribing attitudes, values, beliefs, and behaviors to broad cultural groups, which may lead to stereotyping. Combining knowledge-based training with training in cross-cultural communication allows for a more nuanced understanding of how cultural content may or may not be relevant to individuals. There is some evidence that cultural competence training can lead to increased knowledge and awareness among providers, but it is unclear at this point whether training also improves patient outcomes, and more research is needed in this area.

Cultural competence is not uniformly accepted as a core competency in therapy. Sue and colleagues[25] summarize debates on the utility of cultural competence through a series of questions. These include whether cultural competence stereotypes minorities, discriminates against other types of diverse identities such as social class or sexual orientation, overemphasizes external factors such as discrimination at the expense of intrapsychic factors, and creates pressure on therapists to ascribe to cultural competency in order to be viewed as nonracist. The authors respond to these debates by noting that the debates tend to oversimplify the concept of cultural competence and ignore a more nuanced perspective, which includes a focus on multiple intersecting identities and an acknowledgment of intrapersonal, interpersonal, and societal influences on the lives of our patients. Ultimately, the authors argue that cultural competence is necessary as a response to a historical context that has resulted in systematic bias against the inclusion of culturally specific experiences in therapy.

At the same time, however, research has been limited on how such interventions improve patient outcomes in racial and ethnic minority groups. In one review article, which aimed to evaluate the effect of cultural competence trainings on patient, professional, and organizational outcomes, researchers found no evidence of improved treatment outcomes or evaluations of care based on cultural competence interventions.[26] In addition, they found that none of the studies evaluated potential adverse events of such interventions. Therefore, while there have been initiatives to address these issues of clinician bias and discriminatory behavior within the health care system through education, the efficacy of these interventions is yet to be determined. Future research must focus on how to better design and evaluate cultural competence interventions.

Qureshi and colleagues[27] note that the term "cultural competence" itself may obscure important distinctions in the types of barriers faced by racial, ethnic, and other minority patients. A focus on culture may pertain to differences in understanding and expressing symptoms, as well as how preferences for treatment are developed and communicated. However, the authors also argue that racial and ethnic bias, discrimination, financial or structural barriers presented by poverty, immigrant status, and other experiences linked to minority status are not "cultural" but rather structural challenges disproportionately experienced by members of nonwhite racial and ethnic groups.

Clinicians must therefore be prepared to address a wide range of possible experiences impacting their patients; however, many current training models focus primarily on acquiring knowledge rather than on developing skills or examining attitudes, which ultimately may prove more useful. Thus "cultural humility" is the "ability to maintain an interpersonal stance that is open in relation to aspects of cultural identity that are most important to the patient."[28] Culturally humble clinicians can express respect and a lack of superiority with regard to the patient's culture; they do not assume competence in terms of working with a particular patient simply based on prior experience with other patients from similar backgrounds.

Indeed, providers who self-identify as being of a minority background may understand their own personal culture but may not understand every culture, or even that of an individual patient sharing their same cultural background. Therefore, it is equally fundamental for providers, regardless of identity or background, to cultivate cultural humility as a lifelong practice.

ORIGIN AND DEVELOPMENT OF THE SOCIOCULTURAL CURRICULUM

The Massachusetts General Hospital (MGH)/McLean Hospital Adult Psychiatry Residency's Sociocultural Psychiatry Curriculum had its origins in 1992 under the leadership of Dr. David Henderson, who sought to create a residency didactics curriculum to focus on social and cultural issues with the goal that these aspects would be integrated into every residency lecture—for example, on bipolar disorder, schizophrenia, and anxiety disorders. Dr. Henderson found that most teaching faculty were reluctant to address these topics themselves due to their feeling of not being "experts" on culture. As a result, this curriculum continued, with subsequent course directors adding their specific focus to the series. Dr. Anne Becker, trained in both anthropology and psychiatry, brought an additional focus on global psychiatry; Dr. Siobhan O'Neill meanwhile incorporated her own interest in religion and spirituality. By the time Dr. Nhi-Ha Trinh took the series as a resident in 2002–2006 and then became course director in 2008, the series had grown both unwieldy as well as somewhat "tokenist"—although there was a robust series on religion and spirituality, "cultural issues" writ large were relegated to two lectures on ethnopsychopharmacology by Dr. Henderson as well as three lectures on Asian American, Latino American, and African American mental health. Dr. Trinh was interested in adding a focus on resident self-reflection in the spirit of developing attitudes of cultural humility; she was also interested in making the series more clinically relevant by adding opportunities for resident case discussion.

As part of a curriculum overhaul for the entire residency didactic curriculum in 2013, "content teams" of teaching faculty and interested trainees were formed to reexamine the content, depth, and breadth of residency education. Dr. Trinh was joined by Dr. Justin Chen and Dr. Chris Palmer, as well as trainees at the time, such as Drs. Mimi Owusu, Christine Crawford, and Maithri Amereskere, to critically examine the scope of the series. The content team recommended expanding the scope of the series to become longitudinal, spanning postgraduate year 1 (PGY-1) through PGY-3, and more than doubling the number of hours from 9 to 19. In addition, the arc of the curriculum was developmentally tailored to budding psychiatry residents as they progressed through training.

Box 1.1 lists the course objectives and Box 1.2 lists the lectures for the series. Both course directors (NHT and JC) teach the four PGY-1 lectures, which occur back to back, in order to develop a relationship with residents early on and to foster trust by creating a safe, confidential space where respect for diversity of opinions is encouraged. The course directors attempt to model the type of introspection and vulnerability they hope the residents themselves will demonstrate by using hefty doses of self-disclosure, humor, and validation. The course directors also lead certain PGY-2 and PGY-3 discussions, and one course director endeavors to be present at

Box 1.1.

MGH-MᴄLᴇᴀɴ Aᴅᴜʟᴛ Pꜱʏᴄʜɪᴀᴛʀʏ Pʀᴏɢʀᴀᴍ, Sᴏᴄɪᴏᴄᴜʟᴛᴜʀᴀʟ Sᴇʀɪᴇꜱ: Cᴏᴜʀꜱᴇ Oʙᴊᴇᴄᴛɪᴠᴇꜱ

Course Directors: Nhi-Ha Trinh, MD, MPH, and Justin Chen, MD, MPH

PGY-1 Course Objectives, Sociocultural Series
By the end of the PGY-1 series, residents will be able to recognize personal cultural influences and how these might impact the psychiatric clinical encounter by:

1) Defining the concepts of culture, minority status, and privilege.
2) Describing their multidimensional cultural identity.
3) Applying a multidimensional cultural perspective in clinical encounters.

PGY-2 Course Objectives, Sociocultural Series
By the end of the PGY-2 series, residents will be able to demonstrate the influence of "culture," broadly conceived, on psychiatric practice by:

1) Identifying three challenges of defining psychiatric illness using global psychiatric epidemiology techniques.
2) Listing three social determinants of psychiatric illness in the United States.
3) Understanding and applying the DSM-5's approach to culture, including specific tools such as the Cultural Formulation Interview.

PGY-3 Course Objectives, Sociocultural Series
By the end of the PGY-3 series, residents will be able to reflect on how psychiatry has been impacted by larger systems (historical precedent, medical practice), and the impact of categories of race, ethnicity, sexuality, socioeconomic status, gender, et cetera by:

1) Describing two historical controversies and two current critiques of psychiatry.
2) Defining minority stress theory, internalized prejudice, and their links to psychiatric illness and practice.
3) Utilizing advanced interviewing techniques to address cultural clinical impasses.

---

each of the sessions led by other faculty in an attempt to "keep a pulse" on the series for any given class.

In PGY-1, the focus is on grounding residents in an attitude of cultural humility and self-reflection. In PGY-2, the series focus shifts to grounding residents in the broader base of sociocultural psychiatry knowledge and key concepts in cross-cultural psychiatry, including social determinants of mental health, global psychiatric epidemiology, defining the line between psychiatric health and illness, and a description of how culture is addressed in the *Diagnostic and Statistical Manual of Mental Disorders* (DSM). A final interactive lecture based on the residents' own clinical cases rounds out this year of the series and serves to bring the preceding topics together. As residents become more clinically advanced and sophisticated in their

Box 1.2.

MGH-McLean Adult Psychiatry Program, Sociocultural Series: Lectures

Course Directors: Nhi-Ha Trinh, MD, MPH, and Justin Chen, MD, MPH

PGY-1 lectures (4 hours) (Nhi-Ha Trinh, MD, MPH, and Justin Chen, MD, MPH)

1. Introduction to the Sociocultural Psychiatry Lecture Series: What's in a name?
2. Culture as multidimensional construct
3. Cultural self-reflection
4. Addressing culture through clinical cases

PGY-2 lectures (6 hours)

1. The other side of normal (Jordan Smoller, MD, ScD)
2. Global psychiatric epidemiology (Alexander Tsai, MD, PhD)
3. Social determinants of psychiatric illness (Erin Dunn, ScD)
4. Culture and psychiatry (Justin Chen, MD, MPH)
5. Disparities in mental health: A case for the DSM-5 Outline for Cultural Formulation and Cultural Formulation Interview (Nhi-Ha Trinh, MD, MPH)
6. Clinical cases through the lens of culture (Justin Chen, MD, MPH, and Nhi-Ha Trinh, MD, MPH)

PGY-3 (9 hours, including three 2-hour workshops)

1–2. Religion and spirituality seminar (2-hour workshop) (Siobhan O'Neill, MD)
3. History of mistakes in psychiatry (Harrison Pope, MD, MPH)
4. Criticisms of psychiatry (David Jones, MD, PhD)
5. Minority stress theory and internalized prejudice (Christine Crawford, MD, MPH)
6–7. When race gets personal in the hospital (2-hour workshop) (Nhi-Ha Trinh, MD, MPH, and Justin Chen, MD, MPH)
8–9. Credibility vs. over-identification in the psychiatric encounter, a.k.a. "You don't know my life" (2-hour workshop) (Chris Palmer, MD, and Nhi-Ha Trinh, MD, MPH)

---

understanding during PGY-3, the series once again shifts to address clinical and ethical challenges through experiential workshops that focus on religion and spirituality, cultural dilemmas between clinicians and patients, and discussions on the impact of the checkered history of psychiatry as well as critics of the field—the latter emphasizing the fact that psychiatry itself represents its own culture, with unique historical influences, thought patterns, and behaviors. Taken together, the series endeavors to fulfill the course objectives outlined while providing opportunity for interactive discussion and self-reflection.

OVERVIEW OF THE VOLUME

Mirroring the structure of the longitudinal sociocultural psychiatry curriculum used in this program, this textbook is designed to take the reader along an arc from more conceptual topics at the beginning to more specific exploration of clinical issues and dilemmas toward the end. The opening chapters focus on big-picture concepts: defining culture as a multidimensional construct, reviewing the role of culture in DSM-5, exploring the principles of global psychiatric epidemiology, and providing an overview of the social determinants of mental health. While some of these topics may seem basic, the editors have previously been frustrated by a lack of engaging, accessible, and succinct articles or publications that summarize these key concepts in a manner that can be used among mental health trainees and clinicians in a practical manner. The current textbook attempts to remedy this deficit.

The next several chapters dive into somewhat more controversial and complex territory, with a consideration of the field of psychiatry as a culture unto itself, an introduction to the concepts of minority stress theory and intersectionality, and an overview and practical guide for working with diverse patient explanatory models of illness. This section of the textbook benefits greatly from the traditions of other disciplines such as history of medicine, sociology, and anthropology to expand the understanding and worldview of learners, while still remaining firmly grounded within the context and practice of psychiatry through the use of real-world clinical examples.

Following these discussions, the important sociocultural concepts of religion/spirituality and gender/sexuality are highlighted with their own chapters. In both cases, concepts of "normal vs. abnormal" and the often blurry line between pathology and culturally acceptable behavior are explored. The next chapter delves further into the influential and expanding knowledge base surrounding implicit bias, with a specific emphasis on the role of clinicians' unconscious stereotyping in the care they provide.

The textbook's two penultimate chapters dive headlong into trickier clinical territory. Dr. Reynolds and colleagues explore the challenges that arise when patients request providers of a specific race, religion, gender, or language, and discuss the various historical, ethical, patient-related, and organizational factors that must be considered when deciding whether to accommodate such requests. Meanwhile, Dr. Immanuel and colleagues take a deeper dive into three more in-depth clinical cases that highlight the difficulty of navigating cultural challenges within patient–clinician dyads.

The textbook closes with a chapter that describes sociocultural psychiatry curricula nationwide and proposes a framework for incorporating this important topic into lifelong learning. While this textbook's chapters roughly correspond to the lectures in the MGH/McLean psychiatry residency's longitudinal curriculum, it is by no means meant to serve as the only possible template for educators wishing to establish their own curricula on this topic. Due to the very nature of sociocultural issues in psychiatry, any curriculum on the subject should ideally be tailored to the particular knowledge/readiness of residents, patient populations, community needs, and local context, as well as of course the availability of faculty to facilitate these often confronting and challenging conversations.

FINAL NOTES: STRUCTURAL COMPETENCY AND TERMINOLOGY

Emerging trends in the fields of medical education have increasingly focused on "structural competency" of clinicians as an important framework for addressing disparities in clinical care. Structural competency is defined as "the ability for health professionals to recognize and respond with self-reflexive humility and community engagement to the ways negative health outcomes and lifestyle practices are shaped by larger socioeconomic, cultural, political, and economic forces."[29] This represents a recent shift in medical education "toward attention to forces that influence health outcomes at levels above individual interactions."[30] More work will be needed to fully develop curricula to address structural competency for trainees, as well as continuing education for clinicians in practice. The editors of this volume wholeheartedly agree with and support the emphasis on structural competency; at the same time, this volume intentionally focuses on the enhancement of clinical care and practice through honing skills and attitudes relevant to care of individual patients of diverse cultural backgrounds. While this book does touch upon on some of the social determinants of health, as well as historical, social, and global forces shaping psychiatry, it does not primarily focus on structures. The editors believe this is a case of "both/and" rather than "either/or"; mental health trainees can and should understand both structural and cultural contributions to health and illness.

Finally, although key concepts are defined, some variation in terminology may occur from chapter to chapter, reflecting the diversity of the field and the academic orientations of the chapter authors. For instance, terms such as provider, clinician, or psychiatrist may be used; similarly, Black versus African American, or Hispanic versus Latino may appear in the chapters. As much as possible, chapter authors have been asked to define terms used and to be consistent throughout. As reflected in the diverse terminology and perspectives presented, the field of sociocultural psychiatry is filled with both lively discussion and often fractious commentary. The intent of this volume is to highlight for the reader overarching themes in sociocultural psychiatry to enrich clinical practice, with the intent of illuminating the full spectrum of human experience.

REFERENCES

1. Kleinman, A. (1977). Depression, somatization, and the new cross-cultural psychiatry. *Social Science and Medicine, 11*, 3–10.
2. Colby, S. L., & Ortman, J. M. (2017). Projections of the size and composition of the U.S. population: 2014 to 2060. U.S. Census Bureau. Retrieved from: http://wedocs.unep.org/bitstream/handle/20.500.11822/20152/colby_population.pdf?sequence=1
3. U.S. Census Bureau. (2012). Section 1. Population. In *Statistical abstract of the United States*. Retrieved from: https://www.census.gov/library/publications/2011/compendia/statab/131ed/population.html
4. U.S. Census Bureau. (2018). QuickFacts: United States. Retrieved from: https://www.census.gov/quickfacts/fact/table/US/PST045217
5. Race. (n.d.). In *Merriam-Webster dictionary*. Retrieved from: https://www.merriam-webster.com/dictionary/race

6. Smedley, A. (2008). "Race" and the construction of human identity. *American Anthropologist, 100*(3), 690–702.

7. Barkan, S. E. (2011). 10.2. The meaning of race and ethnicity. In *Sociology: Understanding and changing the social world*. Retrieved from: http://open.lib.umn.edu/sociology/chapter/10-2-the-meaning-of-race-and-ethnicity/

8. Begley, S. (2008, Feb. 29). Race and DNA. *Newsweek*. Retrieved from: http://www.newsweek.com/race-and-dna-221706

9. Ethnicity. (n.d.). In *Merriam-Webster dictionary*. Retrieved from: https://www.merriam-webster.com/dictionary/ethnicity

10. Smedley, B. D., Stith, A. Y., & Nelson, A. R.; Institute of Medicine Committee on Understanding and Eliminating Racial and Ethnic Disparities in Health Care. (2003). *Unequal treatment: Confronting racial and ethnic disparities in health care*. Washington, DC: National Academies Press, 191.

11. Culture. (n.d.). In *Merriam-Webster dictionary*. Retrieved from: https://www.merriam-webster.com/dictionary/culture

12. Minority. (n.d.). In *Merriam-Webster dictionary*. Retrieved from: https://www.merriam-webster.com/dictionary/minority

13. Barzilai, G. (2010). *Communities and law: Politics and cultures of legal identities*. Ann Arbor: University of Michigan Press.

14. Safran, M. A., Mays Jr, R. A., Huang, L. N., McCuan, R., Pham, P. K., Fisher, S. K., . . . Trachtenberg, A. (2009). Mental health disparities. *American Journal of Public Health, 99*(11), 1962–1966.

15. U.S. Census Bureau. (2010). Census 2010 News. Retrieved from: https://www.census.gov/2010census/news/press-kits/demographic-profiles.html

16. American Psychiatric Association. (2018, January 11). 2005-13: Demographics of the U.S. psychology workforce. Retrieved from: http://www.apa.org/workforce/publications/13-demographics/index.aspx

17. American Psychiatric Association. (2018, March 26). CWS Data Tool: Demographics of the U.S. psychology workforce. Retrieved from: http://www.apa.org/workforce/data-tools/demographics.aspx

18. Nivet, M. A., & Castillo-Page, L. (2014). Diversity in the physician workforce: Facts & figures 2014. Association of American Medical Colleges. Retrieved from: https://www.aamc.org/data/workforce/reports/439214/workforcediversity.html

19. Brotherton, S. E., Rockey, P. H., & Etzel, S. I. (2005). US graduate medical education, 2004-2005: Trends in primary care specialties. *Journal of American Medical Association, 294*(9), 1075–1082.

20. Lokko, H. N., Chen, J. A., Parekh, R. I., & Stern, T. A. (2016). Racial and ethnic diversity in the US psychiatric workforce: A perspective and recommendations. *Academic Psychiatry, 40*(6), 898–904.

21. Data USA. (2018, March 26). Social workers. Retrieved from: https://datausa.io/profile/soc/211020/#demographics

22. Maxie, A. C., Arnold, D. H., & Stephenson, M. (2006). Do therapists address ethnic and racial differences in cross-cultural psychotherapy? *Psychotherapy: Theory, Research, Practice, Training, 43*(1), 85.

23. NCCC. (2018, March 26). Curricula enhancement module series. Retrieved from: https://nccc.georgetown.edu/curricula/culturalcompetence.html

24. Betancourt, J. R., Green, A. R., Carrillo, J. E., & Ananeh-Firempong, O. (2003). Defining cultural competence: A practical framework for addressing racial/ethnic disparities in health and health care. *Public Health Reports, 118*(4), 293–302.

25. Sue, D. W. (1994). Asian-American mental health and help seeking be-havior: Comments on Solberg et al. (1994), Tata and Leong (1994), and Lin (1994). *Journal of Counselling Psychology*, *41*, 280–287.

26. Horvat, L., Horey, D., Romios, P., & Kis-Rigo, J. (2014). Cultural competence educa-tion for health professionals. *Cochrane Database Systematic Reviews*, *5*, CD009405.

27. Qureshi, A., Collazos, F., Ramos, M., & Casas, M. (2008). Cultural competency training in psychiatry. *European Psychiatry*, *23*, 49–58.

28. Hook, J. N., Davis, D. E., Owen, J., Worthington, E. L., & Utsey, S. O. (2013). Cultural humility: Measuring openness to culturally diverse clients. *Journal of Counselling Psychology*, *60*(3), 353–366.

29. Bourgois, P., Holmes, S. M., Sue, K., & Quesada, J. (2017). Structural vulnera-bility: Operationalizing the concept to address health disparities in clinical care. *Academic Medicine*, *92*(3), 299–307.

30. Neff, J., Knight, K. R., Satterwhite, S., Nelson, N., Matthews, J., & Holmes, S. M. (2017). Teaching structure: A qualitative evaluation of a structural competency training for resident physicians. *Journal of General Internal Medicine*, *32*(4), 430–433.

2

Culture as a Multidimensional Construct

ANNE EMMERICH AND LESLIE TARVER ■

CASE

Mr. A, a 25-year-old graduate student from China studying in the United States, was brought to the hospital after becoming agitated on a flight, insisting he was an important government official. He was taken to a Catholic hospital, where he was found to be manic and was transferred to the inpatient psychiatric unit, where he was assigned to the team of a Chinese American attending physician. The team appreciated that the attending physician spoke the patient's native language as the patient did not speak English. The physician spoke to the patient's parents in China by phone and communicated that he understood how hard it was for them to acknowledge their son's mental illness as he had also grown up in China and felt this gave him cultural competence. The patient's mania subsided quickly with medication treatment and the team began to discuss discharge. However, at this point the patient became increasingly depressed. One day he was found trying to cut his wrist with a plastic knife from his lunch tray. The team felt this was all an expectable depressive swing in a patient with bipolar disorder, and further medication adjustments were made. However, the patient became increasingly isolative. One day while the attending physician was off the unit at a conference, the medical student interviewed the patient through an interpreter and learned that while in the United States studying the patient had allowed himself to explore his sexual identity and had dated other men. He was nearing the end of his time in the United States and was feeling increasing stress about returning to China, where he felt he would never again be able to live as a gay man. When asked why he had not revealed this earlier to the team, the patient replied that the attending physician had not asked him about his sexual or gender identity. The patient felt that the fact the physician had not asked him about his sexual or gender identity was because the Chinese physician also held negative feelings about homosexuality, the way the patient's Chinese father did.

INTRODUCTION

The United States is becoming an increasingly pluralistic society, with an increasing proportion of younger Americans identifying as racially nonwhite or of mixed-race ancestry.[1] In contrast, the demographic profile of mental health professionals is changing slowly. A 2016 survey showed that the majority of practicing psychologists were white and female (84% and 65%, respectively). Despite advances, rates of Asian, Black, and Latino psychologists remained low (4%, 4%, and 5%, respectively).[2]

Our cultural identity is multifaceted, encompassing our age, race, gender, sexual orientation, religion, national origin, socioeconomic status, body size, health status, and more. Each individual has a unique sense of which aspects of cultural identity are central to sense of self at any particular moment in life. Clinicians and patients bring these dynamic conceptualizations of cultural identity to the clinical encounter, often without conscious awareness that these might influence their interaction.

As we approach the third decade of the 21st century, understanding the multidimensional aspects of cultural identity and developing cross-cultural communication skills are important goals for all Americans. For those of us to whom society has entrusted the work of helping others recover from psychological trauma and illness, these skills are not only desirable but arguably part of our ethical responsibility, explicitly mentioned in the American Counseling Association[3] and American Psychological Association[4] codes of ethics. As clinicians, the first step in this work is understanding ourselves.

In this chapter, we discuss the concepts of culture and cultural self-awareness. First, we offer a discussion of the overall concept of culture. This is followed by a discussion of the relevance of the theme of culture in clinical settings. The third section focuses on cultural identity development and related concepts. In the fourth section, we outline ways that clinicians can undertake their own cultural self-assessment, and offer autognostic prompts that clinicians can use in this regard.

CULTURE

Culture can refer to people who have always lived together in one place, such as an island in the Pacific Ocean, or to people who have only just met but share something in common such as size, sexual orientation, career, or hobby. It can refer to people who have never met but identify with shared traditions of religion or ancestral heritage.

The modern concept of culture originated in the field of anthropology,[5] where culture has been defined as "The system of shared beliefs, values, customs, behaviors, and artifacts that the members of society use to cope with their world and with one another, and that are transmitted from generation to generation through learning."[6] This learning can involve material objects, verbal and written history, and ritual practices.

Although the concept of culture has its origins in anthropology, even within this field there has been an evolution of the definition of culture over time. In the past, culture was thought to be determinative of behavior.[7] A shift in thought has led to the belief that one's individual culture is a replicate of the larger social and cultural entity. Culture is now viewed less as something that integrates people, and more in terms of the outcome of interactions. As Cohen describes, it is the "means by which we make meaning, with which we make the world meaningful to ourselves, and ourselves meaningful to the world."[7]

The term "culture" has been defined and redefined by various disciplines, including sociology, political theory, and minority studies. It is now understood that cultural identity is multidimensional and dynamic, potentially changing many times throughout an individual's lifespan. This concept can be challenging for medical practitioners who have been trained to think of a patient's cultural identity as a static or fixed risk factor for illness.

In the 19th and 20th centuries there was debate over whether cultural characteristics were tied to genetic differences. These ideas appealed to individuals and groups with racist tendencies, such as those who promoted the idea of eugenics, both in the United States and Germany, who hoped this practice would result in the elimination of "undesirable groups" through sterilization.[8] Late in the 20th century, the Human Genome Project proved that the broad racial and ethnic differences that humans notice are not evident at the genomic level. Humans are more alike than different genetically, regardless of striking racial or cultural differences. In a 2002 article "Race, Ethnicity, and Genomics: Social Classifications as Proxies of Biological Heterogeneity," Morris Foster and Richard Sharp wrote, "Today nearly all geneticists reject the idea that biological differences belie racial and ethnic distinctions. Geneticists have abandoned the search for 'Indian' or 'African' genes, for example, and few if any accept racial typologies."[9]

It is now commonly accepted that race is a social construct.[10] How we view or define ourselves and how we view or define others depends on factors such as where we live, when we live, and with whom we live. The American neuroscientist Robert Sapolsky says, "Humans universally make us/them dichotomies . . .We do so with remarkable speed and neurobiological efficiency."[11] In their ethnographic study of Korean American college students, many of whom considered themselves Korean or Korean American rather than American despite living in the United States their entire lives, Euichal Jung and Changho Lee write, "Identity is regarded as a cultural and historical product of constant negotiation processes influenced by specific social and cultural contexts."[12] In this case, the authors felt that an important variable was the heavy emphasis the parents of these students had placed on teaching them about Korean culture during their identity-forming years.[12]

There are many paths to becoming part of a cultural group, or to being seen by others as part of a particular cultural group. These include the following.

Birth

Cultural membership can be something one is born into, such as the tradition within Judaism that the child of a Jewish mother is considered to be Jewish or the tradition of Catholic families to baptize their children shortly after birth. The early home setting is often the site in which cultural heritage is passed down through the celebration of holidays, observance of rituals, eating certain foods, and encouraging the continued use of a particular language at home or in communal settings.

Adoption

When, how, and if adopted children learn about their birth culture usually depends on how adoptive parents feel about this issue, and this can vary depending on where the adoption occurs. Harf and colleagues[13] presented results of a review of studies of international adoption and discussed the tendency for European adoptive families to focus mainly on the adoptee taking on the culture of the adoptive family, in contrast to the United States, where adoptive families are more likely to incorporate elements of the adoptee's birth culture into their family cultural practices.

Choice

Our cultural connections often shift during our lifetime. A 2007 Pew survey, revised in 2011,[14] showed that roughly half of Americans have changed religious affiliation at least once in their life, with 28% reporting having made a committed change to a new religion as an adult through conversion ceremonies such as baptism for Christians or saying the Shahada for those converting to Islam.

Americans are also increasingly taking on new cultural identities through marriage. The rate at which newlyweds married someone of a different race or ethnicity rose from 3% in 1967 to 7% in 1980 and 17% in 2015.[15]

Many choose a new cultural course through immigration. Phinney and colleagues[16] postulate that psychological adaptation to immigration depends on factors particular to the attitude and coping style of the immigrant and on factors such as how accepting the receiving country is to immigrants becoming part of the society. These authors offer a model clinicians can use to evaluate where patients are in the process of adjustment to immigration.

Sometimes a group of people will define and claim a distinct culture for themselves. In their 2009 book *Inside Deaf Culture*,[17] Carol Padden and Tom Humphries explain, "We wrote our first book, *Deaf in America: Voices from a Culture*, to explain the use of 'culture' as a way of describing the lives of Deaf people. The term had long been used to describe the practices of hearing communities around the world but it had never been widely used to describe Deaf people . . . We used a definition of culture that focused on beliefs and practices, particularly the central role of sign language in the everyday lives of the community."[17]

Law

Sometimes cultural membership is defined by a government agency for the purposes of determining eligibility for benefits. The U.S. Department of the Interior's Bureau of Indian Affairs manages services for 1.9 million people recognized as American Indian or Alaska Native. According to the Bureau's website,[18] while factors such as having some degree of Indian ancestry or having extensive knowledge of a tribe's language and customs are relevant, "The protections and services provided by the United States for tribal members flow not from an individual's status as an American Indian in an ethnological sense, but because the person is a member of a Tribe recognized by the United States and with which the United States has a special trust relationship."[18]

Activism

Many Americans participate in activities designed to encourage political or social change. Sometimes this comes from personal experience of oppression, either experienced or witnessed. Other times it comes from an individual's desire to make a difference in the world. Activism can take many forms, such as participating in a political party (e.g., Democrat or Republican) or gathering with other community members to accomplish a shared goal (e.g., Mothers Against Drunk Driving). Within these activities, deep personal bonds can be forged and a sense of a cultural connection can develop and be manifested through slogans, emblems, art, and music. While these material legacies have deep personal meaning for individuals who participate in these activities, some also rise to the level of becoming part of our national landscape. In an article titled "How Social Movements Do Culture,"[19] William Roy discusses the role social justice movements have in creating culture and the ways they do this, such as the folk music of the civil rights movement of the 1960s, which helped bond people together and reduced stress and fear when they were marching. Roy observes:

> As important as *content* of cultural forms is, the effects of art, music, drama, literature, etc. achieved by social movements depend at least as much on the social relations within which culture is embedded. We need to move beyond attending to the *content* of art, music, drama, literature, etc. to examine how people relate to each other while *doing* music, drama, literature, etc.[19]

Other writers have also addressed the role that art can play in helping to form cultural movements as well as arising from them. In her tribute to Honor Moore's book, *Poems from the Women's Movement*,[20] Julie Enszer[21] writes,

> The women's movement was—and is—many things, and poetry was—and is—a necessary part of it. During the 1970s, poetry provided a way for women to find their voices and validate their experiences. Poetry enabled feminists to challenge dominant narratives and begin to think differently. Feminists wrote, circulated and performed poetry to agitate and inspire other women.[21]

John Kenny,[22] writing about Chicano movement mural artists such as Samuel Leyba in the 1960s, observed, "Leyba, speaking for himself, argues that the primary purpose of his painting murals was to educate the people of the barrio about who they were, particularly that they were Americans with the rights and entitlements of every citizen."[22]

Other

Many individuals form connections with groups with whom they share talents (e.g., singing in a choir), hobbies (e.g., hunting), or professions (e.g., being a first responder) and over time come to identify these as part of their cultural self-identity. As clinicians we can often be so preoccupied with our patients' illnesses that we might forget to ask about these other cultural associations, which are often indicators of a patient's capacity for fun and social connection.

CULTURE IN THE CLINICAL SETTING

The ways in which culture is seen as a multidimensional construct in a clinical context have been explored in depth in the medical anthropology literature.[23-26] Explanatory models, introduced by Arthur Kleinman, are an important concept in medical anthropology.[27] This term refers to schemata for understanding illness from the perspective of individual sufferers, their families, and their local network of healers, who have their own ideas about sickness and health that influence the experience of illness. This concept emphasizes the role of *local moral networks*—such as a family, a community, or a health system—on people's own understandings of and solutions to health problems: "Local moral worlds are settings of moral experience which express what is most at stake for people in their local networks of relationships in communities. These worlds . . . extend to networks where everyday life is enacted and transacted, where individuals' inner subjective experience is in interaction with the practices and engagements of other people."[26] Each illness episode and each clinical encounter represents its own local cultural system of meanings, norms, and power. At the same time, these local cultural systems are influenced by factors from the current society, including economic and political forces.

Another important concept from the field of medical anthropology is the distinction between disease and illness. While disease is defined as "malfunctioning or maladaptation of biologic and psychophysiologic processes," illness experience is viewed as culturally constructed and is described as "representing personal, interpersonal, and cultural reactions to disease or discomfort."[24] In other words, our perception of, experience with, and ability to cope with disease is thought to be a result of our own explanations of sickness, which are determined by the systems of meaning we are part of—whether that be our family, social position, or societal views.[24]

The distinction between these concepts is important as we develop our own personal understandings of the illness experience and interpret the experiences of our patients. An individual's cultural beliefs influence how he or she communicates about health issues, describes relevant symptoms, goes for care, and perceives that care. Given this, there can be significant cross-cultural differences in how people present with a health problem and how they cope with it. Physicians' explanations, behaviors, and interpretations of patient's symptoms are also culturally influenced. Kleinman and colleagues[24] describe the importance of eliciting the patient's explanatory model as a way to better understand the set of beliefs, social meanings, and expectations that the patient has about his or her disorder, treatment, and therapeutic goals. An important aspect of this process is for the clinician to be able to compare the patient's explanatory model with his or her own. This enables the clinician to be able to identify discrepancies in expectations regarding care. Kleinman and colleagues note, "Such comparisons also help the clinician grasp which aspects of the clinician's explanatory model need clearer explanation to patients and families and to understand that conflicts in explanatory models may not be related to different levels of knowledge but different values and interests."[24]

This discussion of explanatory models also relates to another important concept known as "social suffering"—the idea that social forces can at times cause illness, and that pain and suffering is not only experienced by the individual but also extends to the family and social network.[28]

The concepts regarding the cultural construction of illness defined above are underscored in situations in which patients' and practitioners' understanding of illness differ. For example, a study by Schoenberg and colleagues[29] found that, across minority ethnic groups disproportionately affected by poor diabetes outcomes, the prevailing perspective was that social stressors, such as inadequate resources, traumatic events, and unstable living environments, could cause or exacerbate diabetes symptoms, as well as undermine diabetes self-care. This patient-centered conceptualization of illness, which takes into account the social realities and life circumstances of the patient, contrasts with the biomedical view of diabetes, which relies on a precise diagnostic definition based on biomarkers and the prescription of complex dietary and medication regimens, in which patients can be seen as "noncompliant" if their blood sugar levels do not improve. This example highlights the contrast between patient and practitioner explanatory models of diabetes: Social stressors play a central role in lay diabetes models, whereas practitioners tend to minimize or disregard the potential influences of social stressors, such as the "food deserts" that cause 13.5 million Americans, mainly in urban areas, to have difficulty accessing healthy foods to alter their nutritional intake.[30,31] Broadening the definition of illness to include understanding the local contexts that influence behavior in diabetes care could help practitioners overcome key challenges in diabetes management.[32]

Beginning in the mid-20th century, health care workers were encouraged to engage in "cultural competency" educational activities, with nurses taking the lead in this effort.[33–35] The concept of cultural competency is now felt to be incomplete as it implies that "culture can be reduced to a technical skill for which clinicians can be trained to develop expertise."[36] Cultural competency training (as opposed to cultural sensitivity training) often coexists with a concept of a static culture that is based primarily on one's ethnicity or nationality. In the clinical context this can lead to inaccurate assessment of patients based on their appearance or language, in which patients are assumed to have a particular set of beliefs or behaviors about illness due to their presumed ethnicity (e.g., believing Hispanic patients always present with "stomach problems" when they are experiencing anxiety). Betancourt[37] warns that in these cases, "Cultural competency becomes a series of 'do's and don'ts' that define how to treat a patient of a given ethnic background" and argues that such a narrow view of culture can lead to a slippery slope in which dangerous stereotyping can occur.

Although a patient may be of a particular ethnic background, cultural factors related to that patient's ethnicity may not be relevant to the central aspect of his or her clinical presentation and might actually hinder accurate understanding or assessment.[36] Awareness of fixed pieces of information such as a person's age or country of birth does not tell us how that person relates to or prioritizes these aspects of his or her cultural identity. In their article "The Changing Racial and Ethnic Composition of the U.S. Population: Emerging American Identities," Perez and Hirschman write

> Many Americans have multiple identities that reflect complex ancestral origins, tribal and communal associations, and varied ideological outlooks on race and culture. In general, people do not change their ethnicities as a matter of fashion, but they may emphasize different aspects depending on the circumstances. For instance, a person who identifies as Mexican among relatives might identify as Hispanic at work and as American when overseas.[1]

Many clinicians currently in practice have had little formal training in the concepts of cultural awareness. In a 2011 article for health care professionals titled "Understanding Your Own Culture First,"[38] Marcia Carteret asserts that "self-reflection is crucial to the cross-cultural learning process" and contrasts the term "ethnocentric" (a view that one's own culture is superior to others) with "ethnorelative" (experiencing our own culture in the context of other cultures). Catoret[38] encourages us, as health care professionals, to examine our own cultural identities, including the culture of being a health care provider, and to examine our relationship to the concept of ethnocentricism as a way of beginning to understand why we respond the way we do in situations of cultural difference.

Returning to the example of diabetes, Dickinson and colleagues[39] note that

> Language lies at the core of attitude change, social perception, personal identity, intergroup bias, and stereotyping. The use of certain words or phrases can intentionally or unintentionally express bias about personal characteristics (e.g., race, religion, health, or gender). . . . How we talk to and about people with diabetes plays an important role in engagement, conceptualization of diabetes and its management, treatment outcomes, and the psychosocial well-being of the individual. For people with diabetes, language has an impact on motivation, behaviors, and outcomes.

Dickinson recommends use of language that is inclusive, person-centered, and strengths-based.

The clinical encounter is a critical arena that highlights the importance of the clinician's ability to develop a capacity for reflection when interacting with patients from different cultures. Katz and Alegria[40] write that this allows clinicians "to recognize and transform assumptions, to notice 'surprises,' and to elicit what really matters to patients in their care."

In working with patients across the cultural spectrum, clinicians might encounter unfamiliar terms and experience uncertainty and inner tension in the clinical encounter as a result. This can be particularly true when working with LGBTQ (lesbian, gay, bisexual, transgender, questioning) patients, as there has been a rapid expansion of available and preferred terminology in recent years. Terms such as nonbinary, cisgender, or pangender are unfamiliar to many clinicians, and some may not be aware of the newer pronouns preferred by some transgender people. Numerous websites offer educational information that clinicians can use to update their knowledge and to gain comfort in asking clients which terms and pronouns they would like the clinician to use. Examples of such websites include the PFLAG National Glossary[41] and the University of Wisconsin LGBT Resource Center Gender Pronouns guide.[42]

Clinicians who have a unidimensional view of culture may not realize how much cultural diversity can be implied by ethnic cultural identifiers and may inadvertently promote stereotypes in their interaction with patients. For instance, the term "Latino" can refer to people from a number of countries in South America, Central America, the Caribbean and North America. People who identify as Latino can be Black, white, biracial, or Mestizo (a blend of Native American and European ancestry), and may speak Spanish or Portuguese. Although Latino people share a cultural heritage, each country of origin has its own unique cultural characteristics, customs, and worldview. Similarly, the terms "African," "Asian," "European," and "Middle Eastern" each refer to people whose origins stem from many countries, each with their own unique customs, religions, and languages.[43]

Our approach to interaction with others can vary widely based on the part of the world we come from. Some cultures value individuality, while others value loyalty to the larger society at the expense of individuality. A U.S. Department of State booklet titled "So You're an American?"[44] describes 11 factors that are consistent with American culture, including the high values placed on individualism, informality, and time efficiency in the United States. The booklet describes the American approach to interpersonal interactions as follows:

> In communication and actions, most Americans believe that a straightforward and direct approach is the best way to ensure that a message is sent and received correctly. Meaning is carried mostly by the words and much less so by contextual clues such as the relative hierarchical position of speaker and listener and where the communication takes place. Professionals often value direct feedback and authenticity over concerns for a relationship as a means to attain efficiency. In other cultures, this can often be perceived as rude.[44]

This emphasis on directness of speech is also part of the health care culture of the United States. Clinicians who do not understand this can fail to recognize the limitations of a direct approach when working with patients who come from cultures in which more emphasis is placed on body language and the development of a relationship before difficult conversations occur.

PERSONAL CULTURAL IDENTITY

As we hope the foregoing discussion suggests, any particular individual's cultural identity is likely to undergo dynamic and constant shifts over time and is influenced by numerous contributing factors. In their book *Raising Biracial Children*,[45] Rockquemore and Laszloffy write, "It is important to emphasize that identity is a social process and not a static fixed end product that has any type of permanence attached to it. Our self-understanding is in a continual state of evolution. Moreover, the process of identity development does not occur through a single interaction, but instead progresses over an ongoing series of highly complex and coded interactions."[45]

In a 2001 article,[46] psychologist Derald Wing Sue describes a model of personal identity that includes three levels: individual, group, and universal. At the individual level, we have our unique genetic makeup and our unique personal experiences. At the group level, we each belong to a variety of groups (ethnic, racial, geographic, religious, gender, interests etc.), with which we share characteristics and attitudes that have influenced our identity development. On the universal level, we share traits with all other human beings, such as a physiologic need to eat and sleep, the experience of birth and death, the fact that we communicate with each other, and the fact that we are each capable of self-awareness. Sue calls his model the Tripartite Model of Personal Identity. Sue proposes that too often clinicians fail in their attempts at cultural competence with clients because they are focusing too much on the individual and universal levels of their clients' life stories and not understanding the importance of group memberships in terms of how patients feel about themselves and others (including the clinician) and how they are treated by others.[46]

For individuals who are members of a majority culture, such as white people in the United States, societal, institutional, and cultural forces often contribute to a life in which there is little cause to think about one's own cultural identity. In her 2014 book *Waking Up White*,[47] Debby Irving describes her own process of realizing her whiteness as an adult and describes the segregation that was the norm in America for much of the 20th century. Most white people lived in neighborhoods with only white neighbors, went to schools, religious institutions, and work settings in which they interacted only with other white people, and watched television shows populated mainly by white actors. Irving says, "The 1960s media-delivered world of white people confirmed my understanding of life as pretty comfortable . . . Normal was a house or two, a car or two, a pet or two, a TV or two." She also says, "I came to view history as something set in stone, printed in books, painted in pictures and taught by teachers who delivered facts. I took it all at face value, constructing for myself a one-dimensional world in which people were right or wrong, good or bad, like me or not." Irving chronicles her journey in which, as an adult, she realized that for many Americans, racial injustice had led to a life far different than the one she thought was the norm in America.[47]

As clinicians, we can be blind to implicit assumptions within ourselves, unaware of the cultural factors that have led to whatever view of "normal" we hold. This often coexists with the influence of the culture of medical settings in which clinicians, after years of training, feel they hold more knowledge than their patients. Combined, these factors can lead clinicians to believe their worldview is more important or valid than the patient's worldview, a dynamic that is often unconscious to the clinician but obvious to the patient, who observes the clinician's body language, speech, and interactions with other members of the clinical team. These internal processes often result in clinicians spending more time talking or looking at the computer, rather than listening, during clinical encounters. In describing the personal decision to confront her own worldview, which led her to a period of learning about racism and white privilege, Debby Irving[47] comments, "I've freed myself from the rigid notion that I have, or will ever have, all the answers."

Cultural Identity Development

Most authors consider Erik Erikson's writings on the developmental stages of life to be the foundation for later theories of cultural identity development. Erickson described eight stages of human development across the lifespan. He called the fifth stage "Identity vs. Role Confusion."[48] In his description of Eriksonian theory, Sokol[49] indicates that the establishment of a sense of cohesive identity is a major task of human development, usually occurring during the adolescent and young adult period. During this stage, individuals ideally develop a sense of themselves as a unique person with a worldview and feelings distinct from those of parents or caregivers. In Erikson's model, this stage precedes development of the capacity for intimacy, but Erikson indicated that identity development can continue over the lifetime.

A number of authors[50–57] have attempted to describe developmental stages of minority identity formation using a particular social grouping as the starting point. These theories offer important perspectives for understanding ourselves and our patients.

Most theories include an early stage in which the individual is not aware of his or her cultural identity as an issue, a stage of "unexamined identity."[50] For those from majority cultures, such as white people in the United States, this phase can last a long time. During the phase of unexamined identity, minority individuals often see the dominant culture as the one they wish to be part of. Examples might be minority children who express preference for white dolls, or children from nonreligious families who want to go to church because all their friends do.

Minority identity theories propose that following a period of unexamined identity (called *pre-encounter* in Cross's Black Identity Model[51] and *conformity* in Atkinson and colleagues' Minority Identity Development Model[52]), individuals progress to other stages of identity development in which they develop awareness of cultural differences. For minority individuals, this often happens in adolescence when the individual encounters difficult social interactions that make him or her feel marginalized. These experiences lead to a phase of recognizing their own culture and investing in learning about it. Individuals in this phase might actively reject other cultures and embrace people like themselves (however they define this) through school clubs or social justice activities related to the oppression they now recognize. Individuals in this phase might actively reject contact with people of other cultures, particularly ones they see as oppressive.

The final stage of identity development is thought to be one of identity integration. In this stage, individuals feel comfortable with themselves as a member of their own culture and feel able to interact in a reciprocal way with people of multiple cultures.

Han and colleagues[53] describe the importance of early childhood educators understanding their own cultural identity and the growth of knowledge of teachers who undertook self-awareness training about white identity development, and how this influenced their interaction with their students. This study used Helms' White Identity Model.[54] Under this framework, white identity in the United States is assumed to involve racism as a core concept because of the constant influence of institutional and structural racism in our society. In Helms' first stage, *contact*, whites are unaware of the existence of racism both within society and within themselves.

In the second stage, *disintegration*, whites begin to have experiences in which they recognize that inequality exists. During this stage there can be feelings of guilt or anxiety. This is followed by a period of *reintegration* when whites again experience feelings that whites are superior to people from minority cultures. In the fourth stage, *pseudo-independence*, whites consciously begin to seek interaction with minority people and intellectually begin to acknowledge the impact of racism. This is followed by a stage of *immersion/emersion* in which whites emotionally connect with the concepts of inequality and prejudice and the impacts of these on people from minority cultures. The final stage, *autonomy*, like the stage of identity integration in minority identity theory, involves a consolidation of what the individual has learned and a comfort with himself or herself and others that allows for meaningful and authentic cross-cultural relationships.[54]

Hud-Aleem and Countryman[55] compare two models of biracial identity development (Poston's 5-Stage Model and Rockquemore and Laszloffy's Continuum of Biracial Identity) and offer recommendations for therapists. Poston's model[56] (Table 2.1) focuses on the pressure biracial individuals feel to choose one or the other racial identity and the guilt they often feel when they do while working toward an integrated identity. Rockquemore and Laszloffy[45] propose that each end of the continuum represents the racial identity of one parent and that biracial individuals move along the continuum throughout their lives as they identify more with one or the other identity. The middle of the continuum represents an equal identity. The authors point out that the middle of the continuum is not necessarily a goal that the biracial individual needs to achieve but rather one point in the continuum that the individual may identify with at times. It is important for clinicians to be open to the fact that one person may identify as biracial while currently embracing just one end of the racial heritage continuum, while another may comfortably blend both sides.

Other cultural identity development models have been proposed. In a chapter titled "Analysis of LGBT Identity Development Models and Implications for Practice," Brent Bilodeau and Kristen Renn[57] review models of LGBT identity, including one by D'Augelli[58] with six identity processes. Carol Gill offers a four-stage model for individuals living with disabilities,[59] and Jean Kim has proposed a five-step model of Asian American identity development.[60]

In 1992 Beverly Tatum[61] wrote of her experience teaching a psychology course on race and racial identity development theory and described that conflict can arise in cross-cultural situations when individuals are at different stages of their cultural identity development. She wrote,

> Sharing the model of racial identity development with students gives them a useful framework for understanding each other's processes as well as their own. This cognitive framework does not necessarily prevent the collision of developmental processes . . . but it does allow students to be less frightened by it when it occurs. If, for example, white students understand the stages of racial identity development for students of color, they are less likely to personalize or feel threatened by an African American student's anger. Conversely, when students of color understand the stages of white racial identity development, they can be more tolerant or appreciative of a white student's struggle with guilt, for example.

Tatum's article provides a thoughtful analysis that clinicians can incorporate into their understanding of interactions with their patients.

Table 2.1 and 2.2 offer a visual comparison of the stages of various cultural identity development models.

Table 2.1 STAGES OF CULTURAL IDENTITY DEVELOPMENT

Asian American Racial Identity Development (Kim)	Biracial Cultural Identity Model (Poston)	Identity Development Model for People Living with Disabilities (Gill)	LGB* Identity Model (D'Augelli)
Ethnic awareness	Personal identity	Integrating into society	Exiting heterosexuality
White identification	Choice of group categorization	Integrating with the disability community	Developing personal LGB identity
Awakening to social political consciousness	Enmeshment/denial	Internally integrating sameness and difference	Developing LGB social identity
Redirection to Asian American consciousness	Appreciation	Integrating how one feels with how one presents oneself	Becoming an LGB offspring
Incorporation	Integration		Developing an LGB intimacy status
			Entering an LGB community

* LGB=Lesbian, Gay, Bisexual

Kim J. Asian American racial identity development theory. In Wijeyesinghe CL, Jackson BW, eds. *New Perspectives on Racial Identity Development: Integrating Emerging Frameworks.* 2nd ed. New York: NYU Press; 2012:138–159.

Poston WSC. The biracial identity development model: A needed addition. *Journal of Counseling & Development.* 1990;69(2):152–155.

Gill CJ. Four types of integration in disability identity development. *Journal of Vocational Rehabilitation.* 1997;9:39–46.

D'Augelli AR. Identity development and sexual orientation: Toward a model of lesbian, gay, and bisexual development. In Trickett EJ, Watts RJ, Birman D, eds. *Human Diversity: Perspectives on People in Context.* San Francisco, CA: Jossey Bass; 1994.

Table 2.2 ADDITIONAL STAGES OF CULTURAL IDENTITY DEVELOPMENT

People of Color Racial Identity Model (Cross)	Racial and Cultural Identity Development (Atkinson, Morten, and Sue)	White Identity Model (Helms)
Pre-encounter	Conformity	Contact
Encounter	Dissonance	Disintegration
Immersion/emersion	Resistance and immersion	Reintegration
Internalization	Introspection	Pseudo-independence
		Autonomy

Cross WE Jr. The psychology of nigrescence: Revising the Cross model. In Ponterotto JG, Casas JM, Suzuki LA, Alexander CM, eds. *Handbook of Multicultural Counseling.* Thousand Oaks, CA: Sage Publications; 1995:93–122.

Atkinson DR, Morten G, Sue DW. A minority identity development model. In Arnold K, Carreiro King I, eds. *College Student Development and Academic Life. Psychological, Intellectual and Moral Issues.* New York: Routledge, Taylor & Francis Group; 2013:193–206.

Helms JE. Toward a model of white racial identity development. In Arnold K, Carreiro King I, eds. *College Student Development and Academic Life. Psychological, Intellectual and Moral Issues.* New York: Routledge, Taylor & Francis Group; 2013:207–224.

Additional Issues and Terminology

Some writers[62–66] have added other elements to cultural identity theory and have pointed out that issues such as minority status, privilege, intersectionality, and white fragility can impact the development of a cohesive sense of identity and the comfort or anxiety an individual may have in cross-cultural situations. These are important concepts for clinicians to be aware of when they undertake an assessment of their own cultural identity and how it impacts their clinical encounters.

Minority status is a term that refers to a culturally, ethnically, or racially distinct group that coexists with but is subordinate to a more dominant group. Examples include Black, Asian, Latino, or Native people living in a majority white culture; Muslim and Jewish people living in a majority Christian culture; and people with limited vision living in a majority sighted population.

Privilege is a term that denotes the advantage that certain members of a society possess compared to others. Sian Ferguson[62] writes that it is important to understand privilege as a systemic issue: "Privileged groups have power over oppressed groups. Privileged people are more likely to be in positions of power . . . Privileged people can use their positions to benefit people like themselves."

The term *white privilege* refers specifically to the privilege white people automatically experience in U.S. society as a result of years of embedded legal and societal frameworks that have favored their race, such as redlining, a policy that allowed whites to purchase houses at a much higher rate than Blacks during the

20th century.[63] In her article "Unpacking the Invisible Backpack,"[64] Peggy McIntosh offers readers a 26-question autognostic exercise to help them understand skin color privilege.

Other forms of privilege in U.S. society include being of male gender, being heterosexual, and being able-bodied. Examples of the effects of those privileges include differences in rates of career advancement and salaries for men versus women, and the ease with which able-bodied people are able to travel to and from work and social gatherings.

Intersectionality, a term derived from feminist sociological theory, was first used by Kimberle Crenshaw[65] in 1989 to refer to the ways in which Black women are victims of the intersection of both racism and sexism in our society. More recently, in popular culture, this term has come to include the many people in our society who have more than one factor that imparts lack of privilege and increases the burden of oppression. Examples include being an older Latino man (who faces both ageism and racism) and being a poor Black transgender woman (who faces classism, racism, and anti-trans prejudice).

White fragility is a term coined by Robin DiAngelo[66] in 2011 to describe the emotional reaction many white people in the United States experience when confronted with experiences of "racial stress" such as conversations about race or diversity trainings. This reaction can manifest as anger, defensiveness, silence, withdrawal, or feelings of guilt and despair. DiAngelo proposes that due to societal factors such as segregation, many white people in the United States have not developed the skills needed for cross-cultural conversations to occur in which people of minority cultures can truly express negative feelings and be heard without the white listener becoming defensive. She calls these skills "psychic stamina."[66] Given that the majority of mental health clinicians in our country are white,[2] DiAngelo's concept of white fragility is an important construct for clinicians to consider when assessing where they are in their own process of cultural identity development and how this impacts both clinical encounters and their patients' ability to express negative emotions.

CULTURAL SELF-AWARENESS

The *Merriam-Webster Medical Dictionary* defines "autognosis" as "an understanding of one's own psychodynamics,"[67] and *The American Heritage Dictionary* defines "self-knowledge" as "knowledge or understanding of one's own nature, abilities, and limitations; insight into oneself."[68] In their book *What Therapists Learn About Themselves and How They Learn It: Autognosis*, Messner, Groves, and Schwartz[69] explain, "Autognosis involves observation, development of a set of procedures for increasing one's knowledge and understanding, and application of that understanding in a constructive way. It is a sweeping spectrum of internal activities . . . In autognosis we have to learn to recognize our responses and find ways of classifying them in order to apply them most usefully."[69] In this way, autognosis represents a process designed to further self-knowledge.

Health care providers benefit from increased self-understanding because naturally occurring blind spots and unconscious biases can exert harm during clinical encounters. Specifically, numerous studies have examined the role of implicit bias in patient–provider interactions[70,71] and indicate an association with health care disparities.[72] The topic of implicit bias will be taken up more fully elsewhere in this textbook, but it is important to note here that this topic relates directly to the critical importance of cultural self-awareness for health care clinicians in general and mental health providers specifically.

Clinicians' deeply held values, which may constitute key aspects of their personal identity, can impact the care they provide. In a study by Hersh and Goldenberg,[73] doctors' political affiliations correlated with the way they evaluated health risk and the kinds of advice they would give to patients. Doctors who were Republican were more apt to rate a patient's use of marijuana or having an abortion as serious concerns. Doctors who were Democrats rated having a firearm in the home or the patient being a sex worker as more serious issues. Similarly, a *Lancet* editorial titled "Physician, Know Thyself"[74] described a study of the correlation between religious beliefs and end-of-life care. According to the report, doctors who were atheist or agnostic are more apt to discuss treatment options that might shorten life expectancy with terminally ill patients as compared to doctors who are more religious. The editorial accompanying this article[74] pointed to the New York Palliative Care Act, which compels doctors to offer patients with terminal illnesses information about hospice care, palliative care, and end-of-life options, and went on to say that the study author suggested that terminally ill patients should ask about the level of religious belief held by their doctors. The editorial authors rightly point out that the burden for this should not be put on the patient, and suggest, "A spell of self-reflection might be the most sensible response. If doctors feel that their beliefs, religious or otherwise, are influencing their ability to fulfill their professional obligations, then they must have the professional integrity and self-awareness to acknowledge this."[74]

For clinicians who wish to undertake a process of cultural self-assessment, there are many tools available, including those already cited in this chapter (e.g., Peggy McIntosh's Invisible Knapsack exercise[64] and Debby Irving's book,[47] which offers many self-reflection prompts). Each of these tools can also be employed by clinicians when undertaking a thorough cultural assessment of patients. The topic of cultural formulation of patients is also taken up at greater length elsewhere in this textbook.

In her book *Addressing Cultural Complexities in Practice*,[75] Pamela Hays suggests the mnemonic ADDRESSING as a way for individuals to begin a cultural self-assessment:

A = age and generational influences
D = developmental disabilities and other disabilities
R = religion and spiritual orientation
E = ethnic and racial identity
S = socioeconomic status and sexual orientation
I = indigenous heritage
N = national origin
G = gender.

For each factor, Hays describes dominant and nondominant groupings. With regard to age, for instance, the dominant group in U.S. society is young and middle-aged adults, while children and older adults are in the minority group.

Dzenowagis,[76] writing for global program managers, says,

Our intercultural competence begins with a reasonable understanding of ourselves. Culture is a pattern for living. It is complex and abstract. It is the dominant shaping force on each of us. As the fish in the water is unaware of the water, we are unaware of the cultural rules that dictate our own patterns of interaction. We are members of multiple cultures. We must first understand ourselves and our own culture.

Dzenowagis offers several examples of how to do this, including a framework called the Cultural Orientations Model that includes 10 factors:

1. *Environment:* How individuals view and relate to the people, objects, and issues in their sphere of influence
2. *Time:* How individuals perceive the nature of time and its use
3. *Action:* How individuals view actions and interactions
4. *Communication:* How individuals express themselves
5. *Space:* How individuals demarcate their physical and psychological space
6. *Power:* How individuals view differential power relationships
7. *Individualism:* How individuals define their identity
8. *Competitiveness:* How individuals are motivated
9. *Structure:* How individuals approach change, risk, ambiguity, and uncertainty
10. *Thinking:* How individuals conceptualize.

The current authors propose that a thorough self-assessment for a health care provider should include all of the following categories. Some of these prompts might also be helpful to use clinically when working with patients who have limited awareness of, or insight into, their own cultural identities.

Where are you from?

1. Where were you born? Where were your parents/grandparents born?
2. What languages were spoken in your home growing up?
3. How did your family make money? What was your family's socioeconomic status?
4. Did you live in a city, suburb, rural area, native reservation?
5. Did you own a home? Did you move often? Who lived with you?
6. What religion did your family practice, if any? What holidays did you observe?

Who are you now?

1. In your adult life, what cultural identities have you acquired? Does your cultural identity include areas of intersectionality?
2. Do you still identify as the gender you were assigned at birth?
3. Do you identify as lesbian, gay, bisexual, heterosexual, or are you still questioning?
4. Do you celebrate the same holidays you did when you were growing up?

5. Do you attend the same religious services you used to? Has your understanding of God or spirituality changed compared to that of your family or cultural group?
6. What kind of jobs have you had? Do you identify yourself through your job? Has your socioeconomic status changed throughout your lifetime?
7. If you are in a relationship, what cultural practices have you acquired through your relationship?

What experiences of privilege/oppression have you had?

1. Have you always lived/worked in places where most people look like you, celebrate the same holidays you do, belong to the same faith group you do?
2. Have you lived/worked in places where you were a minority or spoke a different language or had less power due to oppression? Has this been true your whole life?
3. Have you lived in a place where you were not a citizen of the country?
4. Have you had times when you didn't have enough money for what you needed?
5. Are there parts of your identity you or your family have kept hidden for fear of oppression?

How has culture shaped the way you relate to other people?

1. Did your family welcome meeting strangers, or did you mainly spend time with extended family? Do you know why?
2. Was everyone in your family the same in terms of race, abilities/disabilities, religion, socioeconomic status, worldview? What impact did this sameness or difference have on how you relate to other people?
3. Were there students in your elementary school or high school who were from different cultural backgrounds than yours, such as students from immigrant families, or students with developmental or physical challenges? Were you encouraged to get to know them?
4. When you entered college or the workforce, did you eagerly seek out people from other cultural groups or were you more hesitant?
5. What about now? Do you prefer to spend time with people from a culture you see yourself being part of, such as people who do the same kind of work or share your political leanings or racial/ethnic background? How often do you seek out interaction with people you view as different?
6. Where are you in your own cultural identity development process? Are you in the stage of unexamined identity, integration, or somewhere in the middle?

What has your cultural environment taught you about health care?

1. How did your family access health care when you were growing up? How do you access health care now?

2. Are there people in your family who prefer to avoid Western health care providers? Do they ever seek treatment from other kinds of providers such as faith healers?

3. What factors in your formative cultural environment led to you becoming a health care provider?

4. Do you believe it is every person's right to determine what kind of health care they want or do you feel Western medicine is the only acceptable approach?

5. How do you feel when working with a client from a cultural group with which you have no or limited experience? Are you aware of any implicit biases or stereotypes you might hold when working with people from different racial/ethnic groups? What about when you are working with large-bodied patients, old patients, patients who are hard of hearing, patients who need an interpreter due to not speaking English, etc.?

6. How do you feel when working with colleagues from other cultures or who trained in other countries? Do you trust them? Do you feel they have something to teach you?

Clinicians can undertake these kinds of exercises alone, but having the support of peers is helpful. Cultural self-awareness is an ongoing and lifelong process. It can also be an uncomfortable one. While the ultimate goal of this work is to achieve an integrated cultural identity that allows for effective and meaningful cross-cultural relationships, there may be times when individuals engaged in cultural self-awareness exercises will feel the complex emotions discussed earlier in this chapter such as shame, guilt, or anger. Clinicians can incorporate their knowledge of the stages of cultural identity development theory[51-61] to help them process the difficult emotions they might feel as they grow in their knowledge of themselves and of how they relate to people of other cultures. White clinicians should be aware of the concept of White fragility[66] while undertaking this work, particularly if they are starting from a place of unexamined identity.[54] Tatum's detailed description of a psychology class on race and identity theory[61] offers a useful framework for groups wishing to undertake cultural self-assessment together.

CASE SUMMARY

In the case presented at the beginning of the chapter, the attending physician was surprised to learn that he had missed such a crucial piece of information as the patient's sexual orientation. Although he usually took a careful sexual and gender identity history, he had not done so in this case. On reflection, he realized that he had been viewing the patient through the lens of his own youth growing up in China. Identifying with the patient culturally had given him a blind spot that caused him not to recognize the multidimensionality of the patient's cultural identity. He also recognized that his role as a psychopharmacologist had caused him to be so focused on convincing the patient and his family that the patient needed medication that he had not looked for a possible psychosocial trigger for the episode. In a debrief session the medical student revealed that he had suspected the patient might be gay early in the course of the hospitalization but had felt nervous about mentioning this for fear it would reveal his own gay identity in the Catholic hospital setting in which the case occurred.

CHAPTER SUMMARY

1. Culture is a multidimensional, socially constructed concept. Our cultural identity forms and changes over a lifetime and is multifaceted.
2. Cultural differences between patients and providers can be associated with implicit biases. Clinicians can reduce this risk by incorporating the anthropological concept of illness explanatory models into their work.[24,27]
3. Members of the majority culture may take much longer to recognize themselves as having a "culture" and how it is impacting interpersonal interactions. Cultural identity development models offer a tool clinicians can use when evaluating confusing cross-cultural interactions.[51-61]
4. Cultural self-assessment is an important tool for clinicians who wish to increase their skill in working with patients across the culture spectrum.

CONCLUSION

In this chapter we have outlined models of cultural understanding that can be used as clinical tools by health care providers. Awareness of, and continued attention to, our own illness explanatory models (framed by our personal development and our professional culture), and those of our patients, can shape our clinical interactions in a way that enhances shared vision in treatment planning. Clinicians who evaluate where they are personally in the schema of cultural identity development models, and consider these models with regard to their patients, can bring increased insight to cross-cultural interactions. The use of autognostic, self-understanding exercises can help clinicians identify the often unconscious attitudes they bring to the clinical encounter that can range from how they think about, and use, time and space, to implicit biases that influence their body language, attitudes, and decision-making in the clinical interaction.

Tibetan Buddhist teacher and nun Pema Chodron[77] has said, "Everything that human beings feel, we feel. We can become extremely wise and sensitive to all of humanity and the whole universe simply by knowing ourselves, just as we are." The authors hope that the material presented in this chapter will help readers to know themselves better, so that they can become wiser and more culturally sensitive, as well as more clinically effective, in the work they do every day as health care providers.

REFERENCES

1. Perez AD, Hirschman C. The changing racial and ethnic composition of the US population: Emerging American identities. *Population and Development Review*. 2009;35(1):1–51.
2. American Psychological Association Center for Workforce Studies. Demographics of US psychology workforce. 2015. http://www.apa.org/workforce/data-tools/demographics/aspx. Accessed 4/8/2018.

3. American Counseling Association. *2014 ACA Code of Ethics*. https://www.coun-seling.org/resources/aca-code-of-ethics.pdf. Accessed 05/06/2018.

4. American Psychological Association. *Ethical Principles of Psychologists and Code of Conduct 2017*. https://apa.org/ethics/code/principles.pdf. Accessed 01/28/2018.

5. Stocking GW Jr. Franz Boas and the culture concept in historical perspective. In Stocking GW. *Race, Culture and Evolution: Essays in the History of Anthropology*. New York: Free Press; 1968:195–233.

6. Bates DG, Plog F. *Cultural Anthropology*. New York: McGraw-Hill; 1990.

7. Cohen AP. Culture as identity: An anthropologist's view. *New Literary History*. 1993;24(1):195–209.

8. Lombardo PA. Miscegenation, eugenics, and racism: Historical footnotes to *Loving v. Virginia*. *UC Davis Law Review*. 1987–1988;21:421.

9. Foster MW, Sharp RR. Race, ethnicity, and genomics: Social classifications as proxies of biological heterogeneity. *Genome Research*. 2002;12:844–850.

10. Smedley A, Smedley BD. Race as biology is fiction. Race as a social problem is real. *American Psychologist*. 2005;60(1):16–26.

11. Sapolsky R. Why your brain hates other people. *Nautilus*. 2017;May/June:20–33.

12. Jung E, Lee C. Social construction of cultural identity: An ethnographic study of Korean American students. *Atlantic Journal of Communication*. 2004;12(3):146–162.

13. Harf A, Skandrani S, Sibeoni J, Pontvert C, Revah-Levy A, Moro MR. Cultural identity and internationally adopted children: Qualitative approach to parental representations. *PLoS ONE*. 2015;10(3): e0119635.

14. Pew Research Center. *Faith in Flux*. https://www.pewforum.org/2009/04/27/faith-in-flux. Accessed 04/08/2018.

15. Pew Research Center. *Trends and Patterns in Intermarriage*. https://www.pewsocialtrends.org/2017/05/18/1-trends-and-patterns-in-intermarriage. Accessed 04/08/2018.

16. Phinney JS, Horenczyk G, Liebkind K, Vedder P. Ethnic identity, immigration & well-being: An interactional perspective. *Journal of Social Issues*. 2001;57(3):493–510.

17. Padden C, Humphries T. *Inside Deaf Culture*. Cambridge, MA: Harvard University Press; 2009.

18. U.S. Department of Interior, Bureau of Indian Affairs. Frequently Asked Questions. https://www.bia.gov/frequently-asked-questions. Accessed 01/28/18.

19. Roy WG. How social movements do culture. *International Journal of Politics, Culture, and Society*. 2010;23:85–98.

20. Moore H. *Poems from the Women's Movement*. American Poets Project # 28. New York: Library of America; 2009.

21. Enszer J. National Poetry Month: "Vagina" sonnet and other poems that drove feminism. *Ms. Magazine* [blog] 2012. https://msmagaine.com/blog/2012/04/01/national-poetry-month-vagina-sonnet-and-other-poems-that-drove-feminism. Accessed 04/01/2018.

22. Kenny J. *The Chicano Mural Movement of the Southwest: Populist Public Art and Chicano Political Activism*. New Orleans, LA: University of New Orleans; 2006. https://scholarworks.uno.edu/cgi/viewcontent.cgi?referer=https://www.google.com/&httpsredir=1&article=1492&context=td2006. Accessed 04/01/2018.

23. Farmer P. *Infections and Inequalities*. Berkeley: University of California Press; 1997.

24. Kleinman A, Eisenberg L, Good B. Culture, illness, and care. Clinical lessons from anthropologic and cross-cultural research. *Annals of Internal Medicine*. 1978;88:251–258.

25. Kleinman A. *The Illness Narratives: Suffering, Healing, and the Human Condition.* New York: Basic Books; 1988:96.

26. Kleinman A, Das V, Lock M. *Social Suffering.* Berkeley: University of California Press; 1997.

27. Kleinman A. *Patients and Healers in the Context of Culture: An Exploration of the Borderland Between Anthropology, Medicine and Psychiatry.* Berkeley: University of California Press; 1980.

28. Kleinman A. Four social theories for global health. *Lancet.* 2010;375(9725): 1518–19. 2010.

29. Schoenberg N, Drew E, Stoller E, Kart C. Situating stress: Lessons from lay discourses on diabetes. *Medical Anthropology Quarterly.* 2005;19(2):171–193.

30. Ver Ploeg M, Nulph D, Williams R. *Mapping Food Deserts in the United States.* United States Department of Agriculture Economic Research Service. 2011. https://www.ers.usda.gov/amber-waves/2011/december/data-featire-mapping-food-deserts-in-the-us. Accessed 05/05/2018.

31. USDA Office of Communications. Food Desert Locator. Release No. 0191.11. Modified 06/02/2017. https://www.ers.usde.gov/data-products/food-access-research-atlas/go-to-the-atlas. Accessed 01/27/2018.

32. Hahn RA, Inhorn MC. *Anthropology and Public Health: Bridging Differences in Culture and Society.* 2nd ed. New York: Oxford University Press; 2009.

33. Albougami AS, Pounds KG, Alotaibi JS. Comparison of four cultural competence models in transcultural nursing: A discussion paper. *International Archives of Nursing and Health Care.* 2016;2(4):1–5.

34. Campinha-Bacote J. The process of cultural competence in the delivery of healthcare services: A model of care. *Journal of Transcultural Nursing.* 2002;13(3):181–184.

35. Leininger M. Culture care theory: A major contribution to advance transcultural nursing knowledge and practices. *Journal of Transcultural Nursing.* 2002;13(3):189–192.

36. Kleinman A, Benson P. Anthropology in the clinic: The problem of cultural competency and how to fix it. *PLoS Med.* 2006;3(10):e294.

37. Betancourt JR. Cultural competence—a marginal or mainstream movement? *New England Journal of Medicine.* 2004;351(10):953–955.

38. Carteret M. Understanding the culture of your practice. 2010. In *Dimensions of Culture: Cross-Cultural Communications for Healthcare Professionals.* https://www.dimensionsofculture.com. Accessed 01/28/2018.

39. Dickinson JK, Guzman SJ, Maryniuk MD, et al. The use of language in diabetes care and education. *Diabetes Care.* 2017;40(12):1790–1799.

40. Katz AM, Alegria M. The clinical encounter as local moral world: Shifts of assumptions and transformation in relational context. *Social Science & Medicine.* 2009;68(7):1238–1246.

41. PFLAG National Glossary of Terms. https://www.pflag.org/glossary. Accessed 1/28/18.

42. University of Wisconsin Lesbian, Gay, Bisexual, Transgender Resource Center. Gender Pronouns. http://uwm.edu/lgbtrc/support/gender-pronouns/. Accessed 1/28/18.

43. Jiminez TR, Fields CD, Schachter A. How ethnoraciality matters: Looking inside ethnoracial groups. *Social Currents.* 2015;2(2):107–115.

44. U.S. Department of State. *So You're an American? A Guide to Answering Difficult Questions Abroad.* https://www.state.gov/m/fsi/tc/answeringdifficultquestions/html/app.htm?p=module1_p1.htm Accessed 1/28/18.

45. Rockquemore KA, Laszloffy T. *Raising Biracial Children.* Oxford, UK: Alta Mira Press; 2005.
46. Sue DW. Multidimensional facets of cultural competence. *The Counseling Psychologist.* 2001;29(6):790–821.
47. Irving D. *Waking Up White and Finding Myself in the Story of Race.* Cambridge, MA: Elephant Room Press; 2014.
48. Erikson EH. *Identity and the Life Cycle.* New York: WW Norton & Co; 1980.
49. Sokol JT. Identity development throughout the lifetime: An examination of Eriksonian theory. *Graduate Journal of Counseling Psychology.* 2009;1(2):1–10.
50. Ojha AK. Different fields, similar processes, but how? *Journal of Intercultural Communication.* 2005; issue 10.
51. Cross W E., Jr. The psychology of nigrescence: Revising the Cross model. In Ponterotto JG, Casas JM, Suzuki LA, Alexander CM, eds. *Handbook of Multicultural Counseling.* Thousand Oaks, CA: Sage Publications; 1995:93–122.
52. Atkinson DR, Morten G, Sue DW. A minority identity development model. In Arnold K, Carreiro King I, eds. *College Student Development and Academic Life. Psychological, Intellectual, Social and Moral Issues.* New York: Routledge, Taylor & Francis Group; 2013:193–206.
53. Han HS, West-Olatunji C, Thomas MS. Use of racial identity development theory to explore cultural competence among early childhood educators. *SRATE Journal.* 2010–2011;20(1):1–11.
54. Helms JE. Toward a model of white racial identity development. In Arnold K, Carreiro King I, eds. *College Student Development and Academic Life. Psychological, Intellectual, Social and Moral Issues.* New York: Routledge, Taylor & Francis Group; 2013:207–224.
55. Hud-Aleem R, Countryman J. Biracial identity development and recommendations in therapy. *Psychiatry (Edgmont).* 2008;5(11):37–44.
56. Poston WSC. The biracial identity development model: A needed addition. *Journal of Counseling & Development.* 1990;69(2):152–155.
57. Bilodeau BL, Renn KA. Analysis of LGBT identity development models and implications for practice. *New Directions for Student Services.* 2005;111:25–39.
58. D'Augelli AR. Identity development and sexual orientation: Toward a model of lesbian, gay, and bisexual development. In Trickett EJ, Watts RJ, Birman D, eds. *Human Diversity: Perspectives on People in Context.* San Francisco, CA: Jossey-Bass; 1994.
59. Gill CJ. Four types of integration in disability identity development. *Journal of Vocational Rehabilitation.* 1997;9:39–46.
60. Kim J. Asian American racial identity development theory. In Wijeyesinghe CL, Jackson BW, eds. *New Perspectives on Racial Identity Development: Integrating Emerging Frameworks.* 2nd ed. New York: NYU Press; 2012:138–159.
61. Tatum B. Talking about race, learning about racism: The application of racial identity development in the classroom. *Harvard Educational Review.* 1992;62(1):1–24.
62. Ferguson S. Privilege 101: A quick and dirty guide. https://everydayfeminism.com/2014/09/what-is-privilege/. Accessed 01/28/2018.
63. Badger W. How redlining's racist effects lasted for decades. https://www.nytimes.com/2017/08/24/upshot/how-redlinings-racist-effects-lasted-for-decades.html. Accessed 01/28/2018.
64. McIntosh, P. White privilege: Unpacking the invisible knapsack. *Peace and Freedom Magazine.* 1989;July/August:10–12.

65. Crenshaw K. Demarginalizing the intersection of race and sex: A black feminist critique of antidiscrimination doctrine, feminist theory and antiracist politics. *University of Chicago Legal Forum.* 1989: Issue 1, Article 8.

66. DiAngelo R. White fragility. *International Journal of Critical Pedagogy.* 2011; 3(3):54–70.

67. Definition of "autognosis." *Merriam-Webster Dictionary,* 2014. https://www.merriam-webster.com/medical/autognosis. Accessed 11/7/2017.

68. Definition of "self-knowledge." *American Heritage Dictionary of the English Language,* 5th ed., 2016. https://ahdictionary.com/word/search.html?q=self+knowledge. Accessed 11/7/2017.

69. Messner E, Groves JE, Schwartz JH. *What Therapists Learn About Themselves and How They Learn It: Autognosis.* Lanham, MD: Rowman & Littlefield Publishing Group; 2004.

70. Sabin JA, Marini M, Nosek BA. Implicit and explicit anti-fat bias among a large sample of medical doctors by BMI, race/ethnicity and gender. *PLoS ONE.* 2012;7(11): e48448.

71. Schouten BC, Meeuwesen L. Cultural differences in medical communication: A review of the literature. *Patient Education and Counseling.* 2006;64:21–34.

72. Chapman EN, Kaatz A, Carnes M. Physicians and implicit bias: How doctors may unwittingly perpetuate health care disparities. *Journal of General Internal Medicine.* 2013;28(11):1504–1510.

73. Hersch ED, Goldenberg MN. Democratic and Republican physicians provide different care on politicized health issues. *Proceedings of the National Academy of the Sciences.* 2016;113(42):11811–11816.

74. Physician, know thyself [Editorial]. *Lancet.* 2010;376:743.

75. Hays PA. Doing your own cultural self-assessment. In Hays PA. *Addressing Cultural Complexities in Practice: Assessment, Diagnosis and Therapy.* 3rd ed. Washington, DC: American Psychological Association; 2016:39–60.

76. Dzenowagis A. Who am I? Analyze and understand your own culture first. Paper presented at PMI® Global Congress 2009—EMEA, Amsterdam, North Holland, The Netherlands. Newtown Square, PA: Project Management Institute, 2009. https://www.mi.org/learning/library/analyze-understand-culture-intercultural-communication-6864. Accessed 05/05/2018.

77. Chodron P. *The Wisdom of No Escape and the Path of Loving Kindness.* Boulder, CO: Shambhala Publishing; 2001.

3

Culture in the DSM-5

NHI-HA T. TRINH, MAYA SON, AND
JUSTIN A. CHEN ■

CASE

A faculty member at an academic psychiatry residency training program is scheduled to supervise a PGY-3 resident on an evaluation in the outpatient clinic. In reviewing the patient's medical record, the attending learns that the patient is a 44-year-old woman originally from Haiti who was recently discharged following a 2-week inpatient psychiatric hospitalization for worsening depression and "paranoia." She also learns that the patient repeatedly endorsed a conviction that her symptoms were caused by someone in her greater social network, motivated by envy of her success, who had sent these illnesses to harm her. While the patient's symptoms improved on a low dose of a second-generation antipsychotic medication, she made reference to the fact that she was unlikely to continue taking medications after discharge because "I'm not the sick one, those bad people are." Neither the resident nor attending is from a Haitian cultural background. The attending understands the importance of applying a culturally-informed understanding of the patient's beliefs in order to negotiate the diagnosis and outpatient treatment of the patient's symptoms but is unsure how to elicit these or how to teach the resident to do so.

INTRODUCTION

The *Diagnostic and Statistical Manual of Mental Disorders* (DSM), published by the American Psychiatric Association (APA), is an essential guide, defining and standardizing definitions of psychiatric disorders with the goal of guiding research and clinical practice. However, an unintended consequence of this standardization has been the exclusion of alternative symptom variants and explanations of these disorders, which occur worldwide as a result of cultural and contextual factors.[1] The most recent, fifth edition of the DSM (DSM-5) has sought to address this concern with a renewed emphasis on cultural factors in the experience and interpretation of patients' symptoms, including an additional focus on providing practical clinical tools such as the Outline for Cultural Formulation (OCF) and the Cultural

Formulation Interview (CFI). In this chapter, we will detail the evolution of the focus on culture from the fourth revision of the DSM (DSM-IV) to DSM-5 and describe best practices in using these tools for evaluation and management of patients of diverse populations.

FROM DSM-IV TO DSM-5: A CULTURAL EVOLUTION

DSM-IV first presented the OCF with the intention of capturing the patient's explanatory model of illness.[2,3] The OCF included five sections: (1) cultural identity of the individual, (2) cultural conceptualizations of distress (cultural explanations of the individual's illness), (3) psychosocial stressors and cultural features of vulnerability and resilience (cultural factors related to psychosocial environment and functioning), (4) cultural features (elements) of the relationship between the individual and the clinician, and (5) overall cultural assessment (for diagnosis and care).[2]

Despite wide interest in and use of the OCF, substantial barriers to its adoption and implementation were reported, including the format being too vague and unstructured, as well as a lack of clarity about how the OCF fit into standard clinical practice.[4] The DSM-5 Cultural Issues Subgroup, part of the larger Gender and Cross-Cultural Study Group, was charged with making recommendations on racial, ethnic, and contextual issues to all the DSM workgroups who were responsible for revamping the DSM-IV. As part of this process, the subgroup organized literature reviews of relevant topics as well as a field trial in five continents of the CFI.[1] The subgroup suggested the following recommendations for DSM-5: (1) including a comprehensive introductory chapter providing conceptual and practical guidance on evaluating the role of culture and context in diagnosis, including a revised OCF and CFI, (2) including culture-relevant material in the descriptive text of each disorder, and (3) renaming *culture-bound syndromes* as *cultural idioms of distress*, and including these in a glossary.

Thus DSM-5, published in 2013, proposed significant changes to the way culture is conceived and used by mental health clinicians and others interested in psychiatric diagnosis. DSM-5 explicitly states that "all forms of distress are locally shaped, including the DSM disorders." As such, the discussion of each disorder contains a discussion of multicultural explanations for similar symptoms for direct use by clinicians as a cross-reference. For example, panic disorder contains a discussion of *ataque de nervios*, a cultural idiom of distress.

Furthermore, efforts to operationalize a practical interview tool emphasizing the role of culture in a patient's clinical presentation led to the creation of the CFI for DSM-5.[5] The current CFI is a standardized, manualized interview based on 16 open-ended question stems and probes, which was tested for feasibility, acceptability, and clinical utility in a DSM-5 field trial. The areas addressed in the interview are cultural definition of the problem, causes, stressors and supports, role of cultural identity, self-coping, past help-seeking behaviors, barriers, preferences, and the clinician–patient relationship. In addition to the core CFI for an initial assessment interview, and an informant interview for collateral information, there are 12 supplementary modules to the CFI available for free download online[6] (to expand on these basic assessments, and to address specific groups such as immigrants and refugees).

Differences Between the DSM-IV and DSM-5

Although the OCF in the DSM-IV has been called the most important contribution of anthropology to psychiatry, it has been criticized on several fronts: (1) it may be time-consuming to use, 2) its dimensions may be too indistinct and overlapping, and 3) the use of the OCF may be repetitive with standard clinical assessment.[1] While the DSM-IV only provided five thematic categories through the OCF, the DSM-5 presents the CFI with specific questions pertaining to each category, giving guidance to clinicians on how to specifically probe for these areas. In addition, whereas the DSM-IV gave limited guidance on when the cultural formulation should be used, the DSM-5 is clear: It should be used with every patient, preferably starting with the initial evaluation. Finally, with the DSM-IV's use of culture-bound syndromes (discussed below), there was a risk of stereotyping cultural groups. The DSM-5 focuses on idioms of distress and takes a person-centered approach, emphasizing a collaborative, shared decision-making process.[5] As a result, Section III of DSM-5 contains two updated versions of the OCF and CFI, discussed further below.

OUTLINE FOR CULTURAL FORMULATION

DSM-5 emphasizes that a clinician must take into account an individual's ethnic and cultural context in the evaluation of each DSM-5 disorder. The OCF organizes the relevance of culture within the patient–clinician encounter around five dimensions. One explicit function of the OCF has been to assist clinicians in diagnosing patients whose presentations do not correspond to DSM-IV diagnoses.[7] For the DSM-5, the DSM-IV OCF was edited for comprehensiveness, clarity, and length (e.g. adding other elements of cultural identity, such as religious affiliation and sexual orientation).[1]

Cultural Identity of the Individual

It is important to consider racial, ethnic, and cultural influences, as well as the degree to which an individual is involved with his or her culture of origin (versus the culture in which he or she lives). It is crucial to listen for clues and to ask specific questions concerning a patient's cultural identity. For instance, an Asian American who grew up in the southern United States may exhibit behaviors, preferences, and views of the world more consistent with a white American Southerner. Language ability, preference, and patterns of mental health service use must also be considered to address difficulties accessing care and to identify the need for an interpreter. In addition, attention to religious affiliation, socioeconomic position, country of origin, migrant status, and sexual orientation may be considered important aspects of cultural identity.

Cultural Conceptualizations of Distress

How an individual understands and experiences his or her symptoms is often communicated through cultural syndromes and idioms of distress (e.g., "nerves," possession by spirits, somatic complaints, misfortune). Thus, the meaning and severity of the illness in relation to one's culture, family, and community should be determined. This idea is exemplified in the case discussed at the beginning of the chapter, where our 44-year-old Haitian woman firmly attributed her symptoms to the malicious effects of someone in her social network attempting to harm her, consistent with the cultural conceptualization of distress known as *maladi moun*. This "explanatory model" may be significantly relevant when developing an interpretation, diagnosis, and treatment plan.

Psychosocial Stressors and Cultural Features of Vulnerability and Resilience

It is important to identify psychosocial stressors and supports within a patient's environment, including for example, religion, family, and social circle. Cultural interpretations of social stress and support, and the individual's level of disability and function, must also be addressed. An individual from a collectivistic community may perceive stress differently than one from an individualistic community, as described in a study done by Kononovas and Dallas comparing Japanese, American, and Lithuanian college students' perceptions of stress and self-efficacy.[8] It is the physician's responsibility to determine a patient's level of functioning, resilience, and disability in the context of his or her cultural reference groups.

Cultural aspects of the relationship between the individual and the clinician, as well as of treatment, should also be considered. Common barriers for clinicians include difficulties with language, establishing rapport, and eliciting symptoms or understanding their cultural significance. For example, clinicians working with Hmong women and men should be mindful of how Hmong community members may be mistrustful and fearful of Western physicians and medicine due to the lack of direct translation of medical terms and diagnosis, as well as the differences between Hmong traditional beliefs and Western biomedical beliefs.[9] Similarly, there are well-documented differences in the level of racial and ethnic minority patient trust in medical research and the health care system in general that are linked to sociocultural and historical legacies.[10]

Overall Cultural Assessment for Diagnosis and Care

The formulation concludes with a summary of the implications of each component outlined above for psychiatric diagnosis, treatment, and other clinically relevant issues. This step directly acknowledges the fact that each society establishes its own criteria regarding which forms of behavior are acceptable or abnormal, and which behaviors represent a medical problem—all of which influences the way mental health care is conceived and delivered.

Social theories inform each domain.[4] The emphasis on cultural identity can help clinicians understand how culture shapes everyday practices affecting patient health and illness, such as diet and sleeping arrangements.[11] A focus on clinicians conducting "mini-ethnographies" with patients acting as informants on cause, onset, mechanism, course, severity, and treatment expectations draws on Kleinman's work.[12] The section on psychosocial stressors and cultural features of vulnerability and resilience draws on the theory of help-seeking pathways influencing how patients seek treatments. The section regarding cultural features of the relationship examines how clinicians' power molds patient histories.[13] The DSM-5 version of the OCF thus represents an attempt to acknowledge the centrality of patient narrative within psychodynamic psychiatry and anthropology.[14,15] Working with patients' diverse explanatory models of illness is explored in much greater detail elsewhere in this textbook.

CULTURAL FORMULATION INTERVIEW

As described above, DSM-5 also includes the CFI, a semi-structured interview composed of 16 questions that physicians can use to assess the influence of culture on a patient's clinical presentation and care. Its main goals are to enhance the cultural validity of diagnostic assessment, facilitate treatment planning, and promote patient engagement. In sum, the CFI can be seen as operationalizing aspects of culture.[1] The CFI focuses on four domains of assessment: (1) cultural definition of the problem (questions #1–3); (2) cultural perceptions of the cause, context, and social support surrounding the problem (#4–10); (3) cultural factors affecting self-coping skills and past help-seeking behaviors (#11–13); and (4) cultural factors affecting current help-seeking behaviors (#14–16). The interview aims to avoid stereotyping; questions regarding cultural identity center on the individual rather than inquiring generically about the views of the group(s) the person identifies with or is ascribed to by the clinician. In doing so, the interview incorporates the cultural knowledge of the patient as well as the social context of his or her illness experience. By doing so, this approach takes account of how individuals' perception of the world are shaped by the various cultural influences in their lives; it provides a forum to explore hybrid identities in a person and ultimately allows intracultural heterogeneity of views to emerge, since individuals hold views stemming from a diversity of cultural influence in their lives.[1]

The CFI is intended for use by any clinician with any patient and in any setting, not exclusively for the evaluation of members of nondominant cultural groups. It may be used when physicians experience difficulties in diagnostic assessment due to cultural differences, difficulties in determining illness severity or impairment, disagreements with patients regarding the course of treatment, or difficulties engaging patients in treatment.

Twelve supplementary modules, to be used in conjunction with the CFI, have been created to help clinicians conduct a more comprehensive cultural assessment, and as described earlier are available for free download online.[6] Modules include explanatory models; level of functioning; the influence of a patient's social network on illness course, and the role of psychosocial and economic stressors; role of spirituality, religion, and moral traditions; cultural identity;

coping and help-seeking skills; and the patient–clinician relationship. The 12 supplementary modules address specific areas of interest as well as the special needs of certain populations: explanatory model; level of functioning, social network; psychosocial stressors; spirituality, religion, and moral traditions; cultural identity; coping and help-seeking; patient–clinician relationship; school-age children and adolescents; older adults; immigrants and refugees; and caregivers.[1]

Feasibility, Acceptability, and Utility

For clinicians and patients, pilot-testing of the CFI has suggested that the CFI has facilitated recognition of communication barriers between patients and providers. Initial qualitative interviews with patients (n = 32) and clinicians (n = 7) suggested that use of the CFI enhances rapport through satisfaction with the interview, elicits both information and perspectives from the patient, and facilitates data collection from multiple sources.[3,4] In a subsequent international field trial of 318 patients and 75 clinicians in six countries (United States, five sites; Peru, one site; Canada, two sites; Netherlands, one site; Kenya, one site; India, two sites), the 14-item pilot core CFI was administered to diagnostically diverse psychiatric outpatients during a diagnostic interview.[16] Participants completed two brief questionnaires—the Debriefing Instrument for Patients (DIP) and the Debriefing Instrument for Clinicians (DIC)—as well as separate semistructured qualitative interviews, with patient and clinicians providing more detailed accounts of the impact of the CFI on each evaluation. Mixed-methods data found the CFI feasible ("Can it be done?"), acceptable ("Do people like it?"), and useful ("Is it helpful?") among clinicians and patients. Clinician feasibility ratings were significantly lower than patient ratings and other clinician-assessed outcomes, demonstrating heightened levels of concern about the tool's feasibility as compared with its acceptability or utility. However, after administering one CFI, clinician feasibility ratings improved significantly, and subsequent interviews required less time. According to the study's authors, by the last CFI administration, a full intake assessment including the CFI lasted 50 minutes, with the CFI taking 22 minutes of the interview.[16] For a subsample of 30 monolingual Spanish-speaking adults in the field trial, findings from qualitative interviews further suggest that using the CFI in this population can help establish trust and enable clinicians to focus on social ties important to patients.[17] In addition, the questions in the CFI facilitated discussions on the impact of stigma on mental illness and patients' pressing social needs.[17]

In addition, family members of participants in the field trial were queried about their experience.[18] Including family members and others who accompany patients to clinic visits may help clinicians understand patients from diverse cultural backgrounds unfamiliar to the clinician; this is particularly important when patients cannot provide a coherent or accurate account due to cognitive or psychiatric impairment.[19] Of the patient interviews in the international field trial described above, only 86 included companions, all of whom were family members or other relatives. If companions attended the CFI interview, they also completed a closed-ended debriefing questionnaire and an open-ended, semistructured interview on CFI feasibility, acceptability, and clinical utility. Relatives' perceptions of the CFI's acceptability and clinical utility were generally favorable, as supported by quantitative analysis of completed questionnaires. In qualitative analyses of debriefing interviews, relatives valued the in-depth exploration of the patient's problem and the opportunity to share their own views and to participate in the assessment process. Some relatives found the CFI too time-consuming and questions too personal or difficult to understand, similar to those barriers reported by patients in the qualitative analyses.[4,16]

The CFI represents an important step forward in standardizing the work of cultural psychiatrists, anthropologists, and others in a format accessible to all clinicians. However, the CFI does not result in diagnosis; the information it obtains must be integrated with other available clinical material to produce a comprehensive clinical evaluation.[1]

DSM-5 CULTURAL CONCEPTS OF DISTRESS

The DSM Cultural Issues Subgroup proposed a thorough revision of the DSM-IV *Glossary of Culture-Bound Syndromes* into a new *Glossary of Cultural Concepts of Distress.* Cultural concepts of distress refer to "ways that cultural groups experience, understand, and communicate suffering, behavioral problems, or troubling thoughts or emotions."[5] The new DSM-5 glossary replaces the term "culture-bound syndromes" with three concepts of greater clinical utility: (1) cultural syndromes, (2) cultural idioms of distress, and (3) cultural explanations or perceived causes. These three concepts (described in greater detail below) have been deemed more clinically relevant than culture-bound syndromes and have replaced the term in DSM-5, as the term *culture-bound syndrome* does not take into account that some "syndromes" are actually variations in ways people experience distress rather than distinct collections of symptoms (e.g., *nervios*), while others are causal explanations for a range of symptoms (e.g., *dhat* syndrome). The term *culture-bound syndrome* also overemphasizes the localized nature and limited distribution of cultural concepts of distress.

Cultural syndromes are clusters of symptoms that occur among individuals in specific cultural groups or communities. *Cultural idioms of distress* are shared ways of experiencing, communicating, and expressing personal or social concerns. *Cultural explanations or perceived causes* are labels, attributions, or features that indicate causation of symptoms, illness, or distress.

Although worth distinguishing conceptually, in common practice the same cultural term frequently denotes more than one kind of cultural concept. As an example, "depression" fulfills the criteria for all three concepts as follows: Western clinicians understand major depressive disorder as a "syndrome," or a cluster of symptoms that often appear together. Depression is also a commonly used cultural idiom of distress, used by laypeople in many Western societies to talk about a certain type of emotional distress. Finally, as a cultural explanation of distress or perceived cause, the term *depression* helps imbue a set of behaviors with meaning and associated etiology.

DSM-5 GLOSSARY OF CULTURAL CONCEPTS
OF DISTRESS

While the term *culture-bound syndrome* has been eliminated, the creators of DSM-5 continue to acknowledge the usefulness of certain well-studied examples of cultural syndromes, explanations, and idioms of distress. Many of these concepts included in the glossary cut across DSM diagnoses, so that the relationship between concepts and disorders is not always one to one.[1] Table 3.1 details nine such concepts that were retained in the DSM-5 glossary. These concepts may aid physicians in identifying how individuals from different specific cultures and communities exhibit and explain psychological issues.

A repeated criticism of the DSM is its traditional assumption that Western diagnostic categories are the "default," meaning that any cultural variations have traditionally been relegated to a glossary of "culture-bound syndromes." In doing away with the concept of culture-bound syndromes, DSM-5 also grants greater privilege to cultural conceptualizations of distress by including direct and reciprocal cross-references of multicultural explanations for clusters of symptoms within the descriptions of each DSM-5 disorder. For example, the glossary description of *ataque de nervios* (defined as "an intense emotional upset, including acute anxiety, anger, or grief; screaming and shouting uncontrollably; attacks of crying; trembling; heat in the chest rising into the head; and becoming verbally and physically aggressive") cross-references the related condition of panic disorder in the main text of DSM-5. Similarly, the description of "panic disorder" in the main text of the manual contains a section (labeled "Culture-Related Diagnostic Issues") that describes *ataque de nervios* and references the glossary.[5,20]

By virtue of this increased emphasis on culture-related diagnostic considerations and reciprocal cross-referencing between the main text and the glossary, DSM-5 represents an advancement over DSM-IV in terms of establishing the centrality of culture for appropriate diagnosis and, by extension, treatment.

USE OF DSM-5 MATERIALS IN TRAINING
AND GENERAL PRACTICE

The OCF and CFI are resources that may be helpful in cultural sensitivity training. In a study of six residency programs in the United States and Canada, psychiatry residents were exposed to a one-hour session on the CFI to assess whether this didactic session could improve the cultural competence of general psychiatry residents.[21] The authors reported that this didactic session improved immediate self-reported cultural competence scores in psychiatry residents, but there was no association between cultural exposure (time spent in previous cultural training used as a proxy measure) and the degree of improvement in self-reported cultural competence. However, the study was limited in that self-report scales were used without translation to actual competence using clinical data.

Of course, one didactic session is not enough, either for those in psychiatric training or in continuing education; a combination of modalities may prove more effective. In the CFI field trial, interviews with 75 clinicians were used to understand their views on training preferences after a standardized training session and

Table 3.1 CULTURAL CONCEPTS OF DISTRESS

	Meaning	Description	Countries/ Regions
Ataque de nervios	Attack of the nerves	A cultural syndrome that involves symptoms of distress which include uncontrollable shouting, crying attacks, trembling, a sense of heat in the chest that migrates to the head, as well as verbal and physical aggression. It frequently occurs as a result of a direct event, often related to the family. The fact that *ataques* are associated with a specific event, and that there is often an absence of acute fear, allows it to be distinguished from panic disorder. Many times affected individuals experience amnesia and then rapidly return to their usual functioning.	Caribbean, Latin America, Latin Mediterranean
Dhat Syndrome	Semen loss	A cultural explanation for patients with diverse symptoms, including: anxiety, fatigue, weakness, weight loss, impotence, depressed mood, and somatic complaints. Characterized by anxiety and stress about loss of *dhat* (white discharge noted upon defecation or urination) in absence of any identifiable physiologic dysfunction.	Southeast Asia
Khyâl cap	Wind attacks	A cultural syndrome with symptoms (such as dizziness, palpitations, dyspnea, cold extremities, and neck soreness) similar to those of panic attacks. *Khyâl* attacks involve a catastrophic fear that *khyâl* (a wind-like substance) may rise in the body, along with blood, and cause a range of serious effects, such as shortness of breath, asphyxia, blurry vision, tinnitus, and a fatal syncope.	Cambodia

(continued)

Table 3.1 CONTINUED

	Meaning	Description	Countries/ Regions
Kufungisisa	Thinking too much	A cultural explanation and idiom of distress among the Shona of Zimbabwe. As a cultural explanation, "thinking too much" is considered damaging to mind and body, causing depression, anxiety, and symptoms such as headaches and dizziness. As an idiom of distress, it reflects interpersonal and social difficulties causing emotional and somatic symptoms (e.g., "my heart is painful because I think too much").	Zimbabwe
Maladi moun	Humanly caused illness	A cultural explanation for a range of medical and psychiatric disorders. Involves beliefs that interpersonal envy and ill will cause people to harm their enemies by sending illnesses (e.g., psychosis, depression), social or academic failure, and inability to perform activities of daily living. May be provoked by economic success (new job, expensive purchase) or being attractive, intelligent, or wealthy.	Haiti
Nervios	Nerves	An idiom of distress which refers to a state of vulnerability to stressful and difficult life experiences and circumstances. Encompasses a wide range of symptoms, such as headaches, "brain aches", irritability, GI discomfort, insomnia, nervousness, tearfulness, difficulty concentrating, trembling, paresthesias, and *mareos* (dizziness). Ranges in severity from individuals free from mental disorder to those with presentations similar to anxiety, depressive, dissociative, or psychotic disorders.	Latin America

Table 3.1 CONTINUED

	Meaning	Description	Countries/ Regions
Shenjing shuairuo	Weakness of the nervous system	A cultural syndrome characterized by physical and mental fatigue, dizziness, headaches, pains, poor concentration, sleep difficulties, and memory loss. Individuals may also experience nausea, vomiting, diarrhea, sexual dysfunction, irritability, and agitation.	China
Susto	Fright	A cultural syndrome attributed to a frightening event causing the soul to leave the body. Symptoms include headache, pain, diarrhea, changes in appetite and sleep, sadness, and a lack of interest or motivation. Symptoms may appear from days to years after the event has occurred.	Latin America, Mexico, Central and South America
Taijin kyofusho	Interpersonal fear disorder	A cultural syndrome that refers to an individual's intense fear that one's body parts/function (e.g., appearance, odor, movement, facial expressions) displease, embarrass, or are offensive to others.	Japan

clinicians' first administration of the CFI.[3] Clinicians named case-based behavioral simulations as the "most helpful" and video as the "least helpful" training methods. Most clinicians preferred active behavioral simulations in cultural competence training, and this effect was most pronounced among older clinicians. The authors of this study concluded that training may be best accomplished through a combination of modalities to reach a larger audience: for instance, reviewing CFI written guidelines, video demonstration of the CFI simulated between clinician and patient, and behavioral simulations pairing clinicians with standardized patients to practice applying the CFI to clinical situations.

CASE SUMMARY

Prior to the outpatient psychiatric evaluation of the 44-year-old Haitian woman, the faculty member reviewed the DSM-5 descriptions of the OCF and CFI. Due to her conviction that culture may be a key factor in this patient's care, she decided to print out the CFI for both herself and the resident. She also invited the resident to review the concept of maladi moun *in the DSM-5 glossary. During the intake, the patient seemed surprised by the outpatient treatment team's interest in her beliefs, noting that the inpatient psychiatrist had tended to become impatient with the idea that her misfortunes were induced by someone else, attributing such beliefs to paranoia and psychosis and increasing the dose of her medications. Having felt validated in her convictions, she subsequently exhibited greater flexibility in considering the outpatient treatment team's suggestion that there may be other potential contributors to her symptoms, including a lifelong tendency toward significant ruminations and worry. While she continued to maintain a conviction that others were jealous of her, she also found benefit in some acceptance and cognitive reframing strategies, and agreed to initiate a selective serotonin reuptake inhibitor. Over time, her symptoms greatly improved and the atypical antipsychotic medication was tapered and discontinued without recurrence of the suspicious or paranoid thoughts.*

CONCLUSION

This chapter discussed the evolution of the focus on culture from DSM-IV to DSM-5 and described best practices in using the OCF and CFI for evaluation and management of patients from diverse populations. While more work needs to be done in implementation, training, and education of trainees and experienced clinicians in using these tools, they represent a bold step forward in incorporating key concepts of culture in general psychiatric practice.

REFERENCES

1. Lewis-Fernández R, Aggarwal NK. Culture and psychiatric diagnosis. *Advances in Psychosomatic Medicine.* 2013;33:15–30.
2. American Psychiatric Association. *Diagnostic and Statistical Manual of Mental Disorders, 4th ed., Text Revision (DSM-IV-TR).* Washington, DC: American Psychiatric Association; 2000.
3. Aggarwal N, Lam P, Castillo E, et al. How do clinicians prefer cultural competence training? Findings from the DSM-5 Cultural Formulation Interview field trial. *Academic Psychiatry.* 2015;40(4):584–591.
4. Aggarwal N, Nicasio A, DeSilva R, Boiler M, Lewis-Fernández R. Barriers to implementing the DSM-5 Cultural Formulation Interview: A qualitative study. *Culture, Medicine, and Psychiatry.* 2013;37(3):505–533.
5. American Psychiatric Association. *Diagnostic and Statistical Manual of Mental Disorders, 5th ed. (DSM-5).* Washington, DC: American Psychiatric Association; 2013.
6. American Psychiatric Association. Supplementary Modules to the Core Cultural Formulation Interview (CFI). 2013. https://www.psychiatry.org/FileLibrary/Psychiatrists/Practice/DSM/APA_DSM5_Cultural-Formulation-Interview-Supplementary-Modules.pdf.
7. Lewis-Fernández R, Díaz N. The cultural formulation: A method for assessing cultural factors affecting the clinical encounter. *Psychiatric Quarterly.* 2002;73(4):271–295.

8. Kononovas K, Dallas T. A cross-cultural comparison of perceived stress and self-efficacy across Japanese, U.S. and Lithuanian students. *Psichologija*. 2009;39:59–70.

9. Johnson S. Hmong health beliefs and experiences in the Western health care system. *Journal of Transcultural Nursing*. 2002;13(2):126–132.

10. Boulware LE. Race and trust in the health care system. *Public Health Reports*. 2003;118(4):358–365.

11. Mezzich J, Caracci G, Fabrega H, Kirmayer L. Cultural formulation guidelines. *Transcultural Psychiatry*. 2009;46(3):383–405.

12. Kleinman A. Lessons from a clinical approach to medical anthropological research. *Medical Anthropology Newsletter*. 1977;8(4):11–15.

13. Good B. *Medicine, Rationality, and Experience: An Anthropological Perspective*. Cambridge, UK: Cambridge University Press; 1994.

14. Lewis-Fernandez R. Cultural formulation of psychiatric diagnosis. *Culture, Medicine, & Psychiatry*. 1996; 20:133–144.

15. Kleinman A. *Rethinking Psychiatry*. New York: Free Press; 1988.

16. Lewis-Fernández R, Aggarwal N, Lam P et Al. Feasibility, acceptability and clinical utility of the Cultural Formulation Interview: Mixed-methods results from the DSM-5 international field trial. *British Journal of Psychiatry*. 2017;210(04):290–297.

17. Díaz E, Añez L, Silva M, Paris M, Davidson L. Using the Cultural Formulation Interview to build culturally sensitive services. *Psychiatric Services*. 2017;68(2):112–114.

18. Hinton L, Aggarwal N, Iosif A, et al. Perspectives of family members participating in cultural assessment of psychiatric disorders: Findings from the DSM-5 international field trial. *International Review of Psychiatry*. 2015;27(1):3–10.

19. Estroff S. Subject/subjectivities in dispute: The poetics, politics, and performance of first-person narratives of people with schizophrenia. In: Jenkins J, Barrett R, eds. *Schizophrenia, Culture, and Subjectivity: The Edge of Experience*. Cambridge, UK: Cambridge University Press; 2003:282–302.

20. Cummings, CA. DSM-5 on Culture: A Significant Advance. Thefprorg Blog. June 2013. https://thefprorg.wordpress.com/2013/06/27/dsm-5-on-culture-a-significant-advance/

21. Mills S, Wolitzky-Taylor K, Xiao AQ, et al. Training on the DSM-5 Cultural Formulation Interview improves cultural competence in general psychiatry residents: A multi-site study. *Academic Psychiatry*. 2016;40(5):829–834.

4

Global Psychiatric Epidemiology

MARIA C. PROM AND ALEXANDER C. TSAI ■

CASE 1

Mrs. A, a 58-year-old white woman with a past psychiatric history of depression and anxiety, presented to the emergency department by ambulance after collapsing to the floor in her home and becoming unresponsive after receiving news of her son's unexpected death.

Upon evaluation in the emergency department, the physician was concerned about a persistent change in mental status from baseline. The patient was reportedly awake and alert but was speaking incoherently and not responding appropriately to questions. A computed tomography image of her brain was unremarkable for a hemorrhage or other acute intracranial process that could potentially explain her exam findings. Psychiatry was consulted to evaluate for psychiatric causes of altered mental status. At the time of psychiatric evaluation, she was awake, alert, and oriented and responded to questions appropriately but with tearful and, at times, irritable affect. Her other children were at the bedside and reported that she was back to her baseline mental status. They felt she had simply been very shocked by the news. Her presentation on interview was felt to be an appropriate response to the loss of a loved one only hours prior. She was cleared by psychiatry for safety and then discharged home with a plan to continue her home medications and follow-up in the coming week with her outpatient mental health provider.

At first glance it may seem unclear how this case fits into a discussion of global psychiatric epidemiology. However, it is a fitting example of what is at the heart of this topic and what we will explore in this chapter: namely, how cultural and societal norms and expectations influence our classification, understanding, and treatment of mental illness. We do not need to look further than our own practice to find evidence of these impacts.

INTRODUCTION

Global psychiatry, also commonly conceptualized by the term *global mental health*, broadly refers to the application of global health concepts and practices to the area of mental health. Global mental health, as such, is defined as "an area of study, research, and practice that places a priority on improving [mental] health and achieving equity in [mental] health for all people worldwide."[1] The field of global mental health confronts the challenge of providing equitable access to mental health care, as well as the challenge of improving respect for the human rights and dignity of those living with mental illness.[2] Implicitly, then, there is a focus on implementation science. It is important not to mistake the word *global* for *international*, as the latter could imply a focus on mental health problems solely in countries other than one's own.[3] That said, the field of global mental health does often focus on mental health problems in low- and middle-income countries, as the greatest inequities of resources for mental health care are often observed in these settings.[4]

Historically, mental health has largely been placed at the bottom of the priority list when addressing global disease due to a multitude of factors, one of which is the lack of immediate threat to mortality. The attention given to mental illness on the global agenda is a relatively new phenomenon, first prompted in the 1990s following the Global Burden of Disease (GBD) Study. The GBD Study introduced the measurement of global burden of disease through disability-adjusted life years (DALYs).[5] DALYs represented a profound conceptual shift, as previously published estimates had focused on years of life lost. DALYs instead are calculated by combining the years of life lost due to early mortality with the years of healthy life lost due to living with a disease or disability. In the GBD Study, neuropsychiatric disorders were, for the first time, identified as one of the top contributors to the global burden of disease. In 2010, mental, neurological, and substance use disorders were estimated to constitute 10.4% of global DALYs and 28.5% of global years lost to disability (YLDs) worldwide, making them the leading cause of YLDs.[6] However, the DALY approach to burden of illness has not been without criticism over the years, including concerns about limited measurement reliability due to modeling and extrapolation of data, ambiguity around weighing the impact of illnesses across countries and cultures, and limited sensitivity in reflecting the impact of public health interventions.[7-9] The GBD collaborators have continued to update and revise their estimates over the years to address these criticisms.[10]

This approach to measuring the global burden of illness has been critical to increasing awareness of not only the global burden of mental illness, but also the mental health treatment gap. According to World Health Organization (WHO) estimates, in middle- and low-income countries, 76.3% to 85.4% of serious cases of mental illness do not receive treatment within 1 year of survey.[11] There are many reasons for this disparity, including lack of treaters: In low-income countries, there are 0.1 psychiatrists for every 100,000 people, compared to 0.4 to 1.2 per 100,000 in middle-income countries and 6.6 per 100,000 in high-income countries.[12]

This chapter will focus on our current understanding of *global psychiatric epidemiology*, the study of the distribution and determinants of mental health disorders and the application of that knowledge to the management of mental health globally. We will discuss the basic principles, concepts, and challenges of global psychiatric epidemiology, including mental illness classification, cultural concepts of distress, and our current understanding of global psychiatric epidemiology and its limitations. First we will describe how mental illness is defined and classified in order to better understand the significant impact of cultural and societal norms on classification and, ultimately, our understanding of global psychiatric epidemiology. We also hope to improve the reader's day-to-day approach to the diagnosis and management of mental illness by raising awareness of how cultural and societal norms and expectations influence our understanding and treatment of mental illness.

DEFINING AND CLASSIFYING MENTAL ILLNESS

We must first develop an understanding of how and why we define and classify mental illness (also referred to as *mental disorder*, a term that is often used interchangeably but does not carry any assumption of etiology). The construct of mental illness does not stand alone; it is conceptualized within a social, cultural, and even historical context. This is an important concept in understanding mental illness in a global context, given the wide variety of social and cultural norms worldwide.

Defining Mental Illness

In the psychiatric context, a mental illness is defined by a group of signs and symptoms that represent a change in an individual's prior mental state and lead to the experience of distress and/or a decline in function.[13,14] Conceptualizations of mental illness have historically appealed to signs and symptoms that exceed some implicit threshold level of severity compromising patients' ability to function within their current social and cultural surroundings. Mental illnesses are unlike many other medical diagnoses in that we lack clear diagnostic tools (e.g., biomarkers) for definitively classifying mental states into "diseased" versus "not diseased"; instead, diagnosis is based on clinical evaluation and judgment guided by the use of classification schemes, which are derived through scientific evidence and professional consensus.

Cultural and social expectations determine the threshold of impairment or severity required for one's signs and symptoms to be defined as a disorder. For instance, the concept of *role impairment* refers to the impact of illness on an individual's role within his or her cultural and societal context. As such, the cross-cultural validity and utility of how mental illness is defined is frequently criticized. It brings to light controversies not only across cultures but also within cultures, with many questioning whether the concept of mental illness, rather than serving to classify disease states, implicitly functions to convey social, political, or moral judgments.[15,16] Additionally, there is concern that this type of definition risks pathologizing expressions of distress that vary within a cultural spectrum of *normal*—such as the concept of bereavement, an experience that can vary greatly both across and within cultures and countries.[17–22] This controversy is exemplified in the case described at the opening of this chapter; the patient's level of impairment was sufficiently concerning to the primary medical team that their concern for pathology led them to consult with the psychiatry service. In contrast, the psychiatric consultant determined that the patient's presentation fell within the culturally acceptable spectrum of distress for bereavement.

Despite its limitations, the present system of classifying mental illness is important for several reasons: to facilitate communication using a common language (e.g., between health care providers or between health care providers and health insurers); to improve the acceptance of mental illness as a valid disease process; to determine the most appropriate and effective clinical management for a patient's signs and symptoms; to improve public health interventions, including prevention; and to assist in evaluating and predicting prognosis, treatment response, and outcomes.

Classification of Mental Illness

Disease classification systems may have myriad goals, including maximizing precision, validity, and/or clinical utility. Here *precision* refers to the ability to consistently identify an illness using a single set of criteria, and *validity* refers to the accuracy of a set of criteria in differentiating a diseased state from a nondiseased state. The WHO favors a goal of *clinical utility*, assessing the value of a classification system by its impact on communication, implementation in clinical practice (e.g., accuracy of description, feasibility), and usefulness in selecting interventions and making clinical management decisions.[23]

In the U.S. medical system, we use two classification systems that are also commonly used worldwide, the *Diagnostic and Statistical Manual of Mental Disorders* (DSM) and the International Classification of Diseases (ICD), both of which feature operational definitions of mental illness. The DSM, published by the American Psychiatric Association (APA), is based on an American system of classifying syndromes of signs and symptoms that eventually became widely accepted in the profession as mental disorders. The ICD, published by the WHO and approved by the World Health Assembly, covers a wide range of health conditions, not just mental illness. The ICD categorization of mental illness now overlaps significantly with the DSM, given increased collaboration between the APA and WHO. While both systems rely on a biomedical approach to diagnosis and, like many medical fields, use symptom clustering for diagnosis, the DSM focuses more on diagnostic validity, while the ICD focuses more on clinical utility. Despite the American origin of the DSM, this system is widely accepted and used globally, and has influenced international classification of mental illnesses.

Other countries and world regions have their own classification systems, such as China's *Chinese Classification of Mental Disorders*, Latin America's *Latin American Guide for Psychiatric Diagnosis*, and Cuba's *Cuban Glossary of Psychiatry*. A major limitation in all classification systems, the DSM and ICD included, is that they are inherently ethnocentric in their definitions, and therefore not generalizable worldwide.

Cultural Concepts of Distress

The cross-cultural limitations and ethnocentrism of the major DSM diagnostic categories have over time led to attempts to incorporate other cultural expressions of distress. *Cultural concepts of distress* is the most recent terminology included in the DSM-5 to describe the cultural variability of emotional distress and dysfunction not accounted for in the DSM. This terminology marks a significant change in the DSM cultural formulation section, which describes the ways in which different cultural groups "experience, understand, and communicate suffering, behavioral problems, or troubling thoughts and emotions."[14] The term *cultural concepts of distress* replaces prior terminology, such as *culture-bound syndrome* (used in the DSM-IV), in an effort to eliminate the implication of cultural exclusivity and improve the DSM's relevance to clinical practice. This terminology also serves to better acknowledge the reality that all psychological distress, including mental illness as defined by the DSM, is shaped in local culture.

Cultural concepts of distress can be divided further into three main concepts: *cultural syndromes, cultural idioms of distress*, and *cultural explanations or perceived causes*. *Cultural syndrome* refers to symptom clusters that occur together within cultural groups or contexts and that are viewed as consistent patterns of experience within that culture. *Cultural idioms of distress* are manners of expressing psychological distress that are not specific to any syndrome or cluster of symptoms but that are a shared experience or manner of expressing concern within a cultural group. *Cultural explanations or perceived causes* refer to explanations of illness that are bound in culturally derived beliefs about the meaning or etiology of symptoms, illness, or distress. This concept also acknowledges that it is not only the symptomatic expression of illness that is relevant to patients, but also the experience and the causal explanation of the illness. The emphasis on patients' causal explanations is particularly notable, as these can influence treatment seeking, coping, and attitudes about mental health care.[2,14]

Cultural concepts of distress are distinctly separated from diagnostic categories within the DSM-5 and are infrequently studied in psychiatric research or acknowledged in the application of psychiatric treatment. This separation has raised the question of how to understand them within the context of existing biomedical classification systems. A related concern is how the field can incorporate these forms of psychological distress into the current understanding of psychiatric epidemiology and clinical practice without losing the important aspect of cultural explanations and expectations.

As such, studies have sought to improve our understanding of how cultural concepts of distress relate to existing systems, particularly biomedical diagnostic conceptualizations. These studies have generally demonstrated a poor correspondence between cultural concepts of distress and existing classification systems (e.g., the DSM). One important exception to this general trend is current evidence from U.S.-based studies in which most participants were immigrants to the Americas. Studies in these populations show a stronger association between cultural concepts of distress and existing biomedical categorizations of mental illness,[24] such that cultural concepts of distress in these populations tend to better fit biomedical diagnostic frameworks. It has been suggested that these findings are a result of acculturation, globalization, and reframing of psychological distress to adapt to a culture and language different from one's own.[24] This is an important consideration for those in the United States who care for immigrants from diverse cultures within their practices.

Acculturation and globalization are also important issues globally, as biomedical conceptualizations of mental illness are adapted worldwide in a manner that is frequently referred to as the *globalization of mental illness*. This process can be seen directly through the worldwide use of classification systems such as the DSM and the ICD, and the widespread adoption of treatment recommendations by organizations such as the APA and WHO. Biomedical illness representations are disseminated not only through clinicians, researchers, and health organizations, but also through other exposure channels like popular media. In Becker's[25] classic study of television exposure and eating behaviors and attitudes in Fiji, she found that Fijian schoolgirls had an increased prevalence of disordered eating attitudes and behaviors following the introduction of television in the region. Some argue that the spread of biomedical concepts of mental illness through globalization has led to homogenization in the conceptualization and treatment of mental illness around the world, at the expense of local cultural and religious beliefs.[26] On the other hand, some suggest that globalization can have the opposite effect, such as intensifying local identities, concepts, and beliefs as a reaction to threats to identity.[27]

These studies and critiques illustrate the importance of incorporating cultural concepts of distress into current screening and detection methods, given that those endorsing a cultural concept of distress have a substantially elevated risk of also experiencing clinically significant psychological distress (or having a DSM-consistent psychiatric diagnosis).[24] In addition, cultural concepts of distress should be considered in evaluating illness and developing treatment interventions. If clinicians diagnose and treat only biomedical concepts of psychological distress, then they may miss cultural concepts of distress that also warrant clinical intervention. Patients with ongoing functional impairment will therefore likely continue to seek treatment.[24]

CASE 2

Mrs. B was a 63-year-old married woman who immigrated from the Dominican Republic to the United States in her late 20s, with a history of depression, anxiety, and posttraumatic stress disorder (PTSD) due to past domestic violence from her current partner. Her medical history was significant for hypertension, renal insufficiency, deep venous thrombosis, and chronic pain. She presented for outpatient psychiatric management.

The interview was conducted in Spanish. The patient described that her nervios *were worse due to several recent family stressors, including a more conflictual relationship with her spouse in the setting of her father-in-law's worsened health. She described multiple symptoms, including shortness of breath, fatigue, tremor, poor sleep, anxiety, depression, tearfulness, nightmares, and decreased motivation. The patient was given another trial of a low-dose medication to treat nightmares, which she discontinued out of her concern that it was causing ankle swelling. No changes were made to her long-term antidepressant medication at that time.*

At the next visit a month later, she reported that she was feeling much better following a vacation with her family. She stated that she felt much happier and that most of her symptoms had improved. The interview was notable for brighter and less anxious affect. She also reported that her relationship with her husband had improved as his father's health had improved.

Nervios (nerves) is one of several similar *nervios*-related terms commonly used among Latinos, particularly within Puerto Rican culture. *Nervios* is frequently expressed in association with the distress surrounding stressful life events. The term *nervios* is a cultural idiom of distress within the broader category of cultural concepts of distress that may be used differently among individuals from different regions of Latin America.[14,28] It does not refer to one single emotional state or symptom, but rather can be used to describe symptoms or states of emotional distress that vary widely in their experience and severity. Some examples of symptoms often associated with *nervios* include headaches, gastrointestinal upset, nervousness, sleep difficulties, trembling, tearfulness, and dizziness. Like many idioms of distress, *nervios* can range from a culturally normative reaction (similarly to feeling stressed or nervous in American culture) to a disorder similar to, but not directly corresponding to, DSM-5 diagnoses such as adjustment disorder, major depressive disorder, generalized anxiety disorder, or somatic symptom disorder.

The case described above provides an example of a patient who immigrated to the United States in her early adulthood. She described her condition as *nervios* with several associated symptoms but with no clear correspondence to any single DSM categorization, including depressive and anxious mood symptoms, somatic symptoms, and symptoms of PTSD. Of note, the patient used both the Latino terminology of *nervios* as well as the American terms of *anxiety* and *depression*; this mixed usage of terminology is an example of acculturation or globalization as discussed above and is an increasingly commonly encountered scenario in U.S.-based psychiatric practice. Cases such as this one can be challenging when using a strict DSM framework and biomedical approach to management. In this particular case, the patient's primary symptoms improved with supportive treatment, and many symptoms improved as her life stressors lessened.

Clinicians should be aware of and understand cultural concepts of distress, especially those frequently encountered in their practices (see Chapter 3, "Culture in the DSM," for further discussion of cultural concepts of distress). This knowledge can lead to performing more appropriate screening; avoiding misdiagnosis; obtaining useful clinical information; improving clinical rapport and engagement through understanding of underlying etiological models; and improving therapeutic efficacy, help-seeking patterns, social response, coping, healing, and recovery. When considered in a broader sense, cultural concepts of distress highlight the need to scrutinize current clinical research (which is largely based on biomedical diagnoses and data from industrialized countries) and clarify cultural epidemiology.

GLOBAL EPIDEMIOLOGY OF MENTAL ILLNESS

The prior discussion about defining and classifying mental illness serves as an important context within which to evaluate and understand available data on the epidemiology of mental illness. Much of what is known in global psychiatric epidemiology has been derived from the WHO World Mental Health (WMH) Survey Initiative, which we describe in detail below, including a discussion of the limitations of the data.

The WMH Survey Initiative

Our current understanding of the global burden of mental illness is based primarily on large-scale epidemiologic studies, the most significant of which is the WMH Survey Initiative. Prior to this initiative, our understanding of the epidemiology of mental illness was based on smaller studies limited by their small scale and lack of consistency. The WMH Survey Initiative was an effort on the part of the WHO to create the first uniform, cross-national, epidemiologic survey to estimate the world-wide prevalence of mental illness, understand its correlates, and improve public health efforts to reduce the global burden of mental illness.

The WMH Survey Initiative uses the Composite International Diagnostic Interview (WMH-CIDI),[29] a structured research diagnostic interview developed by the WHO and later revised by a cross-national research consortium. It is the most commonly used, fully structured diagnostic interview in global psychiatric epidemiology. The CIDI is based on the criteria within the DSM-IV and ICD-10 diagnostic systems and covers *common mental disorders*. The *common mental disorders* concept refers to a wide variety of distress states often encountered in the community or at the level of nonspecialist providers, and includes anxiety disorders (generalized anxiety disorder, panic disorder, agoraphobia without panic disorder, specific phobia, social phobia, PTSD, and separation anxiety disorder), mood disorders (major depressive disorder, dysthymic disorder, bipolar I or II disorder, and subthreshold bipolar disorder), disruptive behavior disorders (attention-deficit/hyperactivity disorder, oppositional defiant disorder, conduct disorder, intermittent explosive disorder), and substance use disorders (alcohol and drug use disorders).

The WMH-CIDI was developed in English and then translated into local languages using specific translation protocols.[29] The survey has been carried out by local lay interviewers trained using standardized protocols and quality control methods and has, at the time of this writing, been implemented in 28 countries worldwide. Most of the WMH studies use multistage clustered area probability household samples, but for most sites the data originate only from specific regions, often larger urban areas.[30,31] Sample sizes have varied by country. The average response rate was 72% (range 46–88%). The data have been analyzed separately by country, with some country groupings based on income level (high, upper-middle, and low/lower-middle) or WHO geographic region. More information about the study design can be obtained at www.hcp.med.harvard.edu/wmh.[31,32]

Prevalence of Mental Illness

The data from the WMH Survey Initiative have demonstrated a high worldwide lifetime prevalence of common mental disorders. Considerable variability has been observed across countries, ranging from a 12% lifetime prevalence of common mental disorders in Nigeria to 47% in the United States.[31] The average 12-month prevalence of common mental disorders has been found to be 17%, ranging from 6% in Nigeria to 30% in Sao Paulo, Brazil (see Table 4.1 for 12-month prevalence estimates stratified by symptom cluster and country income level).[33] The most prevalent classes of common mental disorders in the WMH are anxiety and mood disorders. More recently, data pooled from a systematic review and meta-analysis spanning 174 surveys conducted in 63 countries from 1980-2013, including those conducted by investigators not affiliated with the WMH, have shown consistent results.[34] In this review, the 12-month prevalence of common mental disorder has been estimated at 18%, with a lifetime prevalence estimate of 29%. Considerable regional variations have been noted, with the lowest 12-month and lifetime prevalence estimates found in North and Southeast Asia, and the highest lifetime prevalence estimates found in English-speaking countries. Additionally, women have been found to have higher

Table 4.1 Twelve-Month Prevalence of Common Mental Disorders Based on WMH Survey Initiative

	All disorders	Anxiety disorders	Mood disorders	Disruptive behavior disorders	Substance disorders
Low/lower-middle-income countries	14.8	9.2	4.8	2.7	1.9
Upper-middle-income countries	16.7	10.2	5.8	2.5	3.2
High-income countries	16.7	10.8	6.2	2.6	2.4

Data are given as mean percentage.

Adapted from data from Table 5.1 in Kessler RC, Alonso J, Chatterji S, He Y. The epidemiology and impact of mental disorders. In: Patel V, Minas H, Cohen A, Prince M, eds. *Global Mental Health: Principles and Practice.* New York: Oxford University Press; 2014:82–101.

rates of mood and anxiety disorders, while men have been found to have higher rates of substance use disorders.[34]

The WMH-CIDI has not evaluated dementia and nonaffective psychosis. A systematic review and meta-analysis of the literature suggests the estimated prevalence of dementia is 5% to 7% among persons aged 60 years and older, with very little variability between regions of the world. More than half of all people with dementia live in low- and middle-income countries.[35] The overall prevalence of dementia is expected to increase worldwide due to life expectancy improvements and demographic shifts.

Worldwide estimates for nonaffective psychosis are limited. Many of the data have focused on schizophrenia, with the most recent reviews reporting an overall mean lifetime prevalence estimate of 0.5% across countries.[36] Other studies have demonstrated a higher incidence of nonaffective psychosis among men and in migrant populations and a lower incidence in low- and middle-income countries compared with high-income countries.[37]

Socioeconomic Outcomes of Mental Illness

The WMH Survey Initiative has also provided useful information about the adverse socioeconomic outcomes of common mental disorders, including associations with educational attainment, employment, marital status, role impairment, and physical illness.[38] Persons with common mental disorders are less likely to complete their education.[39] Those with early onset of illness are more likely to be unemployed, are less likely to marry, and, in high- and upper-middle-income countries, have lower household income.[40,41] Disorders present prior to marriage predict marital violence, particularly disruptive behavioral disorders and substance use disorders.[41] Persons with common mental disorders report an increased number of days they are unable to work or carry out their normal daily activities due to their illness, particularly those with bipolar disorder, PTSD, panic disorder, generalized anxiety disorder, and social phobia.[38] They are also more likely to have comorbid physical illness.[42] As a result, disparities in life expectancy have increased, with more than a decade of potential life years lost attributable to mental illness.[43,44]

Limitations of Estimates

These estimates represent a significant advancement in global psychiatric epidemiology and have helped to increase visibility for a previously underrecognized contributor to the global burden of disease. However, there are many limitations and criticisms of the current epidemiologic data. Here the focus will be on survey measures and the methodology of implementation, with a focus on cross-cultural diagnostic precision and validity. Some of these limitations have been touched upon earlier in this chapter; further discussion in this section will focus on how cultural and societal differences influence understanding of the current data. Much of the criticism focuses on the survey methodology, including the choice of classification system, use of language, and how and where the survey was implemented.

LIMITATIONS OF SURVEY DESIGN

The WMH-CIDI survey, like many international epidemiologic surveys, is based on DSM and ICD diagnoses and classification systems, which as discussed previously are structured within biomedical frameworks. This design choice could influence the accuracy of diagnoses, the concordance of diagnoses across countries, and the clinical relevance of the diagnoses obtained, particularly in non-Western cultures. As such, the validity of the data from the WMH Survey Initiative has been subject to some criticism, with concern that the high variability in the prevalence of common mental disorders across countries is a result of underestimating the prevalence of mental illness in non-Western countries.[45] Consistent with this hypothesis, results from both the WMH Survey Initiative and the larger literature base have estimated the lowest prevalence rates in both non-Western cultures and low-income countries (most of which have non-biomedical cultural and diagnostic frameworks) (see Table 4.1).[34]

A related criticism holds that the prevalence estimates in countries less reliant on a biomedical framework and low-income countries may be biased downward due to the use of biomedical classification systems that do not address cultural concepts of distress. As covered earlier in this chapter, cultural concepts of distress have variable overlap and comorbidity with existing biomedical classification systems, such as the DSM.[24] As such, there is a nontrivial possibility that epidemiologic surveys that do not incorporate cultural concepts of distress may be missing clinically significant psychological distress.

Prevalence estimates may also be limited by survey language, including translation difficulties and cultural differences in the language of distress. Epidemiologic surveys, such as the WMH-CIDI, are often written in English and then translated into the local language. Translation can be challenging, as the vocabulary of distress can vary greatly due to cultural and language differences. For instance, in some languages the equivalent vocabulary may not exist, or there may be different nosology or idioms of distress not accounted for in translation. From an anthropologic perspective this represents a *category fallacy*: Simply because a biomedical term or category, such as *anxiety*, can be applied to other cultures does not mean that it represents the same concept or is a valid term in that culture.[46] Thus, attempts to establish the construct validity of certain diagnoses across cultural contexts may represent the use of an *etic* approach to answer an *emic* question. That is, taking the biomedical cultural perspective rather than a local perspective may lead investigators to miss information pertinent to understanding the local epidemiology of mental illness. An effort has been made to address these issues through specific translation protocols, in the case of WMH-CIDI, but these procedures may be insufficient. As such, some argue for cultural and regional modifications and revalidation of the WMH-CIDI survey.[47]

Concern has been raised for the clinical relevance of prevalence estimates based on surveys such as the WHM-CIDI, given that the DSM classification system has been criticized not only for its Western bias but also for being too conservative in measuring subthreshold, but potentially clinically significant, illness. For instance, the DSM-IV diagnosis of generalized anxiety disorder requires a six-month duration and at least three specific associated symptoms. Some have argued that based on these criteria, individuals who would benefit from identification and potential treatment go undiagnosed.[48] Questions have also been raised over the consistency of diagnostic thresholds across countries, such that prevalence estimates may vary based on local perception of the severity of illness needed to cross the threshold into mental illness.[49]

Current data are also limited in that surveys such as the WMH-CIDI are designed to detect only some mental disorders to the exclusion of others. However, some argue that achieving adequate coverage of the most common mental disorders should return data reflecting the bulk of the global burden of mental illness and, therefore, is clinically significant in fulfilling the intended purpose.[45] On the other hand, a significant burden of illness may be underestimated in ignoring personality disorders, the psychiatric overlap with neurologic and pain disorders, and severe and persistent disorders (e.g., primary psychotic disorders).[50] Furthermore, somatic presentations of mental illness could also be a significant undetected burden, particularly in primary care settings where physical complaints are the most common presentation of mental illness.[51]

LIMITATIONS DUE TO THE STIGMA OF MENTAL ILLNESS

Finally, there is concern for underreporting of illness worldwide due to stigma, particularly in cultures where the stigma of mental illness is profound. Cross-country studies have consistently shown that the prevalence of anticipated, experienced, and self-stigma among persons with mental illness remains high despite the availability of effective treatment.[52-54] Research exploring the presence, variation, and distribution of stigma across countries and cultures has increased in recent years; however, a standardized worldwide comparison of countries, particularly low- and middle- income countries, has not been completed.[55]

Existing research on the stigma of mental illness is limited by variability in the methodology of stigma measurement and a focus on few illnesses. Much of our knowledge about stigma comes from studies in Western cultures, particularly the United Kingdom, the United States, and Canada. These studies have consistently demonstrated that there have been improvements over time in knowledge about and understanding of mental illness and help-seeking, but that ongoing stigma persists.[55-57] Studies in low- and middle-income countries are more variable and are often limited to specific regions or specific conditions, such as schizophrenia. Nonetheless, the overarching thrust of the literature is that stigma is consistently present around the world, including among providers, with few exceptions.[55,57] Although making comparisons between countries and cultures can be difficult, the current literature suggests that variations of stigma can be understood through historical, cultural, socioeconomic, and religious contexts, as well as explanatory models of mental illness (such as supernatural forces, sorcery, or spirit possession) and treatment strategies (such as spiritual or natural remedies).[57-61]

LIMITATIONS OF SURVEY IMPLEMENTATION

One difficulty in epidemiologic surveys lies in identifying individuals to administer the survey. Like many epidemiologic surveys, the WMH-CIDI is administered by local laypeople who are not clinically trained in the diagnosis of mental illness, which could impact diagnostic thresholds and the reliability and concordance of diagnosis.[62] The WMH Survey Initiative has addressed these concerns by maximizing the consistency of training documents and protocols, providing interviewer supervision, and evaluating concordance. The latter has led to appropriate adjustments to improve concordance; subsequently, the WMH-CIDI as applied by laypersons has achieved reasonable degrees of reliability.[63] However, evaluations of validity and concordance have been conducted primarily in Western and/or high-income countries, and there are few cross-national comparisons involving non-Western and/or low-income countries.

An additional critique has been that in some countries, the data originate only from specific regions, particularly large urban areas.[30,31] While such design decisions may represent difficulties in establishing a robust research infrastructure or simply the realities of conducting complex studies, the systematic exclusion of rural areas is likely to bias prevalence estimates. In high-income countries, the prevalence of mental disorders in urban areas significantly exceeds that in rural areas.[64] Furthermore, data analyses separate the world's population into regions of study and bring into question the cultural relevance or epidemiological validity of larger categories such as "Latin America," "sub-Saharan Africa," or "southeast Asia."[30] Geography may not be the best proxy for culture, as it ignores within-country differences, subcultures, and the heterogeneity of psychological distress.[2,30]

RELEVANCE AND APPLICATION TO PRACTICE

At first glance, the topic of global psychiatric epidemiology may seem disconnected to the everyday clinical practice of psychiatry. However, understanding how cultural and societal norms influence our classification, conceptualization, and treatment of mental illness is important for culturally informed practice. By reflecting on this body of work, clinicians can become more aware of the impact that their own cultural and societal backgrounds have on their interactions with and treatment of patients; second, with increased awareness, clinicians will take deliberate steps toward improving their own cultural competence.

The cultural, societal, and historical context of our practice in psychiatry can often go unrecognized in the context of busy daily practice. It is important to remain aware that all clinicians bring their individual background, culture, and personal beliefs into their practice, such that their approach may be different from that of their colleagues. In addition to individual backgrounds, U.S.-trained clinicians approach psychological distress and mental illness through biomedical perspectives, which greatly influences their perspective of mental illness, including diagnosis and management. A biomedical perspective is the norm in the medical culture in which they practice.

Improving our awareness of how our personal and training background affects the way we practice psychiatry is the first step toward making deliberate changes in improving our cultural awareness and subsequently patient care. Once we are ready, there are many ways that we can improve our cultural approach to practice. One action is to improve our knowledge base and training in cultural concepts of distress, particularly those that may be relevant to patients or populations in our own practice.[65-76] Another action is to improve our use of interpreters; even if patients speak sufficient English to communicate, perhaps using an interpreter will improve their ability to express their distress through their own language. Although this can be challenging to approach, a good rule to avoid ambiguity is simply to use an interpreter with every patient not fully fluent in English. An interpreter can also serve as a cultural broker by helping to provide a cultural context for the patient's presentation and insight into local cultural concepts of distress.

Taking steps toward improving our cultural competence could have an important impact on patient care, such as detection of illness, help-seeking, engagement in care, family and community involvement, and healing. Importantly, treatment outcomes in patients from other countries and cultural backgrounds may not always be consistent with the popular literature, as most research on treatment recommendations is based on a biomedical diagnostic classification, and outcomes typically have been examined in less-diverse white patient populations.

However, we must take care in our approach to cultural competence to appreciate and respect heterogeneity within a cultural group as well as to avoid overgeneralizing and "exoticizing" a cultural group or belief.[2] It is also important to place presentations of distress into local context to avoid medicalizing or pathologizing a cultural concept of distress within the spectrum of normal in any individual patient. This is especially relevant for patients who have immigrated to Western cultures, and may have displaced their native language of distress for a biomedically-based language of distress, through acculturation or globalization. It is important to keep in mind that some presentations, particularly those of immigrants, may not fit within either a biomedical diagnostic concept or a cultural concept of distress, as illness presentations may evolve through acculturation. Alternatively, some patients may more intensely identify with their background culture after immigration,[27] so using biomedical language and illness concepts could at times create more difficulty in building rapport and engaging a patient in care.

An example of this concept is seen in the second case study of this chapter: Mrs. B, the 63-year-old Latino woman who presented with a complaint of *nervios*. Using a strict biomedical approach, such as the DSM framework, presents a challenge for both diagnosis and treatment. The patient's description of *nervios* does not fit easily into any single DSM category; rather, it overlaps with several DSM categories. As such, a clinician may find it difficult to address the patient's symptoms using a biomedical framework. The patient herself seemed to have adapted the biomedical concepts of *anxiety* and *depression* within her expression of distress. Furthermore, for this patient, a biomedical attempt to address nightmares through medication management alone was met with difficulty, partially due to the lack of addressing and incorporating the somatic components of the patient's presentation. Ultimately, the patient improved on her own, with improvement of what she knew to be the etiology of her *nervios*: family conflict.

CONCLUSION

This chapter provides an introduction and discussion of the basic principles, concepts, and challenges of global psychiatric epidemiology, including the classification of mental illness, cultural concepts of distress, and the current understanding of global epidemiology and its limitations. This discussion most importantly brings to light the challenge of understanding global epidemiology through the lens of biomedical diagnostic classification systems, and the importance of understanding how culture and society impacts our knowledge of and approach to the diagnosis and treatment of mental illness.

We have provided recommendations for how readers can improve their awareness of how their personal background and professional training affect their classification, understanding, and treatment of mental illness and how they can improve their cultural competence and ultimately their patient relationships and care management. As readers reflect on this newfound knowledge, it will allow them to grow and improve as clinicians.

REFERENCES

1. Patel V, Prince M. Global mental health: A new global health field comes of age. *JAMA*. 2010;303(19):1976–1977.
2. Gureje O, Stein D. Disorders, diagnosis, and classification. In: Patel V, Minas H, Cohen A, Prince M, eds. *Global Mental Health: Principles and Practice*. New York: Oxford University Press; 2014:27–40.
3. Koplan JP, Bond TC, Merson MH, et al. Towards a common definition of global health. *Lancet*. 2009;373(9679):1993–1995.
4. Tsai AC, Tomlinson M. Inequitable and ineffective: Exclusion of mental health from the post-2015 development agenda. *PLoS Med*. 2015;12(6).
5. Murray CJ, Lopez ADCN-C. *The Global Burden of Disease: A Comprehensive Assessment of Mortality and Disability from Diseases, Injuries, and Risk Factors in 1990 and Projected to 2020*. World Health Organization; 1996:1–43.
6. Whiteford HA, Ferrari AJ, Degenhardt L, Feigin V, Vos T. The global burden of mental, neurological and substance use disorders: an analysis from the Global Burden of Disease Study 2010. *PLoS One*. 2015;10(2):e0116820.

7. Reidpath DD, Allotey PA, Kouame A, Cummins RA. Measuring health in a vacuum: Examining the disability weight of the DALY. *Health Policy Plan.* 2003;18(4):351–356.

8. Mont D. Measuring health and disability. *Lancet.* 2007;369(9573):1658–1663.

9. Üstün TB, Rehm J, Chatterji S, et al. Multiple-informant ranking of the disabling effects of different health conditions in 14 countries. WHO/NIH Joint Project CAR Study Group. *Lancet.* 1999;354(9173):111–115.

10. Murray CJL, Lopez AD. Measuring global health: Motivation and evolution of the Global Burden of Disease Study. *Lancet.* 2017;390(10100):1460–1464.

11. Demyttenaere K, Bruffaerts R, Posada-Villa J, et al. Prevalence, severity, and unmet need for treatment of mental disorders in the World Health Organization World Mental Health Surveys. *JAMA.* 2004;291(21):2581–2590.

12. World Health Organization. *Mental Health Atlas 2014.* 2015. Available at: http://www.who.int/mental_health/evidence/atlas/mental_health_atlas_2014/en/

13. Kendell R. What are mental disorders? In: Freedman A, Brotman R, Silverman I, Hutson D, eds. *Issues in Psychiatric Classification: Science, Practice and Social Policy.* New York: Human Sciences Press; 1986:23–45.

14. American Psychiatric Association. *Diagnostic and Statistical Manual of Mental Disorders, Fifth Edition (DSM-5).* Washington, DC: American Psychiatric Association; 2013:758–759, 833–837.

15. Horwitz A. *Creating Mental Illness.* Chicago: University of Chicago Press; 2002.

16. Elliot C. *Better Than Well: American Medicine Meets the American Dream.* New York: W.W. Norton and Company; 2003.

17. Horwitz A, Wakefield J. *The Loss of Sadness: How Psychiatry Transformed Normal Sorrow into Depressive Disorder.* Oxford: Oxford University Press; 2007.

18. Kendler KS, Myers J, Zisook S. Does bereavement-related major depression differ from major depression associated with other stressful life events? *Am J Psychiatry.* 2008;165(11):1449–1455.

19. Zisook S, Shear K, Kendler KS. Validity of the bereavement exclusion criterion for the diagnosis of major depressive episode. *World Psychiatry.* 2007;6(2):102–107.

20. Wakefield JC, First MB. Validity of the bereavement exclusion to major depression: Does the empirical evidence support the proposal to eliminate the exclusion in DSM-5? *World Psychiatry.* 2012;11(1):3–10.

21. Wakefield JC. DSM-5 grief scorecard: Assessment and outcomes of proposals to pathologize grief. *World Psychiatry.* 2013;12(2):171–173.

22. Kleinman A. Culture, bereavement, and psychiatry. *Lancet.* 2012;379(9816):608–609.

23. Reed GM. Toward ICD-11: Improving the clinical utility of WHO's International Classification of Mental Disorders. *Prof Psychol Res Pract.* 2010;41(6):457–464.

24. Kohrt BA, Rasmussen A, Kaiser BN, et al. Cultural concepts of distress and psychiatric disorders: Literature review and research recommendations for global mental health epidemiology. *Int J Epidemiol.* 2014;43(2):365–406.

25. Becker AE, Burwell RA, Gilman SE, Herzog DB, Hamburg P. Eating behaviours and attitudes following prolonged exposure to television among ethnic Fijian adolescent girls. *Br J Psychiatry.* 2002;180(June):509–514.

26. Watters E. *Crazy Like Us: The Globalization of the American Psyche.* New York: Free Press; 2010.

27. Kraidy M. *Hybridity, or the Cultural Logic of Globalization.* Philadelphia, PA: Temple University Press; 2005.

28. Guarnaccia PJ, Lewis-Fernández R, Marano MR. Toward a Puerto Rican popular nosology: *Nervios* and *ataque de nervios*. *Cult Med Psychiatry*. 2003;27(3):339–366.

29. Kessler RC, Üstün BB. The World Mental Health (WMH) Survey Initiative version of the World Health Organization (WHO) Composite International Diagnostic Interview (CIDI). *Int J Methods Psychiatr Res*. 2004;13(2):93–117.

30. Kirmayer L, Swartz L. Culture and global mental health. In: Patel V, Minas H, Cohen A, Prince M, eds. *Global Mental Health: Principles and Practice*. New York: Oxford University Press; 2014:41–62.

31. Kessler RC, Angermeyer M, Anthony JC, et al. Lifetime prevalence and age-of-onset distributions of mental disorders in the World Health Organization's World Mental Health Survey Initiative. *World Psychiatry*. 2007;6(3):168–176.

32. World Mental Health Survey Initiative. https://www.hcp.med.harvard.edu/wmh/. Published 2005. Accessed August 2, 2017.

33. Kessler RC, Aguilar-Gaxiola S, Alonso J, et al. The global burden of mental disorders: An update from the WHO World Mental Health (WMH) Surveys. *Epidemiol Psichiatr Soc*. 2009;18(1):23–33.

34. Steel Z, Marnane C, Iranpour C, et al. The global prevalence of common mental disorders: A systematic review and meta-analysis 1980–2013. *Int J Epidemiol*. 2014;43(2):476–493.

35. Prince M, Bryce R, Albanese E, Wimo A, Ribeiro W, Ferri CP. The global prevalence of dementia: A systematic review and meta-analysis. *Alzheimers Dement*. 2013;9(1):63–75.

36. Simeone JC, Ward AJ, Rotella P, Collins J, Windisch R. An evaluation of variation in published estimates of schizophrenia prevalence from 1990–2013: A systematic literature review. *BMC Psychiatry*. 2015;15(1):193.

37. McGrath J, Saha S, Chant D, Welham J. Schizophrenia: A concise overview of incidence, prevalence, and mortality. *Epidemiol Rev*. 2008;30(1):67–76.

38. Alonso J, Chatterji S, He Y. *The Burdens of Mental Disorders: Global Perspectives from the WHO World Mental Health Surveys*. Cambridge, UK: Cambridge University Press; 2013.

39. Lee S, Tsang A, Breslau J, et al. Mental disorders and termination of education in high-income and low and middle-income countries: Epidemiological study. *Br J Psychiatry*. 2009;194(5):411–417.

40. Kawakami N, Abdulghani EA, Alonso J, et al. Early-life mental disorders and adult household income in the world mental health surveys. *Biol Psychiatry*. 2012;72(3):228–237.

41. Miller E, Breslau J, Petukhova M, et al. Premarital mental disorders and physical violence in marriage: Cross-national study of married couples. *Br J Psychiatry*. 2011;199(4):330–337.

42. Von Korff M. Global perspectives on mental-physical illness. In: Von Korff M, Scott K, Gureje O, eds. *Global Perspectives on Mental-Physical Comorbidity in the WHO World Mental Health Surveys*. New York: Cambridge University Press; 2009:17–218.

43. Walker ER, McGee RE, Druss BG. Mortality in mental disorders and global disease burden implications: A systematic review and meta-analysis. *Jama Psychiatry*. 2015;72(4):334–341.

44. Hjorthøj C, Stürup AE, McGrath JJ, Nordentoft M. Years of potential life lost and life expectancy in schizophrenia: A systematic review and meta-analysis. *Lancet Psychiatry*. 2017;4(4):295–301.

45. Kessler RC, Alonso J, Chatterji S, He Y. The epidemiology and impact of mental disorders. In: Patel V, Minas H, Cohen A, Prince M, eds. *Global Mental Health: Principles and Practice.* New York: Oxford University Press; 2014:82–101.

46. Kleinman AM. Depression, somatization and the "new cross-cultural psychiatry." *Soc Sci Med.* 1977;11(1):3–9.

47. Ghimire DJ, Chardoul S, Kessler RC, Axinn WG, Adhikari BP. Modifying and validating the Composite International Diagnostic Interview (CIDI) for use in Nepal. *Int J Methods Psychiatr Res.* 2013;22(1):71–81.

48. Ruscio AM, Chiu WT, Roy-Byrne P, et al. Broadening the definition of generalized anxiety disorder: Effects on prevalence and associations with other disorders in the National Comorbidity Survey Replication. *J Anxiety Disord.* 2007;21(5):662–676.

49. Chang SM, Hahm BJ, Lee JY, et al. Cross-national difference in the prevalence of depression caused by the diagnostic threshold. *J Affect Disord.* 2008;106(1-2):159–167.

50. Vigo D, Thornicroft G, Atun R. Estimating the true global burden of mental illness. *Lancet Psychiatry.* 2016;3(2):171–178.

51. Ustun T, Sartorius N. *Mental Illness in General Health Care: An International Study.* Chichester, UK: John Wiley & Sons; 1995.

52. Lasalvia A, Zoppei S, Van Bortel T, et al. Global pattern of experienced and anticipated discrimination reported by people with major depressive disorder: A cross-sectional survey. *Lancet.* 2013;381(9860):55–62.

53. Brohan E, Gauci D, Sartorius N, Thornicroft G. Self-stigma, empowerment and perceived discrimination among people with bipolar disorder or depression in 13 European countries: The GAMIAN-Europe study. *J Affect Disord.* 2011;129(1-3):56–63.

54. Thornicroft G, Brohan E, Rose D, Sartorius N, Leese M. Global pattern of experienced and anticipated discrimination against people with schizophrenia: A cross-sectional survey. *Lancet.* 2009;373(9661):408–415.

55. Pescosolido BA, Olafsdottir S, Martin JK, Long JS. Cross-cultural aspects of the stigma of mental illness. In: Arboleda-Flórez J, Sartorius N, eds. *Understanding the Stigma of Mental Illness: Theory and Interventions.* Chichester, UK: Wiley; 2008:19–35.

56. Pescosolido BA. The public stigma of mental illness: What do we think; what do we know; what can we prove? *J Health Soc Behav.* 2013;54(1):1–21.

57. Mehta N, Thornicroft G. Stigma, discrimination, and promoting human rights. In: Patel V, Minas H, Cohen A, Prince M, eds. *Global Mental Health: Principles and Practice.* New York: Oxford University Press; 2014:401–424.

58. Fabrega H. The culture and history of psychiatric stigma in early modern and modern Western societies: A review of recent literature. *Compr Psychiatry.* 1991;32(2):97–119.

59. Dovidio JF, Major B, Crocker J. Stigma: Introduction and overview. In: Heatherton TF, Kleck RE, Hebl MR, Hull JG, eds. *The Social Psychology of Stigma.* New York: Guilford; 2000:1–28.

60. Ng CH. The stigma of mental illness in Asian cultures. *Aust N Z J Psychiatry.* 1997;31(3):382–390.

61. Lefley HP. Culture and chronic mental illness. *Hosp Community Psychiatry.* 1990;41(3):277–286.

62. Wittchen H-UU. Reliability and validity studies of the WHO—Composite International Diagnostic Interview (CIDI): A critical review. *J Psychiatr Res.* 1994;28(1):57–84.

63. Haro JM, Arbabzadeh-Bouchez S, Brugha TS, et al. Concordance of the Composite International Diagnostic Interview Version 3.0 (CIDI 3.0) with standardized clinical

assessments in the WHO World Mental Health Surveys. *Int J Methods Psychiatr Res.* 2006;15(4):167–180.

64. Peen J, Schoevers RA, Beekman AT, Dekker J. The current status of urban-rural differences in psychiatric disorders. *Acta Psychiatr Scand.* 2010;121(2):84–93.

65. Wig N. Problems of mental health in India. *J Clin Soc Psychiatry.* 1960;17:48–53.

66. Sumathipala A, Siribaddana SH, Bhugra D. Culture-bound syndromes: The story of *dhat* syndrome. *Br J Psychiatry.* 2004;184(3):200–209.

67. Teo AR, Gaw AC. Hikikomori, a Japanese culture-bound syndrome of social withdrawal? *J Nerv Ment Dis.* 2010;198(6):444–449.

68. Kato TA, Kanba S, Teo AR. A 39-year-old "adultolescent": Understanding social withdrawal in Japan. *Am J Psychiatry.* 2016;173(2):112–114.

69. Hinton DE, Pich V, Marques L, Nickerson A, Pollack MH. *Khyâl* attacks: A key idiom of distress among traumatized Cambodia refugees. *Cult Med Psychiatry.* 2010;34(2):244–278.

70. Patel V, Simunyu E, Gwanzura F. *Kufungisisa* (thinking too much): A Shona idiom for non-psychotic mental illness. *Cent Afr J Med.* 1995;41(7):209–215.

71. Kaiser BN, Haroz EE, Kohrt BA, Bolton PA, Bass JK, Hinton DE. "Thinking too much": A systematic review of a common idiom of distress. *Soc Sci Med.* 2015;147:170–183.

72. World Health Organization and Pan-American Health Organization. *Culture and Mental Health in Haiti: A Literature Review.* 2010. http://www.who.int/mental_ health/emergencies/culture_mental_health_haiti_eng.pdf

73. Chang D, Myers H, Yeung A, Zhang Y, Zhao J, Yu S. *Shenjing shuairuo* and the DSM-IV: Diagnosis, distress, and disability in a Chinese primary care setting. *Transcult Psychiatry.* 2005;42(2):204–218. *doi:10.1177/1363461505052660*

74. Kleinman A. Neurasthenia and depression: A study of somatization and culture in China. *Cult Med Psychiatry.* 1982;6(2):117–190.

75. Rubel AJ. The epidemiology of a folk illness: *Susto* in Hispanic America. *Ethnology.* 1964;3(3):268–283.

76. Tanaka-Matsumi J. *Taijin kyofusho*: Diagnostic and cultural issues in Japanese psychiatry. *Cult Med Psychiatry.* 1979;3(3):231–245.

5

Social Determinants
of Psychiatric Illness

KRISTEN NISHIMI, ESTHER HOWE, AND ERIN C. DUNN ■

CASE

A 28-year-old woman presented to a community mental health center for evaluation of symptoms of depression and anxiety following an emergency department visit for suicidal thoughts. She described a chaotic childhood characterized by significant domestic turmoil and frequent verbal and physical altercations between her parents, who eventually divorced. For a time she and her mother were homeless, and she recalled periods of food insecurity, when she did not have easy access to food. Though she never experienced direct physical abuse, she described frightening episodes in which she had to hide from her mother's violent and rageful boyfriend. Her symptoms of depression and anxiety first emerged after college, but she had not sought care at that time due to a lack of health insurance and ability to access mental health care.

INTRODUCTION

The goal of this chapter is to provide readers with an understanding of the social determinants of health, or the "specific features of and pathways by which societal conditions affect health and that potentially can be altered by informed action."[1] These social determinants are the conditions and social contexts in which people are born, grow, work, live, learn, and age, and the wider set of forces and systems shaping the conditions of daily life. Thus, as described below, "social" can describe anything pertaining to society, or the systems of common life, rather than focusing solely on the individual.[1] In this way, social determinants can be thought of not as the causes of disease, but rather as the "causes of causes," or factors that influence the distribution or degree of exposure to the ultimate causes of disease. As we will demonstrate, these social determinants play a pivotal role in shaping the etiology, course, and treatment of mental health.

To help readers develop and apply a "social determinants" lens from which to view their clinical research and practice in psychiatry, this chapter is organized into four main sections. First, we introduce the concept of social determinants by showing how social determinants are related to the field of public health and population health frameworks. Second, we describe ways in which knowledge of the social determinants of health can inform psychiatric clinical practice. Third, we summarize research on four commonly studied social determinants—gender, socioeconomic status (SES), childhood adversity, and school and neighborhood environments—as applied to risk for major depressive disorder. Last, we show how information about social determinants can be integrated with more individual-level factors, using the example of genetic variation and gene–environment interplay (G×E).

LINKS BETWEEN SOCIAL DETERMINANTS AND POPULATION/PUBLIC HEALTH FRAMEWORKS

The roots of work on social determinants of health are primarily based in the fields of sociology and public health, the latter of which could be viewed as a "sister" field to medicine. Whereas medicine is concerned with monitoring, diagnosing, and treating individuals who experience illness or injury, and therefore has as its goal the maintenance of individual health and well-being, public health is concerned with identifying disease patterns, understanding determinants and mechanisms of disease, and ultimately informing policy or practice to alleviate disease, all at the population level. Thus, the goal of public health is to improve the health and well-being of *populations*. This goal is accomplished through theory-guided epidemiologic research, empirically based interventions, and research-informed policy.

How Can We Determine and Monitor the Population's Health?

Within the field of public health, epidemiology is the discipline concerned with capturing the distribution (i.e., disease *prevalence*, or the proportion of cases with disease in the population at a given time; disease *incidence*, or the rate at which new cases of disease occur over a specific period of time)[2] and determinants (i.e., risk and protective factors leading to or protecting from health outcomes) of disease frequency in the population. Knowledge of disease distribution and determinants is then used to identify strategies to prevent or treat disease. Within epidemiology, the subfield of social epidemiology focuses on the social distribution and social determinants of states of health, disease, and well-being.[3] Similarly, psychiatric epidemiology is concerned with understanding the distributions and determinants of mental health and mental illness.[4] These branches of epidemiologic study overlap when the emphasis is on how social factors impact mental health and illness.

What Does "Social" Mean, as in the "Social" Determinants of Health?

As noted earlier, "social" can refer to anything beyond the individual level, though as we will make clear, even individual-level factors can be socially determined or have implications at the societal level. For instance, although gender is an individual-level attribute, or personal characteristic, the manifestations of gender operate at community and society levels by shaping norms and roles that ultimately influence individual behavior. These social factors exist at multiple levels of influence and are commonly organized into "social-ecological" frameworks designed to capture the multiple, hierarchical factors that dynamically interact throughout a person's life to influence his or her health, development, and well-being.[5,6] Figure 5.1 presents one such social-ecological model, which is organized into five levels: *individual, interpersonal, institutional, community*, and *policy*.[6] *Individual* factors include a person's attitudes, beliefs, behaviors, and knowledge, as well as biology. The remaining four levels would be considered "social" determinants. *Interpersonal* factors are the relationships between individuals, such as family members, friends, peers, neighbors, and coworkers. *Institutional* factors involve formal institutions, such as schools, workplaces, and religious organizations, as well as these institutions' culture, climate, social norms, rules, and policies. *Community* encompasses the organizations and informal institutions people belong to and interact with, as well as their cultures and norms. *Policy* factors incorporate local, state, and federal law and policies. Examples of factors shaping risk for psychiatric disorders at each level of the social-ecological model are shown in Figure 5.1. Although social-ecological models have been typically applied to individuals as a way of understanding the multiple levels of influence on individual health, these frameworks can also be applied to understand the wide set of factors contributing to the health of populations.

Why Focus on Populations and Not Just Individuals?

In 1985, the epidemiologist Geoffrey Rose proposed a framework to conceptualize both the risk factors shaping population health and risk for disease and also to identify strategies to prevent disease outcomes in the population.[7] The core features of Rose's model are displayed in Figure 5.2. Rose observed that within a population, most health outcomes were distributed on a continuum, such that prevalence of disease in a population would gradually increase as the level of exposure to a given risk factor increases; this is depicted by the dashed-line curve labeled "disease continuum." However, Rose also observed that most of the risk factors that influence disease are normally distributed in a population, as seen in the curve that represents

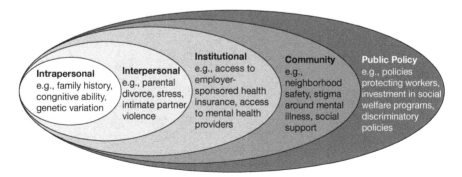

Figure 5.1 The social-ecological model.
Adapted from McLeroy KR, Bibeau D, Steckler A, Glanz K. An ecological perspective on health promotion programs. *Health Educ Q*. 1988;15(4):351–377.

the density of the population across levels of a risk factor. These two observations led Rose to make two important conclusions:

1. At any given time, a small proportion of individuals in the population will have very low and very high levels of exposure to a given risk factor, as seen in the lower and upper tails of the curve.
2. Most of the population has a moderate amount of exposure to a given risk factor, as seen by the peak in the middle of the curve.

The field of medicine focuses on individuals at the highest end of the disease continuum, meaning those individuals with the highest levels of risk factors or worst disease symptoms, depicted by the right-most tail shaded in gray. Rose identified efforts to target this group as the "high risk approach," as such efforts target high-risk individuals through individualized and tailored treatment designed to alleviate exposure to a given risk factor so that symptoms can be reduced and disease can be prevented. However, as Rose observed, the normal distribution of risk factors in the population means that a large portion of people are at low or moderate risk for disease onset, thus falling outside of the purview of traditional medicine. This

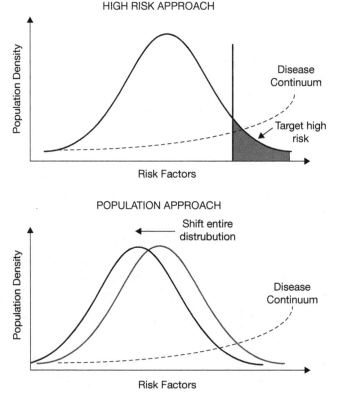

Figure 5.2 High-risk versus population approaches to improving health. Adapted from Rose G. Sick individuals and sick populations. *Int J Epidemiol.* 1985;14(1):32–38.

seemingly contradictory effect is what Rose termed the "prevention paradox," whereby the majority of cases of a disease arise from individuals in a population who are at low or moderate risk and a minority of cases actually arise from those at high risk. He therefore argued that a "population approach" was needed to target the underlying risk factors that impact the entire population, ultimately leading to a slightly lower risk for everyone. Population-based efforts to reduce exposure to risk factors, including the social determinants of health, would therefore shift the entire distribution of the population to a lower level of risk, as depicted by the shifted black curve. Such changes would result in small improvements at the individual level but large improvements at the population level.

Blood pressure is one of the classic examples used to illustrate the differences in interventions that characterize the high-risk versus the population-level approach. Blood pressure is normally distributed in the population. However, only people in the upper tail of the blood pressure distribution are considered to have clinically elevated blood pressure. These individuals may be targeted for "high-risk strategy" treatments, such as being prescribed antihypertensive medications, which help to decrease individual risk for hypertension-related medical sequelae such as heart attack or stroke by lowering their blood pressure. Such interventions would therefore have a potentially large impact on the individual. In contrast, targeting underlying social determinants through a "population approach," such as implementing policies to reduce manufacturers' use of sodium in the food supply, or a worksite intervention designed to promote physical activity, could yield small decreases in blood pressure across larger populations, thereby shifting the entire distribution of blood pressure to a slightly lower risk. Although we describe the high-risk and population-based approaches as separate strategies, they are not mutually exclusive, and both are necessary to promote the overall health of populations. However, the population approach explicitly targets underlying risk factors, or the social determinants of health.

HOW INCORPORATING A SOCIAL DETERMINANTS PERSPECTIVE CAN ENRICH PSYCHIATRIC CLINICAL PRACTICE

There are several ways that incorporating a social determinants lens can enrich psychiatric clinical practice. First, it can expand clinicians' focus beyond individual-level treatment toward considering strategies to prevent the onset of disease. This shift is consistent with the recent emphasis on "preventive psychiatry," which aims to help people develop the cognitive and social skills to cope with stress in an effort to prevent the onset of mental illness.[8] Toward these ends, psychiatrists can promote resiliency skills at multiple social-ecological levels. For instance, at the individual level, psychiatrists can help patients and family members identify situational risk factors and behavior patterns linked to negative mental health symptoms. They can also intervene directly by helping patients acquire the skills and knowledge to develop more adaptive coping strategies, which could reduce symptoms and the likelihood of crossing the diagnostic threshold for a disorder. Similarly, such practices can be applied on a population level by incorporating cognitive and behavioral skills training into early childhood and elementary education programs, which would allow teachers and children to benefit from preventive psychiatry measures regardless of their individual risk level.[8] Recent studies suggest these types of school-based mindfulness programs and social and emotional learning interventions are effective at improving students' cognitive performance and resilience to stress[9] and promoting social and emotional skills, attitudes, behavior, and academic performance.[10]

Second, knowledge of the social determinants of health can inform diagnosis and nosology and provide new insights about the causes of disease, as emerging evidence suggests that disease states may be a unique biological manifestation of a person's social status. Teicher and Samson have proposed that having a history of childhood adversity, which is one of the social determinants we describe later in detail, may represent a clinically and biologically distinct subtype of psychopathology.[11] Their hypothesis is based on the observation that people exposed to child maltreatment, for example, have an earlier age at disorder onset, greater symptom severity, more comorbidities, greater risk for suicide, and worse treatment response than people with depression, anxiety, or substance use disorders who did not experience childhood maltreatment. Based on these findings, they argue that exposure to maltreatment may lead to multiple "ecophenotypes," or distinct subtypes within diagnostic categories. Differentiating between these ecophenotypes may help uncover different biological bases of disorders and inform more targeted treatment practices.

Finally, incorporation of a social determinants lens can help clinicians design better treatments and interventions. For example, in light of evidence showing that exercise protects against the development of depression,[12] a physician may recommend exercise as a treatment to an individual with mild depression; however, if the individual lives in an unsafe neighborhood where outdoor exercise is not possible and cannot afford a gym membership, it will be difficult to adhere to such a recommendation. Thus, attention to the social determinants of health can help clinicians obtain a more complete picture of the constellation of risk and protective factors that shape patients' behavior. Such insights could help patients recognize their social environmental constraints versus possibilities and, in some instances, identify strategies to bolster their social environmental resources (when such resources can be modified) so that these limitations are not barriers to successful psychiatric treatment.

OVERVIEW OF THE MAJOR SOCIAL DETERMINANTS OF DEPRESSION

In this section, we summarize research on four of the most commonly studied social determinants of health—the role of gender, SES, exposure to childhood adversity, and school and neighborhood context—as they relate to major depressive disorder (MDD), which is one of the most common, costly, and burdensome mental disorders worldwide.[13] The estimated lifetime prevalence of MDD is 16.2% in the United States,[14] with global lifetime prevalence estimates ranging from 6.6% in Japan to 21% in France.[13] The average age at first onset of depression is 30 years, with earlier onsets associated with worse illness course and outcome.[15] Depression is also associated with significant morbidity and mortality, including substance use disorders, suicidality, and functional impairment, leading to profound individual, family, and societal costs, and it commonly presents alongside multiple mental and physical health comorbidities.[14,16] Although we limit our discussion to depression, many of the social determinants introduced here also influence other mental illnesses and can be considered in relation to these. Due to space constraints, other important social determinants, including race/ethnicity, sexual orientation, and immigration status, are omitted.

Gender

Epidemiological studies have consistently shown that before puberty, the lifetime prevalence of depression is the same in males and females (estimated at 1.6% among children age 8–11).[17] However, by midadolescence, gender differences emerge, with females outpacing their male counterparts by a ratio of 2:1; specifically, between the ages of 13 and 18, the lifetime prevalence of MDD and dysthymic disorders is 15.9% in females and 7.7% in males.[17,18] Some evidence suggests these gender differences persist until adulthood, through midlife to late life.[18]

Gender differences in the prevalence of depression do not appear to be explained by methodological factors, such as differences in the reporting or experiencing of depression, or recall of depressive symptoms, by gender.[19–21] As summarized in a 2000 review by Piccinelli, researchers have theorized that males may be less inclined than females to report depression or other psychological symptoms.[21] However, multiple studies have found that gender is not linked to underreporting psychological symptoms. Furthermore, despite evidence that males tend to downplay or have difficulty recalling past episodes of depression, even after such factors have been accounted for, females still have a higher lifetime prevalence of depression. Last, though some researchers have hypothesized that gender differences in depression are merely an artifact of depression rating scales that are disproportionately focused on symptoms experienced more frequently by females than males, studies have also not shown this to be the case.[19–21]

Moreover, gender differences in the prevalence of depression do not appear to be a phenomenon specific to the United States. Indeed, researchers have considered the female-to-male ratio of lifetime history of depression in countries all around the world. While the ratios of the gender difference vary to some extent (from a low of 1.6 in Beirut, Lebanon, and Taiwan to a high of 3.1 in West Germany), there is a consistent pattern across all countries studied, revealing an excess risk of depression in women relative to men.[22] Thus, if these gender differences are real, what factors explain how and why they emerge and persist?

Several conceptual models have been proposed to explain gender differences in the prevalence of depression that, consistent with the social-ecological framework, incorporate factors ranging from the individual to the institutional level.[6] For example, Hyde's affective/biological/cognitive model ("ABC model") emphasizes individual-level factors, including genetic variation, pubertal development, and cognitive and affective factors (e.g., ruminative tendencies and emotion regulation skills).[23] Nolen-Hoeksema's stress model emphasizes interpersonal-level factors, including exposure to trauma and stressful life events, which may be more common in women than men.[24] For instance, in childhood and adolescence, girls are up to five times more likely than boys to experience sexual abuse.[25] Nolen-Hoeksema postulates that women may be more vulnerable to depression than men as a result of both increased stress exposure and perhaps different levels of stress reactivity, meaning varying biological and social reactions to stress.[24]

Other conceptual models emphasize community-level factors, such as media portrayals of women and body image, as well as policies and cultural values related to women's roles at home and work.[24,26,27] For instance, researchers have examined the role of women's status at the local and state levels, asking whether gender differences in depression may narrow as the roles and status of men and women become more equal. This theory, often referred to as the gender role theory, asserts that gender differences in the prevalence of depression are due to differences in the allocation of stressors, coping resources, and opportunity structures made available to men and women.[28] Studies testing this theory have found that as opportunities for employment, access to birth control, and other indicators of increasing gender equality improve, fewer gender differences in depression emerge. For example, Seedat and colleagues used data from 15 countries participating in the World Health Organization World Mental Health Survey Initiative to examine the association between country-level measures of female labor force participation, educational attainment, age at marriage, and use of contraception on gender differences in risk for 18 psychiatric disorders in adulthood.[26] Consistent with the gender role and women's status hypothesis, gender differences in rates of depression have narrowed across time as gender role traditionality has decreased, and the status of men and women has become more equal.

Socioeconomic Status

SES is one of the strongest social determinants not only of mental health, but also multiple physical health outcomes. A person's socioeconomic position within a given society is determined by both actual resources and socially determined status or prestige.[29] SES can be measured in terms of *absolute* factors, or tangible resources an individual can access, including indicators of income, education, occupation, and wealth. In contrast, *relative* measures of SES capture the position of individuals or families within a social structure based on their access to and control over wealth, prestige, and power.[30] Both absolute and relative measures of SES can be temporally dynamic. For example, although childhood SES is often a strong predictor of adult SES,[31-33] changes in SES can occur throughout life in response to major life events, including job loss or divorce.

There are multiple pathways by which the material, social, and psychological resources made available through SES can impact mental health, such as access to health care, environmental hazards, lifestyle practices, psychological stress, and discrimination.[3] These pathways operate so that SES is an important determinant of not only whether people will develop depression, but also their likelihood of receiving treatment, as well as the severity and prognosis of their illness. For example, compared to their high-SES peers, individuals with low SES have about 1.18 times the odds of becoming depressed and 2 times the odds of remaining depressed.[34]

Interestingly, the association between SES and depression is not specific to adults. In a systematic review, researchers found that children and adolescents with low SES had more than three times the risk of experiencing mental health problems compared to their high-SES peers.[35] Many experts also argue that early life SES is itself an important predictor of future mental health—and indeed, studies have found

that childhood SES is an important determinant of adult depression even after accounting for adult SES.[36]

A major question often raised about the association between SES and depression
is: Are these associations really causal? In other words, are people of low SES really more likely to *become* depressed, or is there "reverse causation," whereby people
with depression are more likely to *decline* in their SES due to the negative sequelae
of mental illness, including failing to achieve higher levels of education? Bruce
Dohrenwend and others have studied these questions, developing two competing
models to explain the relationship between SES and psychopathology. The first is a
social selection model, which argues that people who are genetically predisposed to
psychopathology will drift down or fail to rise out of low-SES positions.[37] The second
is a *social causation* model, which argues that adversity and stress are associated with
low SES and ultimately lead to poor mental health.[37]

Studies assessing both models have generally shown that among adult samples,
social causation is more consistently supported,[38,39] though there is some evidence
supporting social selection as well.[40,41] However, among children and adolescents,
findings have been more mixed;[37,42-44] these mixed results are likely explained by the
conflation of both current and intergenerational cycles of deprivation and mental illness, which could make social causation and social selection operate simultaneously.[35]

In the strongest test of this association among children, Costello and colleagues
assessed the mental health effects of income changes occurring naturally via random
assignment (i.e., a natural experiment), and their findings supported the social
causation model. Specifically, during an ongoing longitudinal study of children in
the rural southeastern United States, a casino opened on an American Indian reservation that provided an income supplement of about $1,000 annually to every
American Indian resident.[45] Since a portion of these residents were included in the
ongoing study, Costello was able to prospectively assess psychiatric symptoms of
American Indian children who were "randomly" provided an income supplement.
This natural experiment therefore allowed the investigators to study these "ex-poor"
children, who moved out of poverty due to the supplement, as well as children who
were either "never poor" or "persistently poor" over the study period. Costello and
colleagues found that while psychiatric symptoms were higher initially among the
"ex-poor" group, after the casino opened, their psychiatric symptoms decreased by
40% and were comparable to the never-poor children. These findings support the
social causation model, whereby socioeconomic conditions impact future psychiatric symptoms.

Childhood Adversity

In the past decade, there has been growing interest in understanding the effects of
exposure to childhood adversity. Childhood adversities are broadly defined as a
set of stressors or traumas experienced by youth; these events can either be *acute*
(e.g., accidents/injury, natural disaster, illness, or death of a loved one) or *chronic* in
nature (e.g., poverty, divorce/marital discord among parents, child abuse/neglect,
witnessing violence, parent psychopathology).

Efforts to study childhood adversity grew out of observations that these exposures
were quite common in the United States and across the globe. Recent estimates from

population surveys in the United States suggest that about 40% of people report having been exposed to at least one type of childhood adversity by age 13.[46] Moreover, exposure to childhood adversity also appears socially patterned, with prevalence estimates of exposure varying by gender, race/ethnicity, and other factors. For instance, females are more likely than males to experience sexual assault, whereas males are more likely than females to experience physical violence. Similarly, exposure to assaultive violence, including being beaten, mugged, or witnessing fighting at home, is more common among non-Hispanic Blacks and Hispanics compared to whites.[46] These childhood adversities also tend to co-occur, with studies suggesting that nearly one-quarter of youth were exposed to four or more individual types of adversity.[47,48]

Given these collective observations, there has been growing interest in studying the effects of adverse childhood experiences (ACEs), which include childhood abuse and other potentially damaging childhood experiences such as psychological, physical, or sexual abuse, as well as exposure to substance abuse, mental illness, violence between caregivers, and criminal behavior in the household. The Centers for Disease Control and Prevention have developed an ACE survey that totals the number of these experiences into a sum score indicating a cumulative burden of adversity for any individual.[49] In hundreds of studies, this ACE score has been assessed in relation to childhood and adult health and well-being across multiple samples, with studies generally finding a dose–response relationship between ACE score and multiple mental and physical health outcomes, with increasing number of exposures associated with increased risk.[50,51]

The ubiquity of exposure to childhood adversity is especially concerning given its strong association with depression. Exposure to childhood adversity, including trauma and maltreatment, has been consistently linked to increased risk of adolescent and adult psychopathology, about doubling the risk of depression.[52,53] Particular types of adversity, including familial dysfunction, interpersonal forms of trauma exposure, and more chronic or severe exposures, are associated with greater depression risk.[48,53,54]

One of the major unanswered questions in the study of childhood adversity is whether there are developmental stages across the lifespan when exposure to adversity has a greater impact in shaping risk for depression. In other words, knowledge remains limited about the existence of possible "sensitive periods" in development, or biologically determined windows of time when the brain is especially "plastic," and when people are therefore more sensitive to the effects of experience, including exposure to childhood adversity. By determining whether, and when, sensitive periods exist across the lifespan, researchers might better identify the mechanisms underlying risk for psychopathology. Furthermore, clinicians, practitioners, and policymakers could use such knowledge to help determine when to time interventions so they would have their greatest impact. Such insights would be helpful since childhood spans multiple developmental periods when different types of interventions, including home- or school-based programs, could be deployed to minimize the effects of adversity based on the age of the child.

Although many experts agree that the timing of exposure to childhood adversity could influence subsequent risk for depression and other types of psychopathology,[55,56] no consensus has emerged as to whether earlier or later onset of exposure is more harmful. For instance, some studies have found that early exposure to child abuse and neglect, usually defined as occurring prior to age 5 or age 12, is most associated with vulnerability to depression.[57-61] However, other studies have found that later exposure to child abuse and neglect during adolescence (ages 12–17) is most harmful.[62-64] Some studies also found no difference in risk for depression based on the developmental timing of exposure.[56,65,66] Therefore, although childhood adversity is a consistent risk factor for poor mental and physical health, additional work is needed in prospective cohorts to tease apart the effects of the developmental timing of exposure.

Schools and Neighborhoods

If we move to a more macro set of social determinants in the social-ecological model, studies have begun to focus on the role of both schools and neighborhoods in shaping risk for depression. Neighborhoods are typically defined by geographical boundaries, such as census tract block groups, or by municipal units. Researchers have examined a wide array of both *social* and *structural* characteristics of these settings. Neighborhood social factors include indicators of violence and crime, social support and social cohesion, and the notion of "collective efficacy," meaning the willingness of neighbors to intervene on behalf of the common good.[67] Neighborhood structural factors include housing quality, availability of green space, and population density. These social and structural aspects of neighborhoods may exert harmful or protective effects on residents. Prior studies have shown that social and structural aspects of neighborhoods exert both harmful and protective effects on residents' mental health. For example, both social processes (e.g., disorder, social interactions, and violence) and structural features (e.g., SES and racial composition, stability, and the built environment) have been associated with depression among adults.[68,69] Among youth, systematic reviews have shown that neighborhoods influence risk of behavioral problems, with disadvantaged neighborhoods explaining between 1.6% and 11% of variation in behavioral symptoms, even after accounting for individual char acteristics.[70]

However, one of the challenges of this literature is that like SES, neighborhood context cannot be "randomly assigned" by researchers, and it is therefore difficult to determine the directionality or causality of such associations. The Moving to Opportunity study (MTO) was a landmark social experiment designed to examine the impact of neighborhoods on health. In MTO, families with children living in public housing were randomized to the opportunity to move to more affluent neighborhoods through the use of housing vouchers.[71] After 3 years, Leventhal and colleagues found that parents who moved to low-poverty neighborhoods had 20% lower psychological distress levels compared to the control group who remained in high-poverty areas. Similarly, anxiety/depressive symptoms were reduced by 16% among the children who moved.[72] These findings suggest neighborhoods may have a direct effect on mental health.

More recently, researchers have also begun to examine the importance of neighborhoods relative to other social settings, including schools. Such work has been made possible through the advent of advanced statistical approaches such as cross-classified multilevel modeling (CCMM),[73] which allows researchers to model the effects of multiple social contexts simultaneously. For example, when studying youth, it would be natural to ask whether any observed neighborhood effect on risk for depression is at least partly explained by the school environment, as schools have been found to explain between 5% and 28% of the variability in health outcomes (e.g., smoking, well-being, problem behavior, and school achievement).[74] Using CCMM, investigators can ask whether neighborhoods and schools, for example, explain similar levels of variability in depression risk, or whether one context explains more than another. In a recent study, Dunn and colleagues found that when each context was studied on its own, both neighborhoods and schools each explained about an equal amount of the variation in depressive symptoms (3.2–3.6%, respectively).[75] However, after adjusting for the "opposite" context, meaning adjusting for the role of schools when examining the role of neighborhoods and vice versa, the authors found that schools—and not neighborhoods—played a larger role in explaining variability in adolescent depressive symptoms. These findings suggest that for depressive symptoms, schools may be a larger contributor to adolescent depressive symptoms than neighborhoods. However, they also emphasize that a major advantage of CCMM is that it enables researchers to avoid the "omitted context bias," wherein variance in the health outcome is incorrectly "soaked up" by the included context, rather than the context that was missing from study.[76,77]

SOCIAL DETERMINANTS OF HEALTH DO NOT OPERATE IN A VACUUM

The previous sections of this chapter focused on social determinants of health that exist across several ecological levels, including the individual (i.e., gender, SES), interpersonal (i.e., exposure to childhood adversity), and community level (i.e., gender roles; schools and neighborhoods). Although each determinant is described on its own, it is important to recognize that none of these factors operate in isolation. Instead, there is a dynamic interaction among factors *within* the same level (e.g., individual level) as well as *across* levels of the social-ecological model (e.g., individual and interpersonal levels).

A classic example of such complex dynamics can be seen through research on gene–environment interactions (G×E), which acknowledges that neither genetic nor social factors are solely deterministic of disease risk, but rather that genes and environment/lived experience work in concert to shape disease course and outcomes. Research on G×E in depression is especially important, as genetic variation is known to explain only about 40% of the population-level risk for depression.[78] Typical G×E studies assume a diathesis-stress model, whereby a genetic liability, or diathesis, interacts with a stressful life event to give rise to depression.[79] As some have noted, the idea of a diathesis-stress model is that "genes load the gun, but environment pulls the trigger."[80]

Despite the longstanding interest in G×E within psychiatry, research in this area has not yet achieved full success. During the "candidate gene era," investigators tested for G×E using genetic variants hypothesized to play a role in the neurobiology of depression, namely those regulating serotonin and dopamine neurotransmission.[81] The best-known work in this area was performed by Caspi and colleagues, who found that a functional polymorphism in the promoter region (5-HTTLPR) of the serotonin transporter gene (SLC6A4) interacted with stressful life events to increase the risk of depression.[82] However, after numerous subsequent failed attempts by other investigators to replicate these initial findings, many in the field have concluded that such candidate gene findings are false, or that even if true, they have limited generalizability.[83] In the more recent "GWAS era," genome-wide association studies[84] are being performed to identify common genetic variants shaping risk for disease outcomes;[79] this work has been considerably more fruitful, with more than two dozen genetic variants associated with depression now identified.[85–88] Initial work on G×E in the context of GWAS also appears promising,[79] though much more work in this area is needed. As this G×E example illustrates, a multidisciplinary approach may be required to understand the complex etiology of depression and to identify strategies to prevent it.

SUMMARY AND CONCLUSIONS

Efforts to promote mental health and well-being should not be limited to individual-level strategies. As demonstrated through the work of Rose and the framework of population prevention, strategies to improve the underlying determinants of disease in the population will lead to lower overall risk and ultimately fewer cases in the population. These underlying determinants—the social determinants of health—exist at multiple social-ecological levels. Although such underlying determinants are often outside the typical purview of medicine, they need not be. By being aware of the nature and impact of these social determinants of mental health, clinicians can more effectively diagnose and treat patients and ultimately prevent psychiatric illness.

REFERENCES

1. Krieger N. A glossary for social epidemiology. *J Epidemiol Community Health.* 2001;55(10):693–700.
2. Wang MJ, Dunn EC. Epidemiology. In: Braaten E, ed. *SAGE Encyclopedia of Intellectual and Developmental Disorders*. New York: Sage; 2017.
3. Berkman LF, Kawachi I, Glymour MM. *Social Epidemiology*. New York: Oxford University Press; 2014.
4. Susser E, Schwartz S, Morabia A, Bromet EJ. *Psychiatric Epidemiology: Searching for the Causes of Mental Disorders*. New York: Oxford University Press; 2006.
5. Bronfenbrenner U. Toward an experimental ecology of human development. *American Psychologist.* 1977;32(7):513.
6. McLeroy KR, Bibeau D, Steckler A, Glanz K. An ecological perspective on health promotion programs. *Health Educ Q.* 1988;15(4):351–377.
7. Rose G. Sick individuals and sick populations. *Int J Epidemiol.* 1985;14(1):32–38.
8. Trivedi JK, Tripathi A, Dhanasekaran S, Moussaoui D. Preventive psychiatry: Concept appraisal and future directions. *Int J Soc Psychiatry.* 2014;60(4):321–329.
9. Zenner C, Herrnleben-Kurz S, Walach H. Mindfulness-based interventions in schools: A systematic review and meta-analysis. *Front Psychol.* 2014;5:603.
10. Durlak JA, Weissberg RP, Dymnicki AB, Taylor RD, Schellinger KB. The impact of enhancing students' social and emotional learning: a meta-analysis of school-based universal interventions. *Child Dev.* 2011;82(1):405–432.

11. Teicher MH, Samson JA. Childhood maltreatment and psychopathology: A case for ecophenotypic variants as clinically and neurobiologically distinct subtypes. *Am J Psychiatry.* 2013;170(10):1114–1133.

12. Mammen G, Faulkner G. Physical activity and the prevention of depression: A systematic review of prospective studies. *Am J Prev Med.* 2013;45(5):649–657.

13. Kessler RC, Bromet EJ. The epidemiology of depression across cultures. *Annu Rev Public Health.* 2013;34:119–138.

14. Kessler RC, Berglund P, Demler O, et al. The epidemiology of major depressive disorder: Results from the National Comorbidity Survey Replication (NCS-R). *JAMA.* 2003;289(23):3095–3105.

15. Kessler RC, Berglund P, Demler O, Jin R, Merikangas KR, Walters EE. Lifetime prevalence and age-of-onset distributions of DSM-IV disorders in the National Comorbidity Survey Replication. *Arch Gen Psychiatry.* 2005;62(6):593–602.

16. Moussavi S, Chatterji S, Verdes E, Tandon A, Patel V, Ustun B. Depression, chronic diseases, and decrements in health: Results from the World Health Surveys. *Lancet.* 2007;370(9590):851–858.

17. Merikangas KR, He JP, Burstein M, et al. Lifetime prevalence of mental disorders in U.S. adolescents: Results from the National Comorbidity Survey Replication— Adolescent Supplement (NCS-A). *J Am Acad Child Adolesc Psychiatry.* 2010;49(10):980–989.

18. Kessler RC, McGonagle KA, Swartz M, Blazer DG, Nelson CB. Sex and depression in the National Comorbidity Survey. I: Lifetime prevalence, chronicity and recurrence. *J Affect Disord.* 1993;29(2-3):85–96.

19. Cyranowski JM, Frank E, Young E, Shear MK. Adolescent onset of the gender difference in lifetime rates of major depression: A theoretical model. *Arch Gen Psychiatry.* 2000;57(1):21–27.

20. Kessler RC. Epidemiology of women and depression. *J Affect Disord.* 2003;74(1):5–13.

21. Piccinelli M, Wilkinson G. Gender differences in depression. Critical review. *Br J Psychiatry.* 2000;177:486–492.

22. Weissman MM, Bland RC, Canino GJ, et al. Cross-national epidemiology of major depression and bipolar disorder. *JAMA.* 1996;276(4):293–299.

23. Hyde JS, Mezulis AH, Abramson LY. The ABCs of depression: Integrating affective, biological, and cognitive models to explain the emergence of the gender difference in depression. *Psychol Rev.* 2008;115(2):291–313.

24. Nolen-Hoeksema S. Gender differences in depression. *Curr Directions Psychol Sci.* 2001;10(5):173–176.

25. Molnar BE, Buka SL, Kessler RC. Child sexual abuse and subsequent psychopathology: Results from the National Comorbidity Survey. *Am J Public Health.* 2001;91(5):753–760.

26. Seedat S, Scott KM, Angermeyer MC, et al. Cross-national associations between gender and mental disorders in the World Health Organization World Mental Health Surveys. *Arch Gen Psychiatry.* 2009;66(7):785–795.

27. Wichstrom L. The emergence of gender difference in depressed mood during adolescence: the role of intensified gender socialization. *Dev Psychol.* 1999;35(1):232–245.

28. Rieker PP, Bird CE. Rethinking gender differences in health: Why we need to integrate social and biological perspectives. *J Gerontol B Psychol Sci Soc Sci.* 2005;60(Spec No 2):40–47.

29. Krieger N, Williams DR, Moss NE. Measuring social class in US public health research: Concepts, methodologies, and guidelines. *Annu Rev Public Health.* 1997;18:341–378.

30. Shavers VL. Measurement of socioeconomic status in health disparities research. *J Natl Med Assoc.* 2007;99(9):1013–1023.

31. Chaudry A, Wimer C. Poverty is not just an indicator: The relationship between income, poverty, and child well-being. *Acad Pediatr.* 2016;16(3 Suppl):S23–S29.

32. Luo Y, Waite LJ. The impact of childhood and adult SES on physical, mental, and cognitive well-being in later life. *J Gerontol B Psychol Sci Soc Sci.* 2005;60(2):S93–S101.

33. Wagmiller RL, Adelman RM. *Childhood and Intergenerational Poverty: The Long-Term Consequences of Growing Up Poor.* New York: National Center for Chidlren in Poverty. Columbia University, Mailman School of Public Health; 2009.

34. Lorant V, Deliege D, Eaton W, Robert A, Philippot P, Ansseau M. Socioeconomic inequalities in depression: A meta-analysis. *Am J Epidemiol.* 2003;157(2):98–112.

35. Reiss F. Socioeconomic inequalities and mental health problems in children and adolescents: A systematic review. *Soc Sci Med.* 2013;90:24–31.

36. Gilman SE, Kawachi I, Fitzmaurice GM, Buka SL. Socioeconomic status in childhood and the lifetime risk of major depression. *Int J Epidemiol.* 2002;31(2):359–367.

37. Dohrenwend BP, Levav I, Shrout PE, et al. Socioeconomic status and psychiatric disorders: The causation–selection issue. *Science.* 1992;255(5047):946–952.

38. Hudson CG. Socioeconomic status and mental illness: Tests of the social causation and selection hypotheses. *Am J Orthopsychiatry.* 2005;75(1):3–18.

39. Simmons LA, Braun B, Charnigo R, Havens JR, Wright DW. Depression and poverty among rural women: A relationship of social causation or social selection? *J Rural Health.* 2008;24(3):292–298.

40. Breslau J, Lane M, Sampson N, Kessler RC. Mental disorders and subsequent educational attainment in a US national sample. *J Psychiatr Res.* 2008;42(9):708–716.

41. Kessler RC, Foster CL, Saunders WB, Stang PE. Social consequences of psychiatric disorders, I: Educational attainment. *Am J Psychiatry.* 1995;152(7):1026–1032.

42. Johnson JG, Cohen P, Dohrenwend BP, Link BG, Brook JS. A longitudinal investigation of social causation and social selection processes involved in the association between socioeconomic status and psychiatric disorders. *J Abnorm Psychol.* 1999;108(3):490.

43. Ritsher JE, Warner V, Johnson JG, Dohrenwend BP. Inter-generational longitudinal study of social class and depression: A test of social causation and social selection models. *Br J Psychiatry.* 2001;178(40):s84–s90.

44. Wadsworth ME, Achenbach TM. Explaining the link between low socioeconomic status and psychopathology: Testing two mechanisms of the social causation hypothesis. *J Consult Clin Psychol.* 2005;73(6):1146.

45. Costello EJ, Compton SN, Keeler G, Angold A. Relationships between poverty and psychopathology: A natural experiment. *JAMA.* 2003;290(15):2023–2029.

46. Koenen K, Roberts AL, Stone DM, Dunn EC. The epidemiology of early childhood trauma. In: Lanius RA, Vermetten E, Pain C, eds. *The Impact of Early Life Trauma on Health and Disease: The Hidden Epidemic.* Cambridge, UK: Cambridge University Press; 2010:13–24.

47. Finkelhor D, Ormrod RK, Turner HA. Poly-victimization: A neglected component in child victimization. *Child Abuse Negl.* 2007;31(1):7–26.

48. McLaughlin KA, Greif Green J, Gruber MJ, Sampson NA, Zaslavsky AM, Kessler RC. Childhood adversities and first onset of psychiatric disorders in a national sample of US adolescents. *Arch Gen Psychiatry.* 2012;69(11):1151–1160.

49. Felitti VJ, Anda RF, Nordenberg D, et al. Relationship of childhood abuse and household dysfunction to many of the leading causes of death in adults. The Adverse Childhood Experiences (ACE) Study. *Am J Prev Med.* 1998;14(4):245–258.

50. Anda RF, Whitfield CL, Felitti VJ, et al. Adverse childhood experiences, alcoholic parents, and later risk of alcoholism and depression. *Psychiatr Serv.* 2002;53(8):1001–1009.

51. Dube SR, Fairweather D, Pearson WS, Felitti VJ, Anda RF, Croft JB. Cumulative childhood stress and autoimmune diseases in adults. *Psychosom Med.* 2009;71(2):243–250.

52. Gilbert R, Widom CS, Browne K, Fergusson D, Webb E, Janson S. Burden and consequences of child maltreatment in high-income countries. *Lancet.* 2009;373(9657):68–81.

53. Heim C, Binder EB. Current research trends in early life stress and depression: Review of human studies on sensitive periods, gene–environment interactions, and epigenetics. *Exp Neurol.* 2012;233(1):102–111.

54. Kessler RC, McLaughlin KA, Green JG, et al. Childhood adversities and adult psychopathology in the WHO World Mental Health Surveys. *Br J Psychiatry.* 2010;197(5):378–385.

55. Barnett D, Manly JT, Cicchetti D. Defining child maltreatment: The interface between policy and research. In: Cicchetti D, Toth SL, eds. *Child Abuse, Child Development, and Social Policy.* Norwood, NJ: Ablex; 1993;8:7–73.

56. English DJ, Graham JC, Litrownik AJ, Everson M, Bangdiwala SI. Defining maltreatment chronicity: Are there differences in child outcomes? *Child Abuse Negl.* 2005;29(5):575–595.

57. Dunn EC, McLaughlin KA, Slopen N, Rosand J, Smoller JW. Developmental timing of child maltreatment and symptoms of depression and suicidal ideation in young adulthood: Results from the National Longitudinal Study of Adolescent Health. *Depress Anxiety.* 2013;30(10):955–964.

58. Dunn EC, Nishimi K, Powers A, Bradley B. Is developmental timing of trauma exposure associated with depressive and post-traumatic stress disorder symptoms in adulthood? *J Psychiatr Res.* 2017;84:119–127.

59. Kaplow JB, Widom CS. Age of onset of child maltreatment predicts long-term mental health outcomes. *J Abnorm Psychol.* 2007;116(1):176–187.

60. Keiley MK, Howe TR, Dodge KA, Bates JE, Petti GS. The timing of child physical maltreatment: A cross-domain growth analysis of impact on adolescent externalizing and internalizing problems. *Dev Psychopathol.* 2001;13(4):891–912.

61. Thornberry TP, Henry KL, Ireland TO, Smith CA. The causal impact of childhood-limited maltreatment and adolescent maltreatment on early adult adjustment. *J Adolesc Health.* 2010;46(4):359–365.

62. Harpur LJ, Polek E, van Harmelen AL. The role of timing of maltreatment and child intelligence in pathways to low symptoms of depression and anxiety in adolescence. *Child Abuse Negl.* 2015;47:24–37.

63. Khan A, McCormack HC, Bolger EA, et al. Childhood maltreatment, depression, and suicidal ideation: Critical importance of parental and peer emotional abuse during developmental sensitive periods in males and females. *Front Psychiatry.* 2015;6:42.

64. Thornberry TP, Ireland TO, Smith CA. The importance of timing: The varying impact of childhood and adolescent maltreatment on multiple problem outcomes. *Dev Psychopathol.* 2001;13(4):957–979.

65. Jaffee SR, Maikovich-Fong AK. Effects of chronic maltreatment and maltreatment timing on children's behavior and cognitive abilities. *J Child Psychol Psychiatry.* 2011;52(2):184–194.

66. Oldehinkel AJ, Ormel J, Verhulst FC, Nederhof E. Childhood adversities and adolescent depression: A matter of both risk and resilience. *Dev Psychopathol.* 2014;26(4pt1):1067–1075.

67. Sampson RJ, Raudenbush SW, Earls F. Neighborhoods and violent crime: A multilevel study of collective efficacy. *Science.* 1997;277(5328):918–924.

68. Kim D. Blues from the neighborhood? Neighborhood characteristics and depression. *Epidemiol Rev.* 2008;30:101–117.

69. Mair CF, Diez Roux AV, Galea S. Are neighborhood characteristics associated with depressive symptoms? A critical review. *J Epidemiol Community Health.* 2008;62(11):940–946.

70. Sellström E, Bremberg S. The significance of neighbourhood context to child and adolescent health and well-being: A systematic review of multilevel studies. *Scand J Soc Med.* 2006;34(5):544–554.

71. Goering J, Kraft J, Feins J, McInnis D, Holin MJ, Elhassan H. *Moving to Opportunity for Fair Housing Demonstration Program: Current Status and Initial Findings.* Washington, DC: US Department of Housing and Urban Development; 1999.

72. Leventhal T, Brooks-Gunn J. Moving to Opportunity: An experimental study of neighborhood effects on mental health. *Am J Public Health.* 2003;93(9):1576–1582.

73. Goldstein H. Multilevel cross-classified models. *Sociol Methods Res.* 1994;22(3):364–375.

74. Sellström E, Bremberg S. Is there a "school effect" on pupil outcomes? A review of multilevel studies. *J Epidemiol Commun Health.* 2006;60(2):149–155.

75. Dunn EC, Milliren CE, Evans CR, Subramanian SV, Richmond TK. Disentangling the relative influence of schools and neighborhoods on adolescents' risk for depressive symptoms. *Am J Public Health.* 2015;105(4):732–740.

76. Dunn EC, Richmond TK, Milliren CE, Subramanian SV. Using cross-classified multilevel models to disentangle school and neighborhood effects: An example focusing on smoking behaviors among adolescents in the United States. *Health Place.* 2015;31:224–232.

77. Evans CR, Onnela JP, Williams DR, Subramanian SV. Multiple contexts and adolescent body mass index: Schools, neighborhoods, and social networks. *Soc Sci Med.* 2016;162:21–31.

78. Sullivan PF, Neale MC, Kendler KS. Genetic epidemiology of major depression: Review and meta-analysis. *Am J Psychiatry.* 2000;157(10):1552–1562.

79. Dunn EC, Brown RC, Dai Y, et al. Genetic determinants of depression: Recent findings and future directions. *Harv Rev Psychiatry.* 2015;23(1):1–18.

80. Olden K, White SL. Health-related disparities: Influence of environmental factors. *Med Clin North Am.* 2005;89(4):721–738.

81. Corvin A, Craddock N, Sullivan PF. Genome-wide association studies: A primer. *Psychol Med.* 2010;40(7):1063–1077.

82. Caspi A, Sugden K, Moffitt TE, et al. Influence of life stress on depression: Moderation by a polymorphism in the 5-HTT gene. *Science.* 2003;301(5631):386–389.

83. Culverhouse RC, Saccone NL, Horton AC, et al. Collaborative meta-analysis finds no evidence of a strong interaction between stress and 5-HTTLPR genotype contributing to the development of depression. *Mol Psychiatry.* 2018;23(1):133–142.

84. Major Depressive Disorder Working Group of the Psychiatric GWAS Consortium, Ripke S, Wray NR, et al. A mega-analysis of genome-wide association studies for major depressive disorder. *Mol Psychiatry.* 2013;18(4):497–511.

85. Converge Consortium. Sparse whole-genome sequencing identifies two loci for major depressive disorder. *Nature.* 2015;523(7562):588–591.

86. Direk N, Williams S, Smith JA, et al. An analysis of two genome-wide association meta-analyses identifies a new locus for broad depression phenotype. *Biol Psychiatry.* 2017;82(5):322–329.

87. Hyde CL, Nagle MW, Tian C, et al. Identification of 15 genetic loci associated with risk of major depression in individuals of European descent. *Nat Genet.* 2016;48(9):1031–1036.

88. Okbay A, Baselmans BM, De Neve J-E, et al. Genetic variants associated with subjective well-being, depressive symptoms, and neuroticism identified through genome-wide analyses. *Nature Genetics.* 2016;48(6):624–633.

6

Psychiatry and Its Checkered Past

Perspectives on Current Practice

JUDITH PUCKETT AND DAVID SHUMWAY JONES ■

CASE 1

A 25-year-old immigrant presents to her primary care physician requesting an antidepressant. On further questioning, she explains that she has been experiencing depressed mood in the setting of multiple stressors: She and her husband are in the United States without legal status; her children remain in their home country with their grandparents; her husband is often abusive, but she relies on him for financial support and will never be able to return home to her children without his assistance. She had responded well to antidepressants during an episode of depression in the past.

CASE 2

A 58-year-old man is admitted to a psychiatric hospital during an episode of severe depression. Since he had failed to respond to multiple prior courses of antidepressants, his psychiatrist recommended electroconvulsive therapy. The patient refused: "Are you kidding? I've read Cuckoo's Nest, *and you're not doing that to me."*

INTRODUCTION

These cases are likely familiar to any mental health care professional today. Such cases, in which a patient requests a medication for mental distress in the setting of multiple social stresses, or another patient refuses needed care because of stigmatized perceptions of psychiatry, are common yet troubling. They raise difficult questions of psychiatric diagnosis and management. They often fuel critiques that psychiatrists pathologize the human experience and push unwarranted medications. Is this a case of normal situational sadness or a treatable disease? Are there times when treatment is worthwhile even if the diagnosis remains unclear?

It is painfully obvious to psychiatrists, and often their patients, that psychiatry has a reputation problem. The public continues to be skeptical about the integrity of psychiatrists. In a 2016 Gallup poll on honesty and ethics in professions, 65% of Americans surveyed responded that medical doctors had "high" or "very high" ethical standards, while only 40% of respondents felt that psychiatrists met these ethical standards[1]—despite the fact that psychiatrists are in fact medical doctors. These results reflect two problems that psychiatrists experience frequently. First, despite their training as medical doctors, psychiatrists are often viewed as a distinct category. In the Gallup poll, for instance, all other medical doctors were lumped together, and only psychiatrists were singled out, along with other groups such as dentists, chiropractors, lawyers, and police officers.

Psychiatrists themselves are partly to blame for this. The profession originally spent decades attempting to designate itself as different from the other medical professions; many maintain a separatist view today. Second, psychiatry continues to be viewed negatively in the public eye. Their fellow physicians often contribute to this: Even within the medical field psychiatrists are often not perceived as "real doctors"; up to 35% of nonpsychiatrists see psychiatrists as less emotionally stable than other physicians.[2,3] Despite this, psychiatrists tend to maintain an elitist and separatist view of themselves, believing they are more introspective, cultured, and mature than their medical colleagues.[2] Though there is evidence that perceptions are improving in recent decades, this remains a work in progress. Insurers have made matters worse by refusing to cover psychiatric services; now that they must provide coverage, they often impose specific barriers for psychiatric care alone and reimburse at low rates. The skepticism, critique, and dismissal of psychiatry raise important questions: Why do they exist? What can be done to improve the situation?

Negative perceptions of psychiatry are not isolated to the United States. Psychiatrists and patients with psychiatric disorders are subjected to negative stereotypes within medical communities and among the general population worldwide. Zaza Lyons reviewed 32 studies encompassing 12,144 medical students and 74 medical schools across the globe.[4] Most studies found that fewer than 5% of medical students considered psychiatry as a career choice.[4] Their lack of enthusiasm for psychiatry reflected perceptions of the low status and prestige of psychiatry; lack of good psychiatrist role models; perceptions of psychiatry as depressing and/or frustrating; and fears of the loss of clinical skills.[4] It is essential to understand how and why the critiques take place and contribute to the low status of psychiatry, including its knowledge, practices, institutions, and practitioners. The low status, in turn, affects the attitudes of patients, insurers, and other physicians. Only by understanding what has gone wrong can psychiatrists mount effective responses.

THE HISTORY OF PSYCHIATRY

The Intuitive Sense of Mental Illness and the Asylum Movement

The history of critiques of psychiatry is likely as old as the profession itself. Aspects of the critique are well deserved, arising from the many regrettable episodes in the history of the field from phrenology, hysteria, and lobotomy, to more recent phenomena such as recovered memories and conversion therapy. This chapter will not cover the history of all aspects of psychiatry that have been called into question. It will instead focus on two major influences on how psychiatry is practiced and perceived today: the development of asylums as a form of confinement for those who are mentally ill, and the development of psychiatric nosology and diagnosis.

The history of mental illness extends much further than the idea of psychiatry itself, a term coined in 1808 by Johann Christian Reil.[5,6] The first institutions devoted to the care of patients with mental illness opened in the Islamic world in the ninth century.[7] During this time, the treatment and care of the mentally ill remained intertwined with religious practice. Many of those with mental illness were cared for in monasteries or almshouses, or by families in their homes. Many without familial resources, or those with severe illness, were forced into the countryside.[7]

Widespread treatment for the mentally ill did not fully develop until the 1300s and 1400s. During this time, the burden of leprosy began to dissipate; hospitals and other institutions once devoted to leprosy were repurposed to care for those with mental illness.[7] These institutions often left much to be desired: Inmates often received little care and lived in appalling conditions. The most notorious, London's Bethlehem Hospital (source of the term "bedlam") was typical.[8] The hospital became one of London's most famous tourist attractions, rivaling even the Tower of London.[8] Well-heeled aristocrats could tour its wards, with patients on display as if at a zoo. Amariah Brigham described the conditions found at Bedlam and similar asylums: Patients "were confined in badly ventilated apartments where they were never discharged but by death. The quiet, the noisy, and the violent were all congregated together, and a majority were chained to beds by their wrists and ankles. No contemplation of human misery ever affected us so much: the howlings, execrations and clanking of chains gave to the place the appearance of the infernal regions."[9]

Critics and reformers, notably William Pinel in France and William Tuke in England, sought to improve conditions. They released patients from chains and called for "moral treatment."[9] While such reforms helped, they did little to stem the growth of large, custodial asylums over the 19th century. Critiques from within psychiatry intensified as these institutions grew. For instance, Pliny Earle is often credited for his dedicated work and his critique of asylums. He served as superintendent of the State Lunatic Hospital at Northampton, Massachusetts.[10] In his 1887 essay "The Curability of Insanity," Earle reviewed cure rates reported by various asylums around the United States.[10] Skeptical of reported claims—some superintendents reported 100% cure rates—Earle looked more carefully at available data.[10] He realized that hospitals counted every discharge as a cure, even if the patients were soon readmitted, something that happened often.[10] For example, one person admitted and discharged 13 times might have been counted as 13 cures. Earle recognized that such patients were simply being stabilized, and not being cured, a pattern we see often today. Keeping track of which discharged patients were soon readmitted, Earle calculated a revised recovery rate of just 34%.[10] He concluded that many hospitals had simply rigged their numbers to improve their standing in the community.[10] Earle's critiques had a significant impact on public and professional perceptions of psychiatry and the treatment of insanity.

Critiques continued into the 20th century. During World War II, some conscientious objectors were assigned to work in asylums. These were thoughtful outsiders, people of high moral courage, who had not previously been exposed or socialized to asylum conditions, and they were shocked by what they saw. One group, assigned to Pennsylvania State Hospital in Byberry, surreptitiously brought cameras into the asylum to photograph conditions, with naked patients huddled in bare rooms and others restrained in their beds.[11] These photographs, published in *Life* magazine, provoked national outrage and led for calls to reform asylums and improve the training of staff.[11]

The Deinstitutionalization Movement to the Present

In the second half of the 20th century, critiques of "the institution" expanded and many called for the closure of asylums. A number of psychiatrists supported this call, as most had nothing to do with asylums: By 1957, fewer than 20% of members of the American Psychiatric Association (APA) had any affiliation with a mental institution.[12] Over the decades that followed, most psychiatric hospitals did close, forcing the discharge of tens of thousands of psychiatric patients, a process known as deinstitutionalization. Deinstitutionalization was made viable by the advent of the first modern psychiatric medications, including chlorpromazine, which assisted in the treatment of agitated patients, as well as the first antidepressants.[13,14] Federal support for community mental health centers and the new availability of Medicare funding enabled the discharge of many persistently ill patients from long-term hospitalization. Unfortunately, the promised community-based care to support these patients outside the institution rarely materialized. Many who would once have been in asylums are now either homeless or incarcerated (a process some have called "transinstitutionalization"), often going without mental health care. This has shifted the bulk of psychiatric care for those with severe and chronic mental illness to emergency departments.[14] The closure of many hospitals and the neglect of discharged patients have fueled critiques that psychiatrists have abandoned the sickest patients, instead practicing in private clinics catering to what Stuart Kirk and Herb Kutchins describe as "clients who were young, attractive, verbal, intelligent, and successful . . . the worried well—and neglecting the more needy."[15] Long-term institutional care has now largely disappeared in the United States, reserved for a small number of the most disabled patients. Conditions on the inpatient psychiatric units that remain are much improved from the 1950s, at least in the United States. Many problems, however, persist, and investigative journalists continue to do important work documenting problems and highlighting need for resources and reform.

THE DEVELOPMENT OF PSYCHIATRIC DIAGNOSIS

Such critiques, while often both dire and deserving, are not critiques of the goals and theories of psychiatry: They are simply critiques of how psychiatry has been implemented at specific times and in specific places. However, critics have also attacked the foundations of the field itself.

Societies have long worried about how to understand and manage people who suffer from mental illness. Many relied on intuitive notions of madness, lunacy, or insanity. Modern nosology developed in the early 19th century in Europe. Two systems of classification were developed, one focused on symptoms and the other on causation.[16] This division largely persists today, providing one of the major differences in approach between neurology and psychiatry. Most areas of medical theory and practice classify diseases by etiology, recognizing that a specific underlying cause can produce diverse clinical phenomena. Symptoms are clues that doctors use to identify the underlying cause. Once the cause has been recognized, physicians can develop specific treatments that target the underlying cause. When this works, the symptoms resolve.

This approach has not yet been successful in psychiatry. Daniel Hack Tuke, a lecturer at the Charing Cross Hospital Medical School in the late 1800s, described the difficulty of psychiatric nosology, stating, "The wit of man has rarely been more exercised than in the attempt to classify the morbid phenomena covered by the term insanity. The result has been disappointing."[16,17] Causation-based classification has remained difficult in psychiatry because the cause of most disorders remains unknown. In fact, it has been a common development that once the cause of a behavioral syndrome is discovered or defined, the diagnosis and treatment of these syndromes are taken over by other medical specialties.[16] In the late 19th century, for instance, neurology took responsibility for diseases of the brain with identifiable causes (e.g., multiple sclerosis, amyotrophic lateral sclerosis, epilepsy, strokes, cancers), leaving syndromes of uncertain etiology (e.g., depression, mania, hysteria, psychosis) to psychiatry.[18] This persists, more or less, a century later. Psychiatry has become the field that manages the complex, unclear behavioral syndromes and suffering that cannot be clearly linked to direct biological or physiologic cause.

In the absence of broad knowledge of etiology, psychiatric classification relies on symptoms and descriptive pathology. This approach became prominent in France in the early 1800s with the work of Philippe Pinel and Etienne Esquirol, who made the first attempts at what is considered the modern classification of today.[16] Psychiatrists revised classification systems repeatedly over the 19th century.[16] Psychiatric nosology took on a recognizably modern form with the work of German psychiatrist Emil Kraepelin, whose writings particularly about schizophrenia and bipolar disorder remain influential today.[16]

Despite these prominent European contributions to psychiatry, American psychiatrists took a different path. In 1913, the APA set up a committee that created a new nosology.[16] Eventually the APA began cooperating with the National Committee for Mental Hygiene to use nosology to monitor state mental hospital statistics, largely based on psychoneurosis and psychoanalytic theory popular at the time.[16] This focus on psychodynamics and individual human relations would remain prominent in American psychiatric nosology until the 1980 publication of the third edition of the *Diagnostic and Statistical Manual of Mental Disorders* (DSM).[16]

Development of DSM: From Research Tool to Clinical Guide

More than a century after Tuke described the challenge of psychiatric diagnosis, psychiatrists still struggle to classify the disorders of the mind. The evolution of the DSM demonstrates this well. The DSM, designed to set new standards of psychiatric science, is also a political and social document. The first edition, published in 1952, was written by a committee appointed by the APA.[16] It was heavily influenced by a diagnostic manual written by psychoanalyst William Menninger during World War II.[16,19] The second edition, published in 1968, remained similar to the first in its structure and approach to diagnosis, with sections on schizophrenia and its subtypes, mood disorders, Freudian disorders (i.e., neuroses), and personality disorders.[16,20] Such psychoanalytic approaches dominated U.S. psychiatry until the 1970s, by which time the advent of effective pharmaceuticals had begun to shift the focus of psychiatry toward psychopharmacology and new etiologic theories.[16,20] In the late 1970s the World Health Organization updated its international classification of disease.[20] In parallel, a joint project between the New York State Department of Mental Hygiene and the Institute of Psychiatry in London demonstrated that American concepts of diagnosis, in particular schizophrenia, were much broader than those used in Britain.[16,20] This motivated a push to reexamine American nosology. The APA appointed Robert Spitzer to direct a taskforce to update the DSM.[16] Spitzer likely went farther than the APA had intended; he largely abandoned the psychoanalytic orientation that had dominated the first two editions and used his mandate to create a new nosology that sought to standardize diagnostic criteria to provide a stable foundation for clinical research.[16,20] He hoped that this would move psychiatry toward a "medical model," with specific diseases and reliable diagnostic criteria that would (someday) be verified with physical findings and laboratory data, and validated by response to treatment.[16,20]

In 1980, the APA published DSM-III, an event now seen as a major turning point in modern psychiatry.[16,19,20] Many new diagnoses, including attention-deficit disorder and posttraumatic stress disorder, first appeared in this publication.[19] However, despite the aspiration toward a medical model, most of the diagnostic criteria still depended on subjective judgments and the experiences of those in the taskforce who developed the document.[19] Rhetoric and personal appeals played a major role in resolving diagnostic controversies emerging during the committee process, and their decisions often reflected a narrow, American cultural orientation.

With each subsequent revision of the DSM, the number of new diagnoses has grown. This has raised concerns among some psychiatrists and their critics that the DSMs now name and pathologize every uncomfortable feeling that is part of being human. Paul Chodoff in 2005 noted, "I feel concern about a burgeoning *furor diagnosticus*, offering a name and number for every untoward feeling or behavior in the way that trivializes the human condition by denying its inescapable, somber, and even tragic elements."[21]

Despite ever-increasing empirical support, the DSM, even today, remains a document founded on "expert consensus"[19] rather than systematic evidence. Critics have argued that clinicians and experts with divergent views have not been invited to participate in the creation and revision process. Despite recommendations to broaden participation in the process, including votes on specific issues by the APA, concerns have been raised by the idea of members voting on what is supposed to be a scientific issue. One dramatic example occurred in 1973, when the APA voted to eliminate homosexuality from its diagnostic categories.[14,22,23] Such voting likely increased political engagement in the development and revision of psychiatric criteria, even as skeptics raised doubts about the validity of diagnoses created by this engagement.

In spite of its flaws, the DSM continues to guide psychiatric practice in the United States. Why does it remain? Its diagnostic criteria provide useful (if imperfect) descriptions that facilitate communication among doctors, patients, and medical colleagues. As Anthony Clare has discussed, a common framework is required in order to understand and describe individual cases and formulations.[24] Without this framework, it is difficult to make sense of each individual case. Clare also discusses therapists who, despite their preference for avoiding the DSM and other medical models, still need to use shared methods of formulation in order to communicate.[24]

The DSM offers the essentialist view of psychiatric diagnosis, based on the framework that each thing, or in the case of psychiatry, each DSM diagnosis, has a set of unchanging attributes that makes it what it is. Humans are disposed to think about biological categories in terms of an essentialist framework: We learn and synthesize information by classifying and categorizing.[25] Psychiatrists have created a model of brain disorders that was helpful at the time.[25] Despite the natural tendency of humans to think categorically, biology does not actually function in an essentialist framework; this is exemplified by the burgeoning number of diagnoses in the DSM as psychiatrists attempt to further define and categorize the existing holes and variable presentations of psychiatric illness. This remains ever-present in the taxonomy of psychiatry, noted by the popularity of "not otherwise specified" as a diagnosis.

Most psychiatrists understand that the DSM framework, our current diagnostic model, is provisional, and hope to refine the manual as new data narrow the gap between the brain and mind. Different models of classification and clustering of symptoms will be required as we develop future treatment options. As we discover genetic and biological variables that affect mental health, the specificity of diagnosis will improve. However, pathology of the mind often consists of immensely complex phenomena with subtle variability, so it is likely that ambiguity will always be present in psychiatric pathology and diagnosis.[26] Psychiatry is currently at a crossroads.[26] While some researchers work to refine the DSM, others investigate alternative modes of classification and grouping that might include ideas and data beyond the "expert consensus" and involve a broader culture of contribution.

Normal Versus Abnormal: Critiques of Psychiatry

Amid this history of shifting and contested nosologies, an issue fundamental to the validity of psychiatric nomenclature and diagnosis has remained constant: Can psychiatry reliably distinguish abnormal from normal? In the 1950s and 1960s—in parallel with the deepening critiques of psychiatric institutions—psychiatrists, philosophers, and others began both to question whether a distinction between normal and pathological truly existed, and to critique the ability of doctors to identify this distinction.[27,28] In 1961, Michel Foucault, a professor of philosophy and psychology in Paris, published his influential *Folie et Déraison: Histoire de la Folie à l'âge classique* (published in English as *History of Madness*), in which he discussed the construction of madness.[27] He postulated that madness and classification of mental illness were a result of power relations developed within society: Society constructed the definition of madness through cultural, economic, and academic influences.[27] The experience of madness is defined as a departure from rationality, as determined by those whose interests would be served by defining this departure from social norms.[27] For instance, he argued that Enlightenment thinkers developed new ideas about mental disease that differed dramatically from the religious conceptions common in the Renaissance.[27] They defined rationality in distinction to those deemed irrational, and then consigned the irrational to asylums—a process that Foucault named the "great confinement."[27] Subsequent work by historians has challenged Foucault's history (there was no great confinement of the sort he described, at least not until much later).[7] However, his critiques of how culture and society shape the context of insanity, how it is experienced, and how it is perpetuated as a mode of control of individuals, remain influential today.

The strongest critique was articulated by American psychiatrist Thomas Szasz.[28] In his 1960 work, *Myth of Mental Illness*, he argued that psychiatric nosology and diagnosis are simply exercises in arbitrary social labeling: People who differ from social norms are deemed deviant or pathological.[28] By pathologizing the suffering of a group of people, society manages to disguise the inevitable conflicts and disappointments of human life.[28] As Mayes and Horowitz summarize, Szasz also put forth the idea that "psychiatry was an authoritarian extension of the state used for controlling nonconformists. Psychiatric labels are arbitrary designations that, instead of serving the needs of patients, serve professional needs and the needs of dominant groups."[14] These critiques generalize into broad condemnations of the basic assumptions of psychiatry. For instance, sociologist Thomas Scheff argues that mental illness is a behavior that occurs as a response to desperation and distress, a behavior that occurs naturally in people as a last resort.[14,29,30] Psychiatric diagnoses are merely labels "behind which psychiatrists and the public hid their ignorance of the real causes behind deviant behavior."[14] Similarly, Scottish psychiatrist R. D. Laing rejects the distinction between normal and abnormal.[31] He believes that what people label as "psychiatric symptoms" are legitimate, and not pathological, expressions of the consequences of lived experience.[31] In his opinion, insanity itself is "a perfectly rational adjustment to an insane world."[31]

Others have argued that psychiatric care—in particular institutionalization itself—causes pathology, and propose the concept of the learned role of the psychiatric patient. One famous example occurred early in the history of the profession: Jean-Martin Charcot, a neurologist who directed the Salpêtrière Hospital in Paris (where Freud trained) in the 1880s, grew famous for his demonstrations of hysteria in women. Skeptics soon began to suspect that much of this behavior was learned by these institutionalized women who, whether consciously or unconsciously, sought to please Charcot by performing behaviors that he wanted to demonstrate. Decades later sociologist Erving Goffman studied the function of asylums.[32] In a collection of essays published in 1961, he argued that asylums, "total institutions," transformed the patients consigned to them.[32] Through a process of institutionalization, or "mortification," they took on new behaviors that were then interpreted as evidence of their mental illness.[32] According to Goffman, some of the phenomenology of mental illness was actually produced by the asylums themselves.[32]

One of the most interesting critiques came in a controversial article published in *Science* in 1973.[22] Stanford sociologist David Rosenhan recruited seven collaborators: Each of them feigned auditory hallucinations and presented to emergency departments at hospitals throughout the United States and managed to gain admission to 12 hospitals in five states.[33] After admission, they all behaved normally.[33] All but one was diagnosed with schizophrenia in remission, and they were kept in the hospital an average of 19 days.[33] All had to accept the diagnosis and treatment as a condition for discharge.[33] Rosenhan concluded that the ability of his group to deceive psychiatrists exposed psychiatric science as a fraud: "It is clear that we cannot distinguish the sane from the insane in psychiatric hospitals."[33] This study produced a firestorm of controversy: *Science* subsequently published 12 pages of letters to the editor condemning Rosenhan's methodology and conclusions.[34] While many were concerned that hospitals admitted the patients simply for a complaint of auditory hallucinations, they defended the hospitals, whose main error may simply have been that they trusted people (i.e., the researchers) arriving at hospitals seeking aid for a distressing symptom.[34] Regardless of whether Rosenhan or his critics are right, the episode reveals the enormous problem facing psychiatry in the early 1970s: Psychiatric knowledge and institutions had fallen into such disrepute that the country's leading science journal was willing to publish a seriously flawed study adding to the critiques.

In the decades that followed Rosenhan's work, the critiques have continued unabated. Social scientists have published rigorous analyses of psychiatric practice, exposing past errors and the deficiencies of current practice. Andrew Scull's *Madhouse* tells the tale of Henry Cotton, superintendent of the Trenton State Hospital.[35] Cotton knew that some infections could cause mental illness: Neurosyphilis was then a leading cause of admission to psychiatric hospitals.[35] He generalized this observation and argued that all psychiatric disorders were caused by occult infections, and that the goal of psychiatry was to root out these infections, so he removed teeth, gallbladders, and other organs from his patients in hopes of removing foci of infection causing their symptoms.[35] He reported an 85% cure rate, even though 30% of his patients died in the operating room.[35] Prominent psychiatrists, notably Adolph Meyer at Johns Hopkins, were aware yet did nothing.[35] Scull sees this tale not as evidence of Cotton as a rogue psychiatrist, but as evidence of a specialty completely unable to set or defend the most basic standards of conduct.

In a similar light, many argue that psychiatric taxonomy is the labeling of deviant behavior as disease and in itself serves as a form of social control. Jonathan Metzl's *Protest Psychosis* tells how, during the civil rights movement in the 1960s, prominent psychiatrists identified civil rights activists as part of a mass delusion about the existence of racism and race-based persecution in the United States.[36] This pathologized civil rights protestors, some of whom ended up in state psychiatric hospitals.[36] This is but one example of the many ways in which psychiatry has colluded with government officials to defend entrenched interests and preserve the status quo.

Concern about psychiatric labeling as a form of social control also became a pervasive concept in popular culture during this time. *One Flew Over the Cuckoo's Nest*, a film adapted from the novel by Ken Kesey, won Academy Awards for best picture, best director, best actor, best actress, and best screenplay in 1975.[37] Both book and movie reinforced the concept that psychiatrists were "mental police."[14,37] They tell the story of Randle P. McMurphy, a man without psychiatric illness who has himself transferred to a psychiatric hospital in order to avoid prison.[37] During the film, McMurphy refuses to show deference to authority; he is brutally punished with electroconvulsive therapy and lobotomy.[37] The film became an immense hit in the 1970s, grossing $300 million worldwide.[14,37] The film "found a receptive audience with many college students, intellectuals, and the anti-authority ethos of the time."[14] It continues to influence the popular perception of psychiatry today.[37]

The question of when a specific behavior pattern should be classified as a mental disorder continues to be controversial and contested even among psychiatrists. Psychiatrists have participated actively in societal debates about the boundary between normal and pathological, in topics as varied as bereavement, substance use, and sexuality. For instance, as stated by journalist Nathan Emmerich,

> In a relatively short historical time, sex between people of the same gender has gone from sinful act, to a pathological sexuality, to one form of human sexuality. To recognize the role of psychiatry in the production and transformation of sexuality is to recognize the moral and political significance of the discipline and the knowledge it has to offer. We might then reflect on the moral and political significance of transforming the cultural problems of "overeating" and "grief" when we label them "binge-eating disorder" and "major depressive disorder" respectively.[38]

Emmerich here references a widely critiqued and, at the time, highly publicized revolution in the field of psychiatry. In the early 1970s increasing debate occurred regarding homosexuality's status as a disorder in DSM-II. The controversy highlighted the influence of public opinion, politics, and social construction on psychiatric diagnosis. Ultimately, in 1974, the APA voted to confirm the committee's decision to remove homosexuality from DSM-II, replacing it with "sexual orientation disturbance."[14,22,23] This fueled the skepticism surrounding the validity of psychiatric diagnosis when "what had been considered for a century or more a grave psychiatric disorder ceased to exist."[39] Even though these issues are discussed most often in the field of mental illness, debates about the contested definitions of disease, behavior, and environment are not unique to psychiatry; debates regarding obesity and addictions as medical illness have also become prominent in American medicine. The American Medical Association, for instance, voted to classify obesity as a disease in 2013, thereby deeming 78 million American adults to have a new medical diagnosis that required treatment,[40,41] triggering debate nationwide.

Human behavior and experience exist along a spectrum, and it remains unclear if a distinct demarcation between normal and abnormal can be made. We continue to seek but lack the data needed to support the proposed fundamental or essentialist pathology on which many DSM disorders are presumably based. Despite the large expansion of nomenclature, the "not otherwise specified" category is frequently used in general practice. The rapid expansion of DSM and the number of psychiatric disorders identified raise concern regarding whether we are pathologizing "problems of living."[42] Karl Menninger argues that psychiatric illnesses do not exist as discrete disorders, instead noting disorders of the mind as "as reducible to one basic psychosocial process: the failure of the suffering individual to adapt to his or her environment."[14,42,43] He notes that the severity of poor adaptation can range from none to severe in a continuous and nondiscrete process.[14,42,43] Outside of extreme presentations (i.e., no distress vs. psychosis), psychiatry remains on the cusp of being able to truly identify and define when mental illness is a maladaptive response to regular life and when it is pathology.

While there likely is no discrete boundary between normal and abnormal functioning, our current definition of psychiatric illness is not purely arbitrary. This is best exemplified by the identification and management of severe mental illness, where there is both widespread acceptance of schizophrenia as a severe pathology and high interrater reliability with the diagnosis of mania. Despite this confidence, mental health providers should remain active in the debates about what truly is a clinically significant level of distress or impairment, as well as about what domains of functioning we should consider. In this vein, and as discussed below, labeling of distress and the resultant management by psychiatry have been based entirely on Western, and largely American, societal norms. It has been proposed that a system of developing points of demarcation along the spectrum of functioning may be more applicable.[19] For example, the demarcation of mental retardation is an arbitrary point picked along a spectrum of measured intelligence: Intelligence is constructed of multifactorial variables without clear breakpoints between normal and abnormal.[19] However, ongoing measurement and study have enabled the development of more reliable ways of predicting levels of impairment and need for intervention.[19]

Despite a burgeoning culture of distrust, the demand for mental health services continues to rise. There remains a shortage of mental health care providers and facilities across the United States. Psychiatry has been transformed from a discipline focused on treating insanity to one concerned with normality.[14,44,45] Treatment has been expanded to maladaptive patterns of behavior and personal problems. Unlike primary care, where patients present in hopes of being told that everything is okay, or other fields of medicine where patients present hoping for treatment or cure, psychiatry at times can hold a unique role in that patients present because they want a label for their distress, whether pathological or not. Many psychiatrists can easily recall experiences where both the patient and the consulting physician expressed disappointment when the psychiatrist determined that the patient simply struggled with normal life events. It is often easier just to give a diagnosis, leading to unnecessary and inaccurate "soft" diagnoses. New generations of psychiatrists and mental health providers need to be active in the ongoing debates that occur regarding taxonomy and to remain vigilant in their diagnosis of pathology.

FACTORS INFLUENCING PSYCHIATRIC DIAGNOSIS AND PRACTICE

The purpose of diagnosis is to provide explanations to patients, guide treatment, and predict outcomes. As Jutel explains in her book *Putting a Name to It*, "With a diagnosis, things don't necessarily get better, but they become clearer."[46] Diagnosis in medicine is part of the ritual enacted by both doctor and patient, and providing a diagnosis involves far more than providing medical information or definition. The ability to provide a diagnosis is a position of power, and the power is given as part of a social contract with society. Diagnoses can authorize allocation of resources, stigmatize or legitimize behavior and experiences, and act as "social framing devices."[46]

Specific to psychiatry, Walter Reich described the power of diagnosis as a social act that allows patients to be committed, delineates populations to be subjected to care, and defines acceptable treatment.[47] Jutel addresses diagnosis as a social creation, noting that "before a diagnosis can exist, it has to be visible, problematic, and perceived to be related to the field of medicine;"[46] all of these factors exist in social contexts. Social and cultural influences affect not only what diagnoses exist and can be made, but also how and when psychiatrists and psychiatric patients chose to give (the former) and receive (the latter) diagnosis.[26] Influences ranging from insurance coverage and pharmaceutical development to advocacy have a substantial impact on when diagnoses are provided.

The development and advertisement of medications for mental illness remain among the most heavily debated and critiqued components of psychiatry. Imipramine, released in 1959, was the first medication to be marketed as a depression-specific treatment, quickly leading to the new term "antidepressant."[48] Many note that the pharmaceutical industry helped popularize this view and led to an era of disease-specific drugs.[48] David Healy is one of the most influential proponents of this view. In his provocative book *The Antidepressant Era*, he argues that the heavy pharmaceutical marketing of antidepressants has led to the overdiagnosis of depression and the overuse of antidepressant medications to address minor problems of everyday life.[49] He argues that the marketing of depression has influenced current practices of primary care screening and diagnosis of depression, with doctors being quick to prescribe medications that are now household names.[49] Though thought-provoking, Healy ignores much of the research by the National Institute of Mental Health on depression and largely disregards the positive effects antidepressants have also had on the field of psychiatry.[50] Similarly, it is hard to discount the witnessed clinical improvement and reported experience of patients who benefit from antidepressant therapy in clinical practice.

Similar critiques have been made of bipolar disorder. The disease concept is an old one. It was first described as *la folie circulaire* in 1851 and then popularized by the work of Kraepelin in the late 19th century.[51] In 1948 Karl Leonhard introduced the term *bipolarity*.[51] However, the diagnosis was not included in the DSM until the third edition.[51] Since that time, it has become one of the most popular diagnoses in psychiatry and has laid the foundation for the pharmaceutical industry to make millions in the market of "mood stabilizers."[14] The diagnostic criteria have been rapidly broadened into variable forms of mood lability such as rapid cycling and bipolar affective disorder.[49] Suddenly, the prevalence of bipolar disorder has ballooned—and the pharmaceutical industry ballooned in parallel.[49]

Healy has questioned the effect of direct-to-consumer advertising of mental health disorders, particularly in a field that depends on the patient's report of symptoms.[49] Investigative journalists have also written muckraking exposés, condemning, for instance, the overdiagnosis and overmedication of attention-deficit/hyperactivity disorder, childhood bipolar disorder, and other diseases in American children. Prominent researchers at elite institutions have been accused of having financial conflicts of interest with pharmaceutical companies.[52-54] One exposé by Stephen Brill targeted one prominent psychiatrist, suggesting that his enthusiasm for risperidone, fueled in part by funding he had received from Johnson & Johnson, had contributed to an epidemic of gynecomastia among American children.[54] This trend has become even more apparent with recent "awareness" campaigns targeting diseases to market newly developed medications[55] (e.g., pseudobulbar affect and Nuedexta; premenstrual dysphoric disorder and Sarafem). While making valid points, these critiques should be focused on the behavior of pharmaceutical companies and research psychiatrists and do not necessarily reflect the practice of most psychiatrists. And despite allegations of overuse, many of the medications have relieved the suffering of many patients.

Diagnostic practices are not simply influenced by marketing. Advocates and government reports can also influence the attention given to diseases, which, in turn, affects what psychiatrists look for, screen, and, diagnose. For example, DeVilbiss and Lee studied the dramatic increase in attention given to autism spectrum disorders by monitoring the number of Google searches for "autism" and "Asperger's" from 2004 to 2014.[56] The greatest number of searches for "autism" occurred each April, which has been designated National Autism Awareness Month.[56] A particular peak was noted in April 2008: April 1 of that year had been designated as World Autism Awareness Day by the United Nations General Assembly.[56] Peaks also coincided with television specials devoted to autism, including both *The Oprah Winfrey Show* and *The Today Show.*[56] The Centers for Disease Control and Prevention have funded a surveillance network, the Autism and Developmental Disabilities Monitoring Network, across several states since 2000.[57]

Autism spectrum disorder prevalence estimates in the overall population increased 78% from 2002 to 2008,[57] and many have questioned the cause for such a rapid change. Many factors may have contributed, including increased media coverage and widely publicized government research.[55] Shifting (and more inclusive) diagnostic criteria likely played a role as well. Jessica Wright notes that prior to the 1980s many people with autism were institutionalized, with diagnoses of mental retardation or other disorders, and many clinicians and family members remained unaware of the clinical features of ASD.[57] She postulates that both the increasing awareness among families and the 2007 decision by the American Academy of Pediatrics to recommend routine screening for autism have prompted more people to seek diagnosis and care.[57]

The increasing role of health insurers in psychiatric care has also influenced diagnostic practices. Since many third-party payers reimburse for mental health care only if a formal diagnosis has been made, psychiatrists have often resorted to vague diagnoses such as "psychosis NOS" or "mood disorder NOS" in order to be reimbursed for their time, even if the appropriateness of that diagnosis is unclear.

Such phenomena have spread beyond the United States. In *Crazy Like Us* and many articles in the popular media, Ethan Watters discusses the social and political influences that have led to the export of American conceptions of mental illness throughout the rest of the world.[58] He critiques this development and highlights evidence that mental illness is not a universal experience, but instead takes on different forms in different cultures (e.g., the culture-bound syndromes that once existed in DSM).[58] Watters proposes that in the past decade, as part of ongoing "export" of Western medical ideas, the symptoms of Western psychiatric illness have been exported as well, "changing not only the treatments but also the expression of mental illness in other cultures."[58] He describes the response after a teenage girl fainted and died on a public street in Hong Kong, noting that as journalists began reporting on the case, they discovered the symptoms and causes of anorexia nervosa and included this in their reporting.[58] This led to awareness campaigns based on the Western diagnosis, and ultimately the rate of anorexia nervosa increased dramatically.[58] Watters sees this as one example of a broader process of the popularization and advertisement of psychiatric diagnoses based on American definitions, a process that permeates ongoing mental health research, publications, and popular culture.[58]

Although Watters's arguments are thought-provoking, the situation requires greater nuance. Culture-bound syndromes have been identified and described by American and other Western psychiatrists. Watters also disregards the plight of countless psychiatric patients worldwide who have received no treatment or who have been subjected to the abusive treatment methods that remain widespread in many countries. Though flawed, the American standard of care being exported is often far superior to the horrific conditions that often existed in these places previously.

THE LINE BETWEEN NORMAL AND ABNORMAL

Psychiatric care remains a complex and controversial undertaking, one that continues to evolve. Despite increasing research and knowledge, we need to understand the fundamental causes of mental suffering. Despite ongoing progress and new insights into the biological factors that lead to changes in behavior and emotional experience, our knowledge of the pathophysiology of mental illness remains deeply imperfect. For instance, even though we understand that syphilis affects the brain and thus the mind (it was once the leading cause of admission to psychiatric hospitals), we still do not have a clear understanding of how it causes psychosis.

Throughout its historical development, both the science and practice of psychiatry have been subjected to criticism. These critiques of psychiatry continue actively in the 21st century, assailing fundamental tenets of psychiatric knowledge and practice. Their persistence reflects many factors. They are a response to our ongoing ignorance about psychiatric pathophysiology. They are a consequence of our lack of decisive treatments. They are a punishment for past transgressions by psychiatrists. And they may even be an inevitable consequence of the attempt by psychiatry as a field to grapple with phenomena that are so intimately tied to individual identity, belief, and behavior. Patients report what their minds suffer, but we remain unable to map this experience onto the brain, and this limits our ability to provide treatment and solace. Regardless of the origins of the critiques, psychiatrists must understand them and work actively to overcome them. Successful efforts will benefit not only the profession, but also, and more importantly, our patients.

REFERENCES

1. Gallup.com. Honesty/ethics in professions. http://www.gallup.com/poll/1654/honesty-ethics-professions.aspx. Accessed August 7, 2017.
2. Sartorius N, Gaebel W, Cleveland H-R, et al. WPA guidance on how to combat stigmatization of psychiatry and psychiatrists. *World Psychiatry*. 2010;9(3):131–144.
3. Fink PJ. You are the only sane psychiatrist I know. *JAMA*. 1984;251(5):611.
4. Lyons Z. Attitudes of medical students toward psychiatry and psychiatry as a career: A systematic review. *Acad Psychiatry*. 2013;37(3):150.
5. Schochow M, Steger F. Johann Christian Reil (1759–1813): Pioneer of psychiatry, city physician, and advocate of public medical care. *Am J Psychiatry*. 2014;171(4):403.
6. Marneros A. Psychiatry's 200th birthday. *Br J Psychiatry*. 2008;193(1):1–3.
7. Symonds B. The origins of insane asylums in England during the 19th century: A brief sociological review. *J Adv Nurs*. 1995;22(1):94–100.
8. McMillan I. Insight into Bedlam: One hospital's history. *J Psychosoc Nurs Ment Health Serv*. 1997;35(6):28–34.
9. Brigham A. The moral treatment of the insane, 1847. *Am J Psychiatry*. 1994;151(6 Suppl):10–15.
10. Earle P. *The Curability of Insanity: A Series of Studies*. Philadelphia: Lippincott; 1887.
11. Shapiro J. WWII pacifists exposed mental ward horrors. *All Things Considered*. December 2009. http://www.npr.org/templates/story/story.php?storyId=122017757. Accessed August 8, 2017.

12. Grob GN. *Mad Among Us: A History of the Care of America's Mentally Ill.* New York: Free Press; 2011.
13. Healy D. *The Antidepressant Era.* Cambridge, MA: Harvard University Press; 1997.
14. Mayes R, Horwitz A. Correction to "DSM-III and the revolution in the classification of mental illness." *J Hist Behav Sci.* 2007;43(4):419.
15. Kirk SA, Kutchins H. *The Selling of DSM: The Rhetoric of Science in Psychiatry.* New York: A. de Gruyter; 1992.
16. Shorter E. The history of nosology and the rise of the *Diagnostic and Statistical Manual of Mental Disorders. Dialogues Clin Neurosci.* 2015;17(1):59–67.
17. Tuke DH. *A Dictionary of Psychological Medicine.* Vol. 1. London: Churchill; 1892:229.
18. Goetz CG, Bonduelle M, Gelfand T. *Charcot: Constructing Neurology.* Oxford: Oxford University Press; 1995.
19. Widiger TA, Clark LA. Toward DSM-5 and the classification of psychopathology. *Psychol Bull.* 2000;126(6):946–963.
20. Greenberg G. *Book of Woe: The DSM and the Unmaking of Psychiatry.* New York: Plume, published by the Penguin Group; 2014.
21. Chodoff P. Psychiatric diagnosis: A 60-year perspective. *Psychiatric News.* 2005;40(11):17.
22. Bailey JM. Homosexuality and mental illness. *Arch Gen Psychiatry.* 1999;56(10):883.
23. Spitzer RL. The diagnostic status of homosexuality in DSM-III: A reformulation of the issues. *Am J Psychiatry.* 1981;138(2):210–215.
24. Clare A. *Psychiatry in Dissent: Controversial Issues in Thought and Practice.* London: Routledge; 2001.
25. Zachar P. Psychiatric disorders: Natural kinds made by the world or practical kinds made by us? *World Psychiatry.* 2015;14(3):288–290.
26. Rosenberg CE. Contested boundaries: Psychiatry, disease, and diagnosis. *Perspect Biol Med.* 2006;49:407–424.
27. Foucault M. *History of Madness.* London: Taylor and Francis; 2013.
28. Szasz TS. The myth of mental illness. *Am Psychol.* 1960;15(2):113–118.
29. Scheff TJ. The labelling theory of mental illness. *Am Sociol Rev.* 1974;39(3):444.
30. Scheff TJ. *Being Mentally Ill: A Sociological Theory.* New York: Aldine de Gruyter; 1999.
31. Mullan B. *Mad to Be Normal: Conversations with R.D. Laing.* London: Free Association Books; 1995.
32. Goffman E. *Asylums: Essays on the Social Situation of Mental Patients and Other Inmates.* New York: Anchor; 1961.
33. Rosenhan DL. On being sane in insane places. *Science.* 1973;179(4070):250–258.
34. Fleischman PR, Israel JV, Burr WA, et al. Psychiatric diagnosis. *Science.* 1973;180(4084):356–369.
35. Scull AT. *Madhouse: A Tragic Tale of Megalomania and Modern Medicine.* New Haven, CT: Yale University Press; 2005.
36. Metzl J. *The Protest Psychosis: How Schizophrenia Became a Black Disease.* Boston: Beacon; 2011.
37. Wolcott J. Still cuckoo after all these years. *Vanity Fair.* November 2011. https://www.vanityfair.com/news/2011/12/wolcott-201112. Accessed August 8, 2017.
38. Emmerich N. Appreciating the politics of psychiatry: Concerns over the DSM are part of a bigger issue concerning the power of the psychological and neurological sciences. *The Guardian.* https://www.theguardian.com/science/political-science/2013/

may/28/politics-psychiatry#comments. Published May 28, 2013. Accessed August 8, 2017.

39. Shorter E. *A History of Psychiatry: From the Era of the Asylum to the Age of Prozac*. New York: Wiley; 1998.

40. Cornwall J, Stoner L. Did the American Medical Association make the correct decision classifying obesity as a disease? *Australas Med J*. 2014;7(11):462–464.

41. Centers for Disease Control and Prevention. Products—Data Briefs—Number 288—October 2017. https://www.cdc.gov/nchs/products/databriefs/db288.htm. Accessed April 2, 2017.

42. Menninger K. *The Vital Balance*. New York: Viking Press; 1963.

43. Wilson M. DSM-III and the transformation of American psychiatry: A history. *Am J Psychiatry*. 1993;150(3):399–410.

44. Butryn T, Bryant L, Marchionni C, Sholevar F. The shortage of psychiatrists and other mental health providers: Causes, current state, and potential solutions. *Int J Acad Med*. 2017;3(1):5–9.

45. Lunbeck E. *The Psychiatric Persuasion: Knowledge, Gender, and Power in Modern America*. Princeton, NJ: Princeton University Press; 1994.

46. Jutel AG. *Putting a Name to It*. Baltimore, MD: Johns Hopkins University Press; 2015.

47. Shackle EM. Psychiatric diagnosis as an ethical problem. *J Med Ethics*. 1985; 11(3):132–134.

48. Moncrieff J. The creation of the concept of an antidepressant: An historical analysis. *Soc Sci Med*. 2008;66(11):2346–2355.

49. Healy D. *Mania: A Short History of Bipolar Disorder*. Baltimore, MD: JHU Press; 2008.

50. Weissman MM. Book review: *The Antidepressant Era* by David Healy. *N Engl J Med*. 1998;338(20):1475–1476.

51. Akiskal H. Special issue on circular insanity and beyond: Historic contributions of French psychiatry to contemporary concepts and research on bipolar disorder. *J Affect Disord*. 2006;96(3):141–143.

52. Schwartz A. Thousands of toddlers are medicated for A.D.H.D., report finds, raising worries. *New York Times*, May 14, 2014. http://www.nytimes.com/2014/05/17/us/among-experts-scrutiny-of-attention-disorder-diagnoses-in-2-and-3-year-olds.html

53. Insel T. Director's blog: Are children overmedicated? National Institute of Mental Health. 2014;6.

54. Brill S. America's most admired lawbreaker. Huffington Post. 2015. http://highline.huffingtonpost.com/miracleindustry/americas-most-admired-lawbreaker.

55. Wright J. The real reasons autism rates are up in the U.S. *Scientific American*. https://www.scientificamerican.com/article/the-real-reasons-autism-rates-are-up-in-the-u-s/. Accessed August 31, 2017.

56. Devilbiss EA, Lee BK. Brief report: Trends in U.S. national autism awareness from 2004 to 2014: The impact of National Autism Awareness Month. *J Autism Dev Disord*. 2014;44(12):3271–3273.

57. Autism and Developmental Disabilities Monitoring Network Surveillance Year 2008, Principal Investigators and Centers for Disease Control and Prevention. *MMWR Surveill Summ*. 2012;61(3):1–19.

58. Watters E. The Americanization of mental illness. *New York Times*. January 10, 2010. http://www.nytimes.com/2010/01/10/magazine/10psyche-t.html. Accessed August 8, 2017.

7

Minority Stress Theory and Internalized Prejudice

Links to Clinical Psychiatric Practice

CHRISTINE CRAWFORD, LISA SANGERMANO, AND NHI-HA T. TRINH ■

CASE

Mr. C is a 21-year-old African American male student who attends a predominantly white university, where he is member of the school's football team. Throughout Mr. C's childhood, he had high hopes of becoming a professional football player. He was told by his teachers, coaches, and family members that excelling in athletics was his best chance of achieving success. During high school, Mr. C did not perform well academically since he believed that colleges would be interested in his athletic abilities rather than his academic achievements. While in high school, he would often make fun of the African American students who were more studious, telling them that it was a waste of time for them to be so preoccupied with school.

Over the past couple of years, he has become increasingly worried that he is prone to criminality given reports in the media regarding increased homicide rates in predominantly African American communities. As result, he avoids spending time with his family and African American childhood friends out of concern that they would try to hinder his success. Also, whenever Mr. C enters certain stores in the mall, he is under the impression the store workers are monitoring his activity because he is African American, and he does not blame them for doing so. Upon entering college, Mr. C made attempts to avoid the small contingent of African American students on campus, noting that he did not want to be associated with a "gang of thugs."

Mr. C sustained an injury during his second football game in college that resulted in a torn ACL and ultimately placed him on the bench for the rest of the season. His sleep, appetite, and concentration in classes started to deteriorate, and he was unable to get out of bed or tend to his daily routine. He became more irritable and told his peers and family that he was worthless and would never amount to anything in life. He refused to attend any subsequent football games and ultimately dropped out of college the following semester, believing that he did not have the intelligence and discipline to successfully complete college.

INTRODUCTION

Minority groups in this country continuously endure stress placed upon them by the dominant culture. Ethnic and sexual minorities in this country are persistently stigmatized and marginalized by society, consequently being forced to carry the significant burden of the resulting chronic stress of oppression. The ongoing stresses of racism, prejudice, and discrimination have lasting deleterious effects on minorities' physical and emotional well-being. Unfortunately, over time minorities begin to internalize these same prejudices, reinforced by the dominant culture, resulting in reduced self-esteem, demoralization, and hopelessness. Because it can be difficult for many of our patients to articulate the emotional distress that they experience secondary to internalized prejudice, mental health clinicians have an obligation to understand the significant impact that minority stress and internalized racism have on our patients' mental health.

In this chapter, we will first provide an overview of the concept of minority stress theory and describe the various sociological and psychological constructs contributing to its development. We will then examine the various elements of internalized prejudice in ethnic and sexual minorities, and review validated measurement scales used to quantify how internalized prejudice affects minority populations. Additionally, we will review evidence on the role of internalized prejudice in a number of psychiatric conditions, as well as discuss the concept of intersectionality and its implications for mental health. At the end of this chapter, we will provide clinical recommendations on how to address the role of minority stress and internalized prejudice on mental health. A discussion of a relevant clinical case will bring together the complexities of minority stress theory and internalized prejudice contributing to psychiatric illness.

CONCEPTUALIZATION OF MINORITY STRESS THEORY

As mental health clinicians, we are often accustomed to hearing our patients use the term "stress" when referring to their daily struggles. Rather than taking an uncritical approach to interpreting stress, clinicians should explore the various unique factors that may contribute to the stress perceived and experienced by individual patients. It is important for clinicians to delve into what stress means to each patient. In this section, we will discuss theoretical models of stress informing the construct of minority stress theory.

Lazarus and Folkman introduced the Standard Stress Model, demonstrating how stressful events have different outcomes for different individuals.[1] They argue that the effects of stressful events are moderated by our personal interpretation of these events.[1] According to their model, after individuals experience a stressful event, they appraise the event as either positive, negative, or neutral. They then assess their coping strategies and available resources to deal with the event. Depending on the cognitive appraisal of both the event itself and potential response strategies, outcomes will manifest differently. Negative outcomes may result in a vicious cycle;

increased stress can lead to poor health, which in turn reduces coping ability and leads to even greater vulnerability to stress.[1] Lazarus and Folkman emphasize the connection between the social environment, stress, and health. They also describe the conflict experienced by minority individuals and the societal norms that are enacted by the dominant culture as the etiology for social stress.[1] Other theorists have noted that individuals from a stigmatized minority group carry an additional burden of "minority stress," caused by disharmony with the surrounding social environment constructed by the dominant culture.[2-4]

Although this model does not allow for specific cultural considerations, it can be adapted to incorporate the effect of cultural context on cognitive appraisal of stress. Slavin built on Lazarus and Folkman's theory by adapting it into the Multicultural Stress Model.[5] Slavin posits that the experience and interpretation of stressful events is affected by cultural contexts. Specifically, Slavin argues that belonging to a marginalized group inherently increases the likelihood of experiencing stressful events. Furthermore, the individual's minority status affects how he or she interprets these events as well as his or her ability to respond to them.[5] For example, people of color experiencing discrimination may feel they lack the structural support to overcome this form of oppression. Slavin also points out that cultural context can affect overall health outcomes after stressful events, due to factors such as access to care, cultural medical practices, and previous positive or negative experiences with the health care system.[5] Taking culture into consideration provides a more nuanced assessment of how individuals handle stress. This is especially important considering the vulnerability of minority populations to increased stress.

Slavin argues that members of minority groups experience more stressful events due to their marginalized status, and Meyer[6] outlines the specific challenges faced by these individuals. According to Meyer, minority group status leads to chronic stress due to stigma placed upon the group as well as the imposition of differing values and experiences from that of the majority.[6] Deviation from these norms leads to a negative reaction from the majority group and increased risk of experiencing prejudice, which in turn leads to stress and negative outcomes such as internalization of prejudice and increase in perceived stigma.[6] The topic of internalized prejudice will be explored later in the chapter.

Meyer argues that minority stress results from a number of processes experienced by the individual with a minority status, which then lead to negative mental health outcomes.[6] He describes the relevance of the circumstances inherent to a minority individual's environment. Socioeconomic factors such as poverty provide an example of such environmental circumstances that reflect certain elements of privilege and disadvantage pertinent specifically to minorities.[6] Although poverty can be attributed to a number of factors, implications of exposure to this known stressor are onerous given the vulnerable status of minorities. Minorities can also be exposed to general stressors such as a death in the family, applicable to both minority and nonminority groups.

Meyer elaborates on specific minority stress processes described as distal and proximal stressors. He proposes that distal stressors are objective sources of stress targeted toward minority groups, such as discrimination and violence. Proximal stressors are secondary to minority status itself, reflecting a subjective process of the individual's internalization of stigma and appraisal of self as belonging to a "devalued minority."[6,7] Meyer asserts that potential consequences of proximal stressors include "expectations of rejection, concealment, and internalized [prej-udice]."[6] In his minority stress theory, Meyer also acknowledges the potential for various coping strategies and social supports to potentially mitigate the negative consequences of stress.[6] Meyer posits that all of these stressors, including environ-mental circumstances, general stressors, and proximal and distal minority stressors, can impact mental health outcomes. Therefore, his theory suggests that negative mental health outcomes are secondary to an excess burden of societally determined stressors through both external and internal pathways.[6]

INTERNALIZED PREJUDICE

Minority stress theory provides a framework for understanding the clinical implications for how a patient's minority status could potentially contribute to nega-tive mental health outcomes. One element highlighted in this theory is internalized prejudice, classified as a proximal stressor. As mental health clinicians, our role is to gain a better appreciation of how our patients view themselves; thus, we must de-velop a better understanding of internalized prejudice.

Definitions

There is a long-documented history of racism, discrimination, prejudice, and stereotyping directed toward minority populations. Given the pervasiveness and enduring consequences of the stress associated with a minority status, before we move forward, it is important to provide context and define terms used throughout this chapter. According to Williams and Neighbors, "Racism refers to an organized system, based on an ideology of inferiority, that disadvantages groups designated to be inferior compared to those presumed to be superior."[8] Bonilla-Silva note that the idealist view of racism is that it is "a set of ideas or beliefs, which result in having neg-ative *ideas* about a particular race."[9] This conceptualization of how racism manifests in society considers how the negative beliefs regarding a particular race "have the po-tential to lead individuals to develop prejudice which is defined as 'negative *attitudes* towards an entire group of people."[9]

Furthermore, discrimination within this framework is defined as "negative *actions* against members of a race," and it is the behavioral manifestation of preju-dice.[8-10] According to Fredrickson, there have been variable definitions of racism, as its manifestation has changed over the course of modern society.[11] He describes moments in history in which the expression of racism predominated within the American South; for example, when Jim Crow laws were enacted to ensure that African Americans remained in a lower social class as a result of racial segregation and discrimination. Despite a longstanding tradition of practices that would now be described as racist throughout history, Fredrickson notes that the term "racism" was coined during the 1930s when Nazis in Germany were persecuting Jews and exerting dominance and power over this particular group.[11] Fredrickson defines racism as not only a set of negative attitudes or beliefs toward another race, but as encompassing two components: difference and power. He goes on to state that "racism exists when one ethnic group or historical collectivity dominates, excludes,

or seeks to eliminate another on the basis of differences that it believes are heredi-
table and unalterable."[11]

Stereotype, as defined by Carter, is the "racial ideology of out-group inferior
status." According to social psychologists, stereotypes "are generalizations about
social groups—characteristics that are attributed to all members of a given group,
without regard to variations that must exist among members of that group."[12-15]

Dominant cultures have long used racism as a form of oppression to disempower
minority groups, which reinforces their inferior status.[16,17] Continuous exposure to
negative societal images, attitudes, beliefs, and stereotypes about minority groups
can have dire psychological consequences on oppressed minority groups; over time
an individual is at increased risk of internalizing racial oppression. Bailey has defined
internalized racial oppression as "the process by which minority groups internalize
and accept the dominant culture's oppressive actions and beliefs toward minority
groups while at the same time rejecting their own worldview and cultural motifs."[15]
Williams and Williams-Morris note that internalized racism refers to acceptance of
the negative stereotypes placed on a minority population by the dominant culture.[18]
The internalization of these negative stereotypes can result in self-hatred, as well as
hatred toward one's own racial group, further perpetuated by the minority group's
inferior status within society.[19] Cokley identified two negative consequences of this
process of internalizing negative stereotypes, noting that acceptance of these beliefs
reinforces the marginalized group's inferiority to the dominant culture, and that
furthermore the minority group may in turn start to exhibit negative attitudes and
behaviors toward members within their own group.[19]

Internalized racism differs from other forms of racism, such as structural racism
and personally mediated racism, in that it ultimately results in an erosion of an
individual's sense of value and self-worth. Public health researcher Jones goes on
to state that members of stigmatized groups experiencing internalized racism lack
a belief in themselves as well as members of their own cultural group.[20] Researchers
have postulated that internalized racism can occur in the absence of awareness
from the individual belonging to the stigmatized group.[15,21] The extent of individual
experiences of internalized racism may occur on a spectrum and can reflect an
individual's exposure to discrimination, prejudice, and racism. The varying degrees
of internalized racial oppression demonstrate the significant range of erosion of self-
esteem and self-worth.[16,22]

Bailey expands upon the concept of the internalization of negative stereotypes by
identifying multiple dimensions of racial oppression (Fig. 7.1), with a particular focus
on African Americans, including the "self-destructive behaviors, devaluation of the
African worldview and motifs, belief in the biased representation of history, and alteration of physical appearance."[23] This conceptualization of racial oppression provides a
framework for understanding the mental health consequences of an individual's internalization of negative feelings about himself or herself and his or her race.

Internalized Homophobia and Transphobia

The internalization of negative stereotypes can also be seen in sexual minorities
in the form of internalized homophobia, defined by Meyer as the internalization
of anti-homosexual attitudes and beliefs.[6] Negative views of sexual minorities can

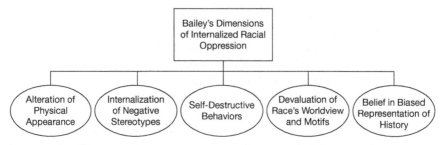

Figure 7.1 Bailey's Dimensions of Internalized Racial Oppression
Adapted from Bailey TKM. Construct Validation of the Internalized Racial
Oppression Scale. Doctoral dissertation. Available from ScholarWorks @ Georgia State
University, 2008.

result in prejudice and ultimately discrimination toward this population, which is perpetuated by society through various institutions such as the media, the workforce, and the legal system. Individuals could develop negative views about themselves with the perception that homosexuality is consistent with deviant and abnormal behavior, resulting in a sense of self-hatred, shame, guilt, and worthlessness. Researchers have noted that this perception of internalizing a deviant identity could be damaging to the psychological well-being of a sexual minority.[24-26]

Meyer noted that inherent to minority stress are three elements: "internalized homophobia, expectations of rejection and discrimination (perceived stigma), and prejudice events."[6] In addition to internalized homophobia, the chronic stress of perceived stigma, assuming that an individual would be treated in a discriminatory manner, could exacerbate and contribute to psychological distress. Meyer performed a survey of 741 gay men in New York City and found that internalized homophobia is strongly associated with various measures of distress, including demoralization, guilt, and suicidality.[6] Results of his study also suggested that gay men with internalized homophobia are more likely to experience increased psychological distress when faced with discrimination, since with the acceptance of negative beliefs toward their sexuality, they also may harbor an element of self-blame regarding discrimination.[6]

Hendricks adapted the Minority Stress Model to incorporate the role of internalized transphobia. The word "transphobia" is used to signify negative attitudes, beliefs, and stereotypes imposed by society on transgender individuals. Using the language of the Minority Stress Model, Hendricks describes transphobia as a proximal stressor with "direct negative effects on the individual's ability to cope with external stressful events" that "ultimately reduces the individual's resilience in the face of negative events."[27] He also discusses the distal stressors experienced by transgender individuals, including victimization, violence, discrimination, and rejection from others, noting that it can result in a negative appraisal of the self. As a result of this negative appraisal, transgender individuals view themselves with a negative lens, resulting in lowered self-esteem and self-worth.[27]

Validated Scales to Measure Internalized Prejudice

A number of measurement scales have been developed and validated over the years to help quantify the degree to which internalized prejudice affects minority populations. These instruments have been used in various studies examining the link between internalized prejudice and a range of psychiatric conditions.

MEASUREMENT SCALES FOR INTERNALIZED RACISM AMONG AFRICAN AMERICANS

The most widely used scale to measure internalized racism specifically within the African American population is the Nadanolitization Scale (NAD) developed by Taylor, Wilson, and Dobbins.[28] The NAD is a 24-item self-report questionnaire measuring the degree to which African American individuals internalize negative stereotypes of their race through the perception of whites, "based on assumptions of biological inferiority and inaccurate perceptions of whites," such as being "mentally defective" or "physically gifted" as compared to whites.[28] Examples of items in the NAD include: "Blacks are born with greater sexual lust than Whites," and "Blacks are just not as smart as Whites."[28] Each item in the NAD is rated on a 0-to-8 scale; studies have demonstrated that higher NAD scores are associated with an increase in depressive symptoms, problematic alcohol use, lower self-esteem, and psychological distress.[29,30]

The Internalized Racial Oppression Scale (IROS) is a self-report instrument developed by Bailey that is "intended to measure the degree to which racial oppression is internalized and replicated by Black individuals in the United States (U.S)."[15] The IROS is based on Bailey's conceptualization of racial oppression, expanding upon internalization of negative stereotypes, while also identifying five domains that he posits better encapsulate the complexity of the negative components of African American racial identity: internalization of negative stereotypes, self-destructive behaviors, devaluation of the African worldview and motifs, belief in the biased representation of history, and alteration of physical appearance.[15] Bailey developed and validated the IROS in studies involving African American college students attending a combination of historically Black universities and predominately white institutions in the southeastern U.S. Bailey used the Racial Identity Attitudes Scale (RIAS-B) developed by Helms and Parham, as well as the African Self-Consciousness Scale developed by Baldwin and Bell, to validate the criteria used in the IROS.[31,32] Bailey identified four factors demonstrating good reliability (internalization of negative stereotypes, devaluation of the African worldview and motifs, belief in the biased representation of history, and alteration of physical appearance [e.g., changing hair]) while excluding the factor of self-destructive behaviors. This led Bailey to conclude that these four factors represent the dimensions of internalized racism. As a result of the study, the IROS was reduced from a 58-item to a 36-item questionnaire; each dimension of internalized racial oppression is divided into subscales.[15] A criticism of the IROS is that the scale focuses on attitudes and beliefs, but neglects to measure the emotional response of the individual.[33]

MEASUREMENT SCALES FOR INTERNALIZED RACISM AMONG LATINOS

Hipolito-Delgado examined internalized racism within the Latino community by modifying the NAD to reflect negative stereotypes about Chicanos and Latinos.[33,34] Hipolito-Delgado reviewed the original 49 items of the NAD to assess which items could be generalized to reflect stereotypes specific to the Latino and Chicano culture, replacing items specific to African Americans with those representative of the Latino and Chicano experience. This modified scale was reviewed by a panel of experts in

Chicano and Latino culture to provide face validity. This scale, called the Mochihua Tepehuani Scale after the Aztec phrase "to become conqueror," conveys that "the internalization of racism in Chicanas/os and Latinas/os is acceptance of European or the conqueror's beliefs."[34] Administered to 258 students to assess internal validity, the scale was eventually reduced to 25 items using a seven-point Likert scale, determining the degree to which the individual agrees with the stereotype listed in each item. The scale has four subscales: racism, a "Latin lover" stereotype, "La Familia" stereotype, and abilities and characteristics stereotypes (e.g., "Whites are superior to Chicanos and Latinos"; "Chicanos have more children than Whites"; "The school dropout problem among Latinos is due to their not having the mental power of Whites"; and "Chicanos and Latinos are mentally unable to contribute toward the progress of the US").[34]

MEASUREMENT SCALES FOR INTERNALIZED RACISM AMONG ASIAN AMERICANS

David and Okazaki developed the Colonial Mentality Scale (CMS) for Filipino Americans (the Philippines was a U.S. colony until 1946, with U.S. presence in military bases until 1992).[33,35] The CMS examines various dimensions of colonial mentality conceptualized as a form of appropriated racial suppression. The CMS was validated in a study with 603 Filipino Americans and includes 36 items examining five factors: within-group discrimination (tendency to discriminate against less-Americanized Filipinos); physical characteristics (tendency to perceive Filipino physical traits as inferior to white physical traits); colonial debt (tendency to feel fortunate at having been colonized and feel indebted toward their colonizers); cultural shame and embarrassment (feelings of shame and embarrassment toward Filipino culture); and internalized cultural/ethnic inferiority (feelings of inferiority toward their ethnicity and culture).[33,35] Studies have found that Filipinos with higher levels of colonial mentality are more likely to have higher levels of internalized racism, which the authors describe as internalized oppression that leads to decreased self-esteem.[35,36]

Choi and colleagues expanded upon David and Okazaki's work on Filipinos by developing the Internalized Racism in Asian Americans Scale (IRAAS) to measure the degree to which a heterogeneous Asian American population experiences internalized racism. The scale was administered to 655 Asian Americans ages 18 to 64 years old from multiple ethnic backgrounds (primarily Chinese, Filipino, Korean, Japanese, Vietnamese, and Indian). The questionnaire comprises 14 items mapping to three factors: self-negativity, weakness stereotypes, and appearance bias.[36]

MEASUREMENT SCALES FOR SEXUAL MINORITIES

There is a growing body of literature regarding scales developed to measure internalized homophobia within sexual minority populations. Grey and colleagues performed a comprehensive literature review of instruments measuring attitudes toward homosexual men.[37] Grey identified six validated scales measuring internalized homophobia: Nungesser Homosexual Attitudes Inventory, Internalized Homophobia Scale, Reactions to Homosexuality Scale, Internalized Homophobia Scale, Internalized Homonegativity Inventory, and Short Internalized Homonegativity Scale.[38-43] Herek's Internalized Homophobia Scale is a nine-item questionnaire based on a five-point Likert scale that assessing an individual agreement with a particular item.[41] This scale is applicable to both lesbians and gay men and was administered to 75 women and 75 men recruited at a lesbian, gay, bisexual, trans, and queer/ questioning (LGBTQ) event. Herek found gay men had higher internalized homophobia scores and reported lower self-esteem than lesbians. The authors commented that this discrepancy could be attributed to society having more negative attitudes toward gay men than lesbians, leading gay men to internalize more negative attitudes toward themselves.[41] Szymanski developed the Lesbian Internalized Homophobia scale, which includes 52 items such as "I hate myself for being attracted to other women" and "I feel bad for acting on my lesbian desires."[44] It comprises five subscales: connection with the lesbian community, public identification as a lesbian, personal feelings about being a lesbian, moral and religious attitudes toward lesbianism, and attitudes toward other lesbians.[44]

There is currently a dearth of research related to the development and use of measurement scales quantifying internalized transphobia. However, a number of researchers have incorporated several scales into their measurement of both external and internal stressors experienced by transgender individuals. The Gender Minority and Resilience Measure (GMSR) measures internalized transphobia, examining both external and internal stressors and assessing for an individual's negative expectations of future events.[45] The internalized transphobia scale included in the GMSR features seven items, including questions such as, "I feel that my gender identity or expression is embarrassing."[45] In a study with 816 transgender individuals who completed the Trans Health Survey, the internalized transphobia scale in the GMSR was positively associated with thwarted belongingness and perceived burdensomeness indirectly leading to an association with suicidal ideation.[45]

This section has defined internalized prejudice and reviewed validated measurement scales used in research studies to quantify this concept in a range of minority groups. As mental health clinicians, our primary role is to understand the clinical implications of internalized prejudice on our patients; the following section will discuss research supporting the known physical and mental health effects of internalized prejudice.

INTERNALIZED PREJUDICE AND EFFECTS ON MENTAL HEALTH

As described in the previous section, a number of studies have incorporated measurement tools to assess the degree of internalized prejudice experienced by minority individuals. Numerous studies have found internalized prejudice to be associated with negative physical health outcomes.[46–48] Given that internalized prejudice is a known stressor, a number of physical conditions typically exacerbated by stress would also be affected by internalized prejudice. The majority of research examining effects of internalized prejudice on physical health has focused on African Americans, a reflection of the longstanding history of oppression on this group in the U.S. Evidence suggests that the internalization of inferiority stigma has been associated with elevated blood pressure.[49] Obesity, increased waist circumference, and higher blood glucose levels have been found to be more common in African Americans reporting higher levels of internalized prejudice.[50–53] Research has also supported changes in various neuroendocrine processes as a result of stress associated with internalized prejudice. Adam and colleagues followed 112 people for 20 years starting around age 12 to understand the association between perceived racial discrimination and diurnal cortisol levels in adulthood. They found that compared to whites, African Americans demonstrated a stress-related change in their diurnal cortisol rhythm during the day, a finding that is associated with obesity, cardiovascular disease, various pain syndromes, and impaired immunity response.[54]

Psychological Factors and Internalized Prejudice

In addition to compromised physical health secondary to internalized prejudice, there is a tremendous burden on minority psychological well-being. Researchers[55-61] have identified several pathways by which racism may contribute to compromised health, including

> reduced access to employment, housing, and education, and/or increased exposure to risk factors (e.g., avoidable contact with police); adverse cognitive/emotional processes and associated psychopathology; allostatic load and concomitant pathophysiological processes; diminished participation in healthy behaviors (e.g., sleep and exercise) and/or increased engagement in unhealthy behaviors (e.g., alcohol consumption) either directly as stress coping, or indirectly, via reduced self-regulation; and physical injury as a result of racially motivated violence[59]

Multiple ethnic minorities experience what has been described as "everyday discrimination" or "interpersonally mediated racism," which is pervasive, persistent, and "cognitively burdensome and psychologically taxing."[55,62] The detrimental effects of internalized prejudice on minority individuals include a diminished sense of self and self-esteem.[12,63,64] Endorsement of negative stereotypes of both oneself and one's minority group as a whole can lead to lower self-esteem and impaired psychological well-being, potentially increasing the likelihood of poor mental health outcomes.[65,66] The psychosocial stress of interpersonally mediated racism has been associated with demoralization and an increased risk for depression.[3,20,62] These psychosocial stressors are compounded by physical impairments along with demoralization and low self-esteem, potentially placing minorities at an elevated risk of mental health conditions. The following section will delineate various mental health conditions associated with internalized prejudice within specific minority groups.

African American Mental Health and the Role of Internalized Racism

Studies have examined the effects of various moderators of racism and their link to mental health, finding that ethnicity significantly moderates internalized racism's negative impact on mental health.[55] Mouzon used secondary data from the 2001–2003 National Survey of American Life to examine the effects of internalized racism on mental health and serious psychological distress among African Americans and Afro-Caribbeans. Internalized racism was measured using a six-item Stereotypes

Scale, including questions featuring six different adjectives (intelligent, lazy, hardworking, give up easily, are proud of themselves, and are violent); response options measured the degree to which the respondent agreed with the statement. Serious psychological distress was also measured in a six-item scale focusing on non-specific psychological distress, which included symptoms of depression and anxiety within the past 30 days."[67-69]

DEPRESSION

Researchers reviewed the results from a survey of 3,570 African American adults and 1,418 Afro-Caribbean adults called the National Survey of American Life, which was administered to U.S. households of African Americans, Afro-Caribbeans, and non-Hispanic white adults. Diminished self-esteem through internalized racism was found to mediate the rates of major depressive disorder (MDD) within the past year.[62] The African Americans who reported higher levels of internalized racism also reported increased levels of interpersonally mediated racism, all of which were found to be associated with an increased risk of MDD.[62]

Although there is a breadth of literature examining the role of racism in physical health outcomes, there are limited reports in the literature investigating the association between internalized racism and mental health. The internalization of negative stereotypes is psychologically damaging and results in negative mental health outcomes for African Americans.[17] Early studies by Taylor, who developed the NAD, found that higher levels of internalized racism are associated with increased risk for alcohol consumption and lower levels of marital satisfaction.[70,71] Taylor and colleagues expanded upon this research; in a study of 289 African American women, Taylor found an association between internalized racism (as measured by higher NAD scores) and depressive symptoms.[72]

Internalized racism is associated with both an increased severity of depressive symptoms and serious psychological distress. U.S.-born African Americans and U.S.-born Afro-Caribbeans were found to have higher levels of internalized racism compared to foreign-born Afro-Caribbeans. U.S.-born African Americans and U.S.-born Afro-Caribbeans had worse overall mental health, as measured by the number of depressive symptoms and the degree of psychological distress.[69] The internal group variation suggests that American society has more negative stereotypes of Africans, presumably increasing the likelihood that U.S.-born African Americans would internalize the negative representation of their race. This is in contrast to foreign-born Blacks, who originate from predominantly Black countries: They are less likely to be inundated by negative images of their race propagated by society, thus resulting in a lower degree of internalized racism. This lower degree of internalized racism becomes a protective effect for foreign-born Black individuals who subsequently move to the U.S.[69,73]

ANXIETY

African Americans' ongoing exposure to racist experiences, discrimination, and negative stereotypes supported by the dominant culture in the U.S. can contribute to a heightened state of arousal and anxiety. Studies have indicated that racial discrimination predicts generalized anxiety disorder among African Americans; meanwhile, a similar relationship has not been found among non-Hispanic whites or Afro-Caribbeans. In a 2016 survey of 173 African American adults recruited from an urban university using a questionnaire assessing anxiety symptoms, internalized racism, and exposure to racist experiences within the past year, Graham found a correlation between anxiety symptoms and frequency of past-year racist experiences; internalized racism as measured by the Cross Racial Identity Scale mediated this relationship.[74,75]

Latino Mental Health and the Role of Internalized Racism

In addition to African Americans, Latinos have also endured racism and subsequent negative mental health effects. Fortes de Leff noted that the conquest and subsequent colonization of the Aztec Empire and other indigenous cultures by Spaniards introduced the concept of domination by whites, and ultimately racism and discrimination, into the Latino population. The presence of the Spaniards in Mexico and their crusade to "civilize" the indigenous people by imposing their religious and cultural values resulted in a stratified class system, placing the "Indios" (indigenous people) in an inferior position to that of the Spaniards and their descendants, who were phenotypically different, with blue eyes and blond hair. Fortes de Leff notes that during that time in Mexico, those who were in power were typically light-skinned and came from a higher class than those who were darker and deemed as inferior and thus deserving of fewer privileges.[76]

Discrimination experienced by the Indios in Mexico during the time of the Aztec Empire persists in current Mexican culture. Finch examined the association between perceived discrimination and depression in a study of 3,012 adults of Mexican origin in Fresno County, California. Perceived discrimination was measured using a three-item questionnaire: "How often do people dislike you because you are Mexican?"; "How often do people treat you unfairly because you are Mexican?"; and "How often have you seen friends treated unfairly because they are Mexican?"[77] Depression symptomatology was measured by the CES-D scale, a 20-item questionnaire assessing neurovegetative symptoms of depression one week prior to the interview. Finch found that those who were born in Mexico had higher levels of perceived discrimination and higher levels of depressive symptoms.[77] The discrepancy in the levels of perceived discrimination and degree of depressive symptoms could reflect the undue burden of immigrant status, as well as the struggle with the untenable tension of maintaining their cultural identity while also embracing the new American culture.

The degree of acculturation to American culture, of which racism has been proposed to be an essential component, and exposure to interpersonal racism and discrimination are directly related to the degree of internalization of racism by Latinos.[70,71,78–80] In a study of 500 undergraduate Latinos, both U.S.- and foreign-born, who attended public, private, and community colleges throughout the U.S., the Mochihua Tepehuani Scale was used to measure internalized racism, and the Abbreviated Multidimensional Acculturation Scale was used to assess the degree of acculturation. Latinos who reported higher levels of U.S. cultural identity were more likely to have higher levels of internalized racism.[80] The results suggest that because acculturation is directly associated with internalized racism, "promoting assimilation in higher education also promotes ethnic self-hatred," potentially "damag[ing] the inner well-being of Latino students" and leading to subsequent "negative implications for the psychological well-being of Latinos."[80] Given this association between acculturation and internalized racism, adopting U.S. culture could be a potential stressor and burden for minorities of immigrant backgrounds. Hovey investigated the association between acculturative stress, depressive symptoms, and suicidal ideation among 70 immigrant and second-generation Latino-American high school students in California and found that one-fourth of the adolescents reported depressive symptoms and suicidal ideation; symptoms were positively correlated with the degree of acculturative stress.[81] Acculturation for immigrants has the potential to highlight the sense of "otherness," resulting in a vilification of their native culture; over time, these feelings may evolve into internalized hate and depression.

Asian American Mental Health and the Role of Internalized Racism

There is also evidence that internalized racism has negative implications for mental health for the Asian American population. The historical context of Asian Americans is important to note when discussing racism and discrimination. The influx of Asian immigrants to the U.S., particularly around 1965 following favorable changes in immigration laws, resulted in a spike in the number of Asian immigrants from China, Japan, and other Asian and Pacific countries. Tensions heightened in the workplace, since the majority of these immigrants competed with white workers for low-wage jobs. A number of whites became angry at the influx of Asian immigrants, whom they viewed as threatening their sense of job security, fueling racially motivated contentious relationship between the two groups.[82] Asian immigrants were ultimately "racialized as others and excluded from the white mainstream," subsequently placing them in the position of ongoing oppression and discrimination.[83-87]

Over time, the perception of Asian Americans has changed in American society, so much so that they have more recently been labeled as the "model minority"— a stereotype constructed by the dominant white culture and imposed upon this minority group, further crystallizing their sense of otherness.[82] The "model minority" is defined as a minority group that aspires to achieve the "American dream" while possessing a hard work ethic and being academically successful, law-abiding, and financially secure.[82] Ogbu distinguishes between voluntary and involuntary minority groups in discussing the "model minority" concept.[88] Minorities who voluntarily immigrated to the U.S. have done so in search of a better life, in contrast to the experiences of African Americans, Mexicans, and other ethnic groups that were brought involuntarily to the U.S. through slavery or conquest. According to Ogbu, voluntary minorities ascribe to the concept of social mobility and have a sense of optimism and hope regarding their future prospects. This sense of optimism and pursuit of the American dream is evident in the use of education as a vehicle for attaining upward social mobility.[89] Researchers have found the stereotype of the highly academic-achieving model minority is perpetuated through the U.S. college educational system as well as mass media, reinforcing this stereotype.[90] Asian Americans are inundated by stereotypical images of themselves as a uniformly high-achieving group, which they potentially internalize, resulting in significant pressures to conform to this perception. Studies of Asian American college students examining academic achievement secondary to the model minority stereotype have found that the stereotype has a negative impact on their psychological well-being, including increased anxiety and depression.[91-96]

Given the dearth of scholarly research on the concept of internalized racism among Asian Americans, Szymanski examined this group's attitudes toward their own ethnicity as a way of measuring internalized racism. He postulated that Asian Americans place "a greater importance on ethnicity than race because of current living contexts and their unique socio-cultural histories."[98] Asian Americans who demonstrate negative attitudes toward their own ethnicity are more likely to have poor psychological well-being, as evidenced by reports of depression and low self-esteem.[99,100] Studies have found that Filipinos with higher levels of colonial mentality are more likely to have higher levels of internalized racism, which the authors described as internalized oppression that leads to decreased self-esteem.[35,36]

Gender and Sexual Minority Mental Health and the Role of Internalized Homophobia

The experience of internalized homophobia among sexual minorities results in negative attitudes toward themselves as differing from the heteronormative dominant culture; this internalized homophobia has the potential to result in inner conflicts and subsequent low self-esteem.[101,102] Meyer found that internalized homophobia among sexual minorities predicted negative mental health outcomes and psychological distress, including demoralization, guilt, and suicidal ideation.[6] Hammelman found that those who discovered their sexual identity in early adolescence were more likely to engage in suicidal behavior and have higher rates of substance use disorder; the latter was seen as a coping mechanism for their sexual minority status.[103] Hammelman's research suggests that identifying as a sexual minority in early adolescence, when one is likely to have negative experiences disclosing one's sexual orientation in a strongly heteronormative environment, may further contribute to isolation and increased internalized homophobia.[104] Research has also found an association between higher levels of internalized homophobia and eating disorders, primarily bulimia nervosa.[104]

Many studies have also shown that internalized homophobia has a direct association with depressive symptomatology. Sexual minorities who have negative attitudes toward themselves and other sexual minorities are more likely to have higher rates of depression and anxiety. Igartua administered the Nungesser Homosexual Attitudes Inventory to 220 adults as well as a self-report questionnaire of psychiatric symptoms and found that possessing negative attitudes toward one's own sexual orientation predicted depression and anxiety symptoms. Igartua also identified a relationship between internalized homophobia and suicide and noted that an individual is at increased risk for suicidality during the period immediately after disclosure of sexuality identity to family and friends.[105] McLaren found that higher levels of internalized homophobia are directly related to higher levels of suicidal ideation and depressive symptoms.[106]

Mental Health of Transgender Individuals and Impact of Internalized Prejudice

Transgender individuals are also at risk for developing psychiatric symptoms secondary to the effects of minority stress related to their nonconforming gender identity. Cisgenderism is defined as "assuming that the gender assigned at birth based on ascribed sex should be the gender with which they identify."[107] Transgender individuals could internalize cisgenderism along with the negative attitudes and stereotypes associated with nonconforming gender identities, resulting in a diminished sense of worth and self-esteem.[30,107] Studies have found that transgender older adults have an increased risk of developing depressive symptoms compared to individuals who identify as gay or lesbian.[108] Hoy-Ellis examined the role of minority stress among older transgender adults and noted that 48% experienced significant depressive symptomatology that could be attributed to the stress of being a minority.[107] Internalized cisgenderism has been found to have a significant indirect effect on depressive symptoms, suggestive of the additive effects of both perceived general stress and minority stress.[107]

IMPLICATIONS OF INTERSECTIONALITY ON MENTAL HEALTH

Throughout this chapter we have discussed the impact of minority stress in the form of internalized prejudice on the impact of mental health among discrete minority groups. However, minority status expands beyond the confines of race and sexuality and can encompass multiple minority identities, and individuals with multiple minority status can experience compounding effects of internalized prejudice from multiple social identities. The concept of intersectionality provides a framework for understanding the meaning and consequences for individuals who identify with multiple minority categories in terms of race/ethnicity, gender, social class, and sexuality.[109] Intersectionality, according to Bowleg, is a "theoretical framework which posits that multiple social categories (race, ethnicity, gender, sexual orientation, socioeconomic status) intersect at the micro level of individual experience to reflect multiple interlocking systems of privilege and oppression at the macro, social-structural level (racism, sexism, heterosexism)."[109]

The historical concept of intersectionality dates back to the early 19th century; activists advocating for nondiscrimination laws toward African Americans also tried to draw attention to the additive effects of gender discrimination experienced by African American women.[110,111] Political movements in the early 20th century focused on gender and racial discrimination but rarely examined the compounded effects on the experiences of African American women. Throughout the 1980s and 1990s, scholars began to investigate the implication of identifying with multiple minority categories, ultimately leading to the theorist Crenshaw coining the term "intersectionality."[111]

Earlier parts in this chapter examined the association between internalized prejudice among various ethnic groups and mental illness. However, as Banks eloquently states, "Psychopathology could be characterized as a field of interactions rather than direct linear relationships."[112] The construct of intersectionality complicates investigations regarding the etiology, potential risk factors, and epidemiology of psychiatric conditions, but the interaction of multiple categories of minority status must be taken into consideration when examining the implications of minority stress theory and its association with mental illness.

Intersectionality also reduces the risk of assuming that various ethnic groups are homogenous, which discounts the inherent variability of individuals identifying with multiple social identities within a specific group.[112] For example, the increased risk of depression among African American women is based on the multiplicative effects of minority stress related to gender, race, socioeconomic status, and perceived discrimination.

Sexual minorities also experience intersectionality via prejudice related to identifying with other marginalized groups. Meyer described minority stress among sexual minority individuals as the "combined experience of internalized homophobia, perceived stigma due to an individual's sexual orientation, and sexual orientation-based victimization[6]," in addition to the stigma associated with identifying with another minority group.[6,102] For example, racial minority lesbians may internalize multiple negative stereotypes; this has an additive effect that could worsen mental health outcomes, compared to someone who identifies with a single minority group.[113]

CLINICAL RECOMMENDATIONS AND SUMMARY

The case of Mr. C, presented at the beginning of the chapter, encapsulates the complexities of internalized racism and its consequences. His diminished self-esteem and self-worth led to the development of depressive symptoms in the context of internalizing multiple negative stereotypes, including that African American males are not intelligent, are prone to criminality, and are respected and highly regarded only for their athletic pursuits. Individuals such as Mr. C have unconsciously internalized both negative and "positive" stereotypes; they may have difficulty recognizing that these negative feelings toward themselves and other members of their minority group are the result of ongoing oppression by the dominant society. External sources of oppression are often easy to recognize as being discriminatory, prejudiced, and hostile, but minority individuals who accept stereotypes as unavoidable truths may miss how much they have internalized this oppression in their own attitudes and beliefs. Minority stress theory and its associated components place an undue burden on individuals, making minorities more vulnerable to negative health outcomes.

Mr. C could have benefitted from early recognition of his conflict with his identity, given that he is constantly inundated with messages from society reflecting stereotypes of African American men. His negative appraisal of his minority status hindered him from expanding his perception of success beyond athletics. Because of his negative appraisal and internalization of prejudices toward African American men, he found himself struggling in the face of adversity, succumbing to limitations reinforced by society. Mental health clinicians might claim that reframing his perception of himself and his circumstances would provide him with sufficient ego strength to overcome the tremendous setback in his career. However, this would place the burden on Mr. C to conform to society's standards in a way that would continue to perpetuate prejudice within our society. Although a lofty task, the burden should be placed on society, which is after all the perpetrator of victimizing minorities through the stressors society continuously places on "the other".[6]

Mr. C would have benefitted from mental health care once he started to exhibit severe neurovegetative symptoms, which eventually led to his departure from college. The following are strategies that a clinician could use if Mr. C sought mental health care:

1. **Elicit the patient's narrative of how he views himself in the world.** Exploring his personal narrative could give him an opportunity to understand the choices he made that led to his current trajectory.
2. **Invite the patient to reflect on how he views the most important people in his life.** Elicit his perspective of how he views his family, friends, and those from his community, possibly generating a discussion of his perception of stereotypes of African American males.
3. **Create a safe space to discuss themes related to racism and internalized prejudice.** If Mr. C doesn't raise themes of racism or internalized prejudice, invite him to explore such difficult topics by fostering a safe space for such conversations. Express a sense of interest and curiosity while maintaining a nondefensive, nonconfrontational stance.
4. **Explore origins for the patient's low self-esteem and self-worth.** If Mr. C expresses low self-esteem and low self-worth throughout his narrative, explore where those feelings could have originated. This discussion could elicit themes of internalized racism.

As clinicians, we often encounter individuals who present with psychiatric symptoms exacerbated by the burdens of internalized racism and the intersectionality of multiple minority statuses. It is critical for us to recognize the negative implications of internalized racism, while also developing a sense of awareness of the mental health implications of this form of oppression. Clinicians can and should take an inquisitive and curious stand and directly inquire about a patient's experience with racism, prejudice, and discrimination.

We should not assume that such an experience affects only certain minority groups. Clinicians must ask all patients about these experiences, given that individuals may identify with multiple social categories that may not be apparent at first glance. Addressing the role of minority stress and internalized prejudice among our patients has the potential to have a tremendous impact on their well-being and mental health. The ability for clinicians to recognize and appreciate the implications of minority stress can ultimately prevent minorities from suffering in silence from psychiatric illnesses exacerbated by oppression.

REFERENCES

1. Lazarus RS, Folkman S. *Stress, Appraisal and Coping.* New York: Springer; 1984.
2. Allison KW. Stress and oppressed social category membership. In: Swim JK, Stangor C, eds. *Prejudice: The Target's Perspective.* San Diego, CA: Academic Press; 1998:145–170.

3. Clark R, Anderson NB, Clark VR, Williams DR. Racism as a stressor for African Americans: A biopsychosocial model. *American Psychologist.* 1999;54(10):805–816.

4. Selye H. Stress and holistic medicine. In: Sutterley DS, Donnelly GF, eds. *Coping with Stress: A Nursing Perspective.* Rockville, MD: Aspen Systems; 1982:69–72.

5. Slavin LA, Rainer KL, McCreary ML, Gowda KK. Toward a multicultural model of the stress process. *Journal of Counseling & Development.* 1991;70(1):156–163.

6. Meyer IH. Minority stress and mental health in gay men. *Journal of Health and Social Behavior.* 1995;36(1):38–56.

7. Miller CT, Major B. Coping with stigma and prejudice. In: Heatherton TF, Kleck RE, Hebl MR, Hull JG, eds. *The Social Psychology of Stigma.* New York: Guilford Press; 2000:243–272.

8. Williams DR, Neighbors H. Racism, discrimination and hypertension: Evidence and needed research. *Ethnicity and Disease.* 2001;11(4):800–816.

9. Bonilla-Silva E. Rethinking racism: Towards a structural interpretation. *American Sociological Review.* 1997; 62(3):465–480.

10. Schaefer RT. *Racial and Ethnic Groups,* 4th ed. London: Longman Higher Education; 1990.

11. Fredrickson G. *Racism: A Short History.* Princeton, NJ: Princeton University Press; 2002.

12. Carter RT. Racism and psychological and emotional injury: Recognizing and assessing race-based traumatic stress. *The Counseling Psychiatrist.* 2007;35(1):13–105.

13. Babad EY, Birnbaum M, Benne KD. *The Social Self: Group Influences on Personal Identity.* Beverly Hills, CA: Sage; 1983.

14. Seiter E. Stereotypes and the media: A re-evaluation. *Journal of Communication.* 1986;36(2): 14–26.

15. Bailey TKM, Chung YB, Williams WS, Singh AA, Terrell HK. Development and validation of the Internalized Racial Oppression Scale for Black individuals. *Journal of Counseling Psychology.* 2011;58(4):481.

16. Poupart L. The familiar face of genocide: Internalized oppression among American Indians. *Hypatia.* 2003;18:86–100.

17. Speight SL. Internalized racism: One more piece of the puzzle. *The Counseling Psychologist.* 2007;35:126–134.

18. Williams DR, Williams-Morris R. Racism and mental health: The African American experience. *Ethnicity and Health.* 2000;5(3-4):243–268.

19. Cokley KO. Testing Cross's revised racial identity model: An examination of the relationship between racial identity and internalized racialism. *Journal of Counseling Psychology.* 2002;49(4):476.

20. Jones CP. Levels of racism: A theoretic framework and a gardener's tale. *American Journal of Public Health.* 2000;90(8):1212.

21. Padilla LM. "But you're not a dirty Mexican": Internalized oppression, Latinos & law. *Texas Hispanic Journal of Law & Policy.* 2001;7:59–113.

22. Prilleltensky I, Gonick L. Polities change, oppression remains: On the psychology and politics of oppression. *Political Psychology.* 1996;17(1):127–148.

23. Bailey TKM. Construct Validation of the Internalized Racial Oppression Scale. Doctoral dissertation. Available from ScholarWorks @ Georgia State University. 2008.

24. Goffman E. *Stigma: Notes on the Management of Spoiled Identity.* Englewood Cliffs, NJ: Prentice-Hall; 1963.

25. Hetrick ES, Martin AD. Ego-dystonic homosexuality: A developmental view. In: Hetrick ES, Stein TS, eds. *Innovations in Psychotherapy with Homosexuals.* Washington, DC: American Psychiatric Association Press; 1984:2–21.

26. Stein TS, Cohen CJ. Psychotherapy with gay men and lesbians: An examination of homophobia, coming-out, and identity. In: Hetrick ES, Stein TS, eds. *Innovations in Psychotherapy with Homosexuals.* Washington, DC: American Psychiatric Association Press; 1984:59–73.

27. Hendricks ML, Testa RJ. A conceptual framework for clinical work with transgender and gender noncomforming clients: An adaptation of the minority stress model. *Professional Psychology: Research and Practice.* 2012;43:460–467.

28. Taylor J, Wilson M, Dobbins J. *Nadanolitization Scale.* Unpublished manuscript. University of Pittsburgh, 1972.

29. Taylor J, Grundy C. Measuring Black internalization of White stereotypes about African Americans: The Nadanolitization Scale. In: Jones RL, ed. *Handbook of Tests and Measurements of Black Populations.* Hampton, VA: Cobb & Henry; 1996: Vol. 2: 217–226.

30. Taylor J. Relationship between internalized racism and marital satisfaction. *Journal of Black Psychology.* 1990;16:53–54.

31. Parham TA, Helms JE. Attitudes of racial identity and self-esteem of Black students: An exploratory investigation. *Journal of College Student Personnel.* 1985;26(2):143–147.

32. Baldwin JA, Bell YR. The African Self-Consciousness Scale: An Africentric personality questionnaire. *The Western Journal of Black Studies.* 1985;9:61–68.

33. Rangel Campon R. The Appropriated Racial Oppression Scale development and preliminary validation. *Cultural Diversity and Ethnic Minority Psychology.* 2015;21(4):497–506

34. Hipolito-Delgado CP. Internalized Racism and Ethnic Identity in Chicana/o and Latina/o College Students. Doctoral dissertation. Available from ProQuest Dissertations and Theses database. 2007.

35. David EJR, Okazaki S. Colonial mentality: A review and recommendation for Filipino American psychology. *Cultural Diversity and Ethnic Minority Psychology.* 2006;12(1):1–16.

36. Choi AY, Israel T, Maeda H. Development and evaluation of the Internalized Racism in Asian Americans Scale (IRAAS). *Journal of Counseling Psychology.* 2017;64(1):52–64.

37. Grey JA, Robinson BBE, Coleman E, Bockting WO. A systematic review of instruments that measure attitudes toward homosexual men. *Journal of Sex Research.* 2013;50:329–352.

38. Nungesser L. *Homosexual Acts, Actors, and Identities.* New York: Praeger. 1983.

39. Wagner G, Serafini J, Rabkin J, Remien R, Williams J. Integration of one's religion and homosexuality: A weapon against internalized homophobia? *Journal of Homosexuality.* 1994;26:91–110.

40. Ross MW, Rosser BRS. Measurement and correlates of internalized homophobia: A factor analytic study. *Journal of Clinical Psychology.* 1996;52:15–21.

41. Herek GM, Cogan JC, Gillis JR, Glunt EK. Correlates of internalized homophobia in a community sample of lesbians and gay men. *Journal of the Gay and Lesbian Medical Association.* 1998;2:17–26.

42. Mayfield W. The development of an internalized homonegativity inventory for gay men. *Journal of Homosexuality.* 2001;41:53–76.

43. Currie MR, Cunningham EG, Findlay, BM. The Short Internalized Homonegativity Scale: Examination of the factorial structure of a new measure of internalized homophobia. *Educational and Psychological Measurement.* 2004;64(6):1053–1067.

44. Szymanski DM, Barry CY. The Lesbian Internalized Homophobia Scale: A rational theoretical approach. *Journal of Homosexuality.* 2001;41:37–53.

45. Testa RJ, Michaels MS, Bliss W, Rogers ML, Balsam KF, Joiner T. Suicidal ideation in transgender people: Gender minority stress and interpersonal theory factors. *Journal of Abnormal Psychology.* 2017;126(1):125.

46. Williams DR, Mohammed SA. Discrimination and racial disparities in health: Evidence and needed research. *Journal of Behavioral Medicine.* 2009;32(1):20–47.

47. Williams DR. Race, socioeconomic status, and health: The added effects of racism and discrimination. *Annals of the New York Academy of Sciences.* 1999;896:173–188.

48. Frost DM, Lehavot K, Meyer IH. Minority stress and physical health among sexual minority individuals. *Journal of Behavioral Medicine.* 2015;38(1):1–8.

49. Blascovitch J, Spencer SJ, Quinn D, Steele C. African Americans and high blood pressure: The role of stereotype threat. *Psychological Science.* 2001;12(3):225–229.

50. Butler C, Tull ES, Chambers EC, Taylor J. Internalized racism, body fat distribution, and abnormal fasting glucose among African-Caribbean women in Dominica, West Indies. *Journal of the National Medical Association.* 2002;94(3):143–148.

51. Chambers EC, Tull ES, Fraser HS, Mutunhu NR, Sobers N, Niles E. The relationship of internalized racism to body fat distribution and insulin resistance among African adolescent youth. *Journal of the National Medical Association.* 2004;96(12):1594–1598.

52. Tull ES, Cort MA, Gwebu ET, Gwebu K Internalized racism is associated with elevated fasting glucose in a sample of adult women but not men in Zimbabwe. *Ethnicity & Disease.* 2007;17(4):731–735.

53. Tull ES, Wickramasuriya T, Taylor J, et al. Relationship of internalized racism to abdominal obesity and blood pressure in Afro-Caribbean women. *Journal of the National Medical Association.* 1999;91:447–452.

54. Adam EK, Heissel JA, Zeiders KH, et al. Developmental histories of perceived racial discrimination and diurnal cortisol profiles in adulthood: A 20-year prospective study. *Psychoneuroendocrinology.* 2015;62:279–291.

55. Paradies Y, Ben J, Denson N, et al. Racism as a determinant of health: A systematic review and meta-analysis. *PLoS ONE.* 2015;10(9):e0138511.

56. Gee GC, Ro A, Shariff-Marco S, Chae D. Racial discrimination and health among Asian Americans: Evidence, assessment, and directions for future research. *Epidemiologic Reviews.* 2009;31(1):130–151.

57. Priest N, Paradies Y, Trenerry B, Truong M, Karlsen S, Kelly Y. A systematic review of studies examining the relationship between reported racism and health and wellbeing for children and young people. *Social Science and Medicine.* 2013;95:115–127.

58. Pascoe EA, Richman LS. Perceived discrimination and health: A meta-analytic review. *Psychological Bulletin.* 2009;135(4):531–554.

59. Harrell CP, Burford TI, Cage BN, et al. Multiple pathways linking racism to health outcomes. *Du Bois Review.* 2011;8(1):143–157.

60. Brondolo E, Brady N, Libby D, Pencille M. Racism as a psychosocial stressor. In: Baum A, Contrada R, eds. *Handbook of Stress Science.* New York: Springer; 2011:167–168.

61. Paradies Y. A systematic review of empirical research on self-reported racism and health. *International Journal of Epidemiology.* 2006;35(4):888–901.

62. Molina KM, James D. Discrimination, internalized racism, and depression: A comparative study of African American and Afro-Caribbean adults in the US. *Group Processes and Intergroup Relations*. 2016;19(4):439–461.

63. Fisher CB, Wallace SA, Fenton RE. Discrimination distress during adolescence. *Journal of Youth and Adolescence*. 2000;29(6):679–695.

64. Brown TN, Sellers SL, Gomez JP. The relationship between internalization and self-esteem among black adults. *Sociological Focus*. 2002;35(1):55–71.

65. Williams DR, Mohammed SA. Racism and health. *American Behavioral Scientist*. 2013;57(8):1152–1173.

66. Kwate NA, Meyer IH. On sticks and stones and broken bones: Stereotypes and African American health. *Du Bois Review*. 2011;8(1):191–198.

67. Kessler RC, Andrews G, Colpe LJ, et al. Short screening scales to monitor population prevalences and trends in non-specific psychological distress. *Psychological Medicine*. 2002;32(6):959–976.

68. Kessler RC, Berglund P, Demler O, et al. The epidemiology of major depressive disorder: Results from the National Comorbidity Survey Replication (NCS-R). *Journal of the American Medical Association*. 2003;289(23):3095–3105.

69. Mouzon DM, McLean JS. Internalized racism and mental health among African-Americans, US-born Caribbean Blacks, and foreign-born Caribbean Blacks. *Ethnicity & Health*. 2017;22(1):36–48.

70. Taylor J, Jackson B. Factors affecting alcohol consumption in black women: Part I. *International Journal of the Addictions*. 1990;25(11):1287–1300.

71. Taylor J, Jackson B. Factors affecting alcohol consumption in black women: Part II. *International Journal of the Addictions*. 1990;25:1407–1419.

72. Taylor J, Henderson D, Jackson BB. A holistic model for understanding and predicting depressive symptoms in African-American women. *Journal of Community Psychology*. 1991;19:306–320.

73. Waters MC. *Black Identities: West Indian Immigrant Dreams and American Realities*. New York: Harvard University Press; 2001.

74. Graham JR, West LM, Martinez J, Roemer L. The mediating role of internalized racism in the relationship between racist experiences and anxiety symptoms in a Black American sample. *Cultural Diversity and Ethnic Minority Psychology*. 2016;22(3):369.

75. Vandiver BJ, Cross WE, Worrell FC, Fhagen-Smith PE. Validationg the Cross Racial Identity Scale. *Journal of Counseling Psychology*. 2002;49(1):71–85.

76. Fortes de Leff, J. Racism in Mexico: Cultural roots and clinical interventions. *Family Process*. 2002;41:619–623.

77. Finch BK, Kolody B, Vega WA. Perceived discrimination and depression among Mexican-origin adults in California. *Journal of Health and Social Behavior*. 2000; 41(3): 295–313.

78. Bell D. *Silent Covenants: Brown v. Board of Education and the Unfulfilled Hopes for Racial Reform*. New York: Oxford University Press; 2005.

79. Asanti T. Suffering internalized racism. *Lesbian News*. 1996;21:51.

80. Hipolito-Delgado CP. Exploring the etiology of ethnic self-hatred: Internalized racism in Chicana/o and Latina/o college students. *Journal of College Student Development*. 2010;51:319–331

81. Hovey JD, King CA. Acculturative stress, depression, and suicidal ideation among immigrant and second-generation Latino adolescents. *Journal of the American Academy of Child & Adolescent Psychiatry*. 1996;35(9):1183–1192.

82. Chou R, Feagin J. *Myth of the Model Minority: Asian Americans Facing Racism*. Boulder, CO: Paradigm Publishers; 2017.

83. Zhou M. Coming of age: The current situation of Asian American children. *Amerasia Journal*. 1999;25:1–27.

84. Espiritu YL. *Asian American Panethnicity*. Philadelphia: Temple University Press; 1992.

85. Gans HJ. Symbolic ethnicity: The future of ethnic groups and cultures in America. *Ethnic and Racial Studies*. 1979;2:1–20.

86. Waters MC. *Ethnic Pptions*. Berkeley: University of California Press; 1990.

87. Pyke K, Dang T. "FOB" and "Whitewashed": Identity and internalized racism among second-generation Asian Americans. *Qualitative Sociology*. 2003;26(2):147–172.

88. Ogbu JU. The individual in collective adaptation: A framework for focusing on academic underperformance and dropping out among involuntary minorities. In: Weis L, Farrar E, Petrie HG, eds. *Dropouts from Schools: Issues, Dilemmas and Solutions*. Buffalo: State University of New York Press; 1989:181–204.

89. Ogbu J. Variability in minority school performance: A problem in search of an explanation. *Anthropology and Education Quarterly*. 1987;18(4):312–334.

90. Suzuki BH. Asian-American as the model minority. *Change*. 1989;21(6):13–19.

91. Wong P, Lai CF, Nagasawa R, Lin T. Asian Americans as a model minority: Self-perceptions and perceptions by other racial groups. *Sociological Perspectives*. 1998;41(1):95–118.

92. Lee SJ. Behind the model-minority stereotype: Voices of high-and low-achieving Asian American students. *Anthropology & Education Quarterly*. 1994;25(4):413–429.

93. Shih FH. Asian-American students: The myth of a model minority. *Chinese American Forum*. 1989;4:9–11.

94. Hartman JS, Askounis AC. Asian-American students: Are they really a "model minority"? *The School Counselor*. 1989;37:109–112.

95. Ahn Toupin E, Son L. Preliminary findings on Asian Americans: "The model minority" in a small private East Coast college. *Journal of Cross-Cultural Psychology*. 1991; 22:403–417.

96. Sue S, Okazaki S. Asian-American educational achievements: A phenomenon in search of an explanation. *American Psychologist*. 1990;45:913–920.

97. Lee RM, Yoo HC. Structure and measurement of ethnic identity for Asian Americans. *Journal of Counseling Psychology*. 2004;51:263–269.

98. Szymanski DM, Gupta A. Examining the relationships between multiple oppressions and Asian American sexual minority persons' psychological distress. *Journal of Gay & Lesbian Social Services*. 2009;21(2-3):267–281.

99. Crocker J, Luhtanen R, Blaine B, Broadnax S. Collective self-esteem and psychological well-being among White, Black, and Asian college students. *Personality and Social Psychology Bulletin*. 1994;20:503–513.

100. Lee RM. Do ethnic identity and other-group orientation protect against discrimination for Asian Americans? *Journal of Counseling Psychology*. 2003;50(2):133.

101. Meyer IH, Dean L. Internalized homophobia, intimacy and sexual behaviour among gay and bisexual men. In: Herek G, ed. *Stigma and Sexual Orientation*. Thousand Oaks, CA: Sage Publications; 1998:160–186.

102. Newcomb ME, Mustanski B. Internalized homophobia and internalizing mental health problems: A meta-analytic review. *Clinical Psychology Review*. 2010;30(8):1019–1029.

103. Hammelman TL. Gay and lesbian youth: Contributing factors to serious attempts or consideration of suicide. *Journal of Gay and Lesbian Psychology*. 1993;2(1):77–89.

104. Williamson IR. Internalized homophobia and health issues affecting lesbians and gay men. *Health Education Research*. 2000;15(1):97–107.

105. Igartua KJ, Gill K, Montoro R. Internalized homophobia: A factor in depression, anxiety, and suicide in the gay and lesbian population. *Canadian Journal of Community Mental Health*. 2009;22(2):15–30.

106. McLaren S. The interrelations between internalized homophobia, depressive symptoms, and suicidal ideation among Australian gay men, lesbians, and bisexual women. *Journal of Homosexuality*. 2016;63(2):156–168.

107. Hoy-Ellis CP, Fredriksen-Golden KI. Depression among transgender older adults: General and minority stress. *American Journal of Community Psychology*. 2017;59(3-4):295–305.

108. Fredriksen-Goldsen KI, Cook-Daniels L, Kim HJ, et al. Physical and mental health of transgender older adults: An at-risk and underserved population. *The Gerontologist*. 2013;54:488–500.

109. Bowleg L. The problem with the phrase women and minorities: Intersectionality—an important theoretical framework for public health. *American Journal of Public Health*. 2012;102(7):1267–1273.

110. Giddings, P. *When and Where I Enter: The Impact of Black Women on Race and Sex in America*. New York: Morrow; 1985.

111. Cole ER. Intersectionality and research in psychology. *American Psychologist*. 2009;63(3):170–180.

112. Banks KH, Kohn-Wood LP. Gender, ethnicity and depression: Intersectionality in mental health research with African American women. *Scholarship*. 2002; Paper 6.

113. Velez BL, Moradi B, DeBlaere C. Multiple oppressions and the mental health of sexual minority Latina/o individuals. *The Counseling Psychologist*. 2015;43(1):7–38.

8

Identifying and Working with Diverse Explanatory Models of Mental Illness

TONY B. BENNING AND JUSTIN A. CHEN ∎

CASE 1

Manny is a 30-year-old male from Ethiopia who presents with a six-month history of persecutory delusions, ideas of reference, and derogatory verbal hallucinations. Prior to arriving in Canada as an asylum seeker, he spent two years in a refugee camp in Kenya. In the initial psychiatric evaluation Manny disclosed that he is a devout Christian, a member of the Ethiopian orthodox church. He expressed to the psychiatrist his belief (one that was corroborated by his wife) that his illness is considered in his culture to have been caused by "bad spirits" and that the remedy is to undergo a "holy water" ceremony in church.

WHY IS IT IMPORTANT TO IDENTIFY PATIENTS' DIVERSE EXPLANATORY MODELS OF MENTAL ILLNESS?

As a result of their training, most psychiatrists privilege biomedical and psychological explanatory paradigms in their approach toward addressing and treating mental illness. But Pat Bracken and Philip Thomas, authors of *Postpsychiatry: Mental Health in a Postmodern World* (2005) and leading exponents of the contemporary critical psychiatric movement in the United Kingdom, point out that contemporary psychiatry's "technological framework of psychopathology and neuroscience" has all but marginalized and stamped out "spiritual, moral, political, and folk understandings of mental illness."[1,p725] This poses a challenge when attempting to forge productive therapeutic alliances with patients, whose subjective report of symptoms remains the primary source of information. Yaseen Ally and Sumaya Laher,[2] psychologists in South Africa, suggest that if effective treatments are to be provided to diverse populations in a multicultural context, clinicians must develop an understanding

of diverse belief systems pertaining to the etiology of mental illness. That senti-
ment is also expressed by British psychiatrist and anthropologist Simon Dein,[3] who
encourages health professionals to familiarize themselves with traditional and indigenous models of illness across cultures, as well as with traditional systems of healing.

Indeed, it has been suggested that the incompatibility between the explanatory
models of specific cultural groups versus mainstream psychiatry might be one factor
contributing to the underutilization of mainstream mental health services by people
from those groups in the West.[4] For Patel,[5] clinicians' clearer knowledge of and willingness to advocate for indigenous systems of healing and culturally-specific explanatory models will translate into a more intimate knowledge of patients' actual
experience, which will result in more considered and useful recommendations regarding care pathways. An emerging literature[6,7] alludes to the range of good clinical
outcomes—including an enhanced therapeutic alliance—that stem from patients'
confidence that the clinician understands their explanatory model. Indeed, a recent study[8] from Jamaica examining supernatural ideas of illness causation among
psychiatric patients found that patients' satisfaction and adherence to treatment
were increased when clinicians' conceptualizations of the causes of mental illness
matched their own, or when there was an acknowledgment of the patients' ideas
about causality.

In this chapter, we review key concepts from the medical anthropology and cross-
cultural psychiatry literatures as they relate to working with diverse explanatory
models of mental illness. Next, we briefly review a representative sample of these
explanatory models from different religious and cultural groups around the world.
Finally, we describe both theoretical and conceptual considerations when working
with diverse explanatory models of mental illness, using representative case vignettes
to illustrate these points.

DEFINITIONS/KEY TERMS

Explanatory models and conceptualizations of mental illness are understood in
terms of an influential definition by Kleinman.[9,10] The term "explanatory model"
encompasses the beliefs that individuals hold about illness, the personal and social
meaning attached to the disorder, and expectations about what will happen to them,
what the doctor will do, and so on. Eliciting patients' narratives is a cornerstone of
culturally sensitive psychiatry for Kleinman,[10] and asking the following "anthropological questions" in the "History of Present Illness" section of the psychiatric evaluation can help draw out that narrative:

> What do you call your problem?
> What names does it have?
> What do you think has caused your problem?
> Why do you think it started when it did?
> What does your sickness do to you?
> How does it work?
> How severe is it?
> Will it have a short or long course?
> What do you fear most about your sickness?

What are the chief problems the sickness has caused for you?
What kind of treatment do you think you should receive?
What are the most important results you hope to receive from the treatment?

Mitchell Weiss acknowledged that Kleinman's explanatory model framework motivated the development of his own much-cited Explanatory Model Interview Catalogue (EMIC),[11] a semistructured tool that has been used in psychiatric and medical research to elicit patients' beliefs regarding their symptoms. The EMIC acronym was chosen intentionally to honor the so-called emic framework of illness experience, one that is "rooted in the ideologies of local communities"[11,p237] and that therefore aspires to understand conceptualizations of illness within local contexts. The EMIC instrument was designed to operationalize the study of explanatory models of illness to permit comparison of illness meanings both intra- and inter-culturally.

Acknowledging their indebtedness to Kleinman's and Weiss's seminal work with explanatory models, Yeung and colleagues[12] developed the Engagement Interview Protocol (EIP) in the context of their own experience with depressed Chinese immigrants in the United States. In the EIP, the patients' illness beliefs are explored within the "History of Present Illness" section using Kleinman's questions listed above. One of the advantages of the EIP is that it can be efficiently integrated into the standard psychiatric assessment even within clinical time constraints.

The American Psychiatric Association's Cultural Formulation Interview (CFI) purports to offer a comprehensive set of guidelines for clinicians in psychiatric as well as general medical settings to integrate cultural considerations into clinical assessments. In their description of the CFI's conceptual foundations, development, and aims in the latest edition of the *Diagnostic and Statistical Manual of Mental Disorders* (DSM-5),[13] Aggarwal and Lewis-Fernández[14] explain, first, that the CFI represents the fulfillment of a developmental trajectory with respect to mainstream American psychiatry's engagement with culture that has been ongoing for the last 30 years or more. Second, the authors assert that the CFI's mission is a radical one insofar as it encourages clinicians to engage with patients' "experience-of-illness" and "life-world," with the aim of recognizing patients' perspectives as equally important as "the signs and symptoms of disease."[14,p430] Clearly, the imperative to honor the subjectivities of patients, whatever their cultural backgrounds may be, constitutes a thread that runs through the work of Kleinman, Weiss, the CFI, and beyond.

In this chapter, we will use the term "diverse explanatory models of mental illness" (DEM) to encompass, on the one hand, conventional biomedical explanatory models of mental illness, be they couched in biomedical or psychological paradigms, and on the other hand, religious, spiritual, indigenous, and/or folk conceptualizations of mental illness. The term "diverse conceptualizations of mental illness" will be used interchangeably with DEM and is synonymous with it. The term "non-biomedical explanatory model" (NBEM) will be used as a shorthand for religious, spiritual, indigenous, and/or folk explanatory models. Of note, biomedical explanatory models are often referred to as "Western," when in fact many "Western" cultures (of European derivation) privilege non-biomedical understandings of mental illness, and non-Western cultures may also subscribe to biomedical explanatory models. For this reason, we avoid using the relatively vague and inaccurate term "Western" in this chapter.

LITERATURE REVIEW ON NBEMS

By drawing on relevant literature, this section gives examples of NBEMs. Though the review encompasses religious and indigenous folk models of mental illness, it is a representative rather than an exhaustive sampling, one that is intended to bring attention to the divergent character of non-biomedical mental illness conceptualizations. It would not be feasible or useful to review here the full scope of NBEMs that one might encounter either clinically or in the literature.

Religious Explanatory Models

It has been posited that Protestant Christians' religious understandings of mental illness exist on a spectrum, with fundamentalist Protestants at one end and liberal Protestants at the other.[15] Given the widely held belief among fundamentalist Protestants that mental illness is caused by sin, the notion of forgiveness is accorded much importance in therapy. This contrasts with liberal Protestants' views that not all personal problems are spiritual problems.[15] Hartog and Gow's[16] study of Protestants in Australia revealed that 38% of participants endorsed a demonic etiology of major depression and 37% endorsed a demonic etiology for schizophrenia.

The relative dearth of literature on religious Jewish conceptualizations of mental illness may reflect a reticence about discussing mental illness that Wikler[17] observed in the Jewish community in general. In Wikler's review of traditional Jewish scriptural resources such as the Tanakh and the Talmud, he identified a multifactorial causal origin for mental illness, encompassing both spiritual and secular etiological factors. One of the points he emphasized was that a bicausal association is posited to exist in the Jewish religious texts between sin and mental illness. That is, sin triggers the wrath of God (*Ha-Shem*), who is thought to inflict mental illness "by punishing the sinner."[17,p342] However, the reverse pathway may exist as well: "the Torah sees mental illness, in some form, as the cause of sin."[17,p343]

Islamic conceptualizations of illness can be traced directly to the Qur'an. Al-Issa[18] described a holistic concept of health in the Qur'an that gives central importance, in the maintenance of health, to the harmonious integration between the soul (*ruh*), the connection between the soul and the body (*qalb*), the mind (*aql*), and the self (*nafs*). Al-Mateen and Afzal[19] and Farooqi[20] contend that from the Islamic perspective, religious doubt or uncertainty, as well as actions that contravene that which is proscribed, are important etiological factors for mental illness. Ally and Laher[2] undertook a qualitative study of six Muslim faith healers in South Africa. Echoing Al-Issa,[19] these faith healers conceptualized the emergence of mental illness as being related to an imbalance between the four interacting components of the self: mind (*aql*), body (*jism*), self (*nafs*), and soul (*ruh*). Another finding was that the Muslim faith healers distinguished between mental illness and so-called spiritual illness. They described causes of mental illness such as a chemical imbalance in the brain, the stress of everyday life, and childhood trauma. Spiritual illness was conceptualized as being causally related to one of two factors: *jadoo* (black magic) and *najar* (ill will). All of the faith healers expressed an interest in collaborating with mainstream medical or psychological practitioners, and all agreed that the decision of whether a given problem ought to be addressed by a faith healer or mainstream professional would be determined by the precise cause (i.e., medical/psychological vs. spiritual).

With reference to the Hindu tradition, Padayachee describes the line distinguishing mental and spiritual illness as "thin"[21,p14] and says that although each can exist in isolation, one may also develop into the other. Padayachee goes so far as to assert that "most Hindus perceive mental illness as having a supernatural etiology,"[21,p19] with the evil eye, witchcraft, and spirit possession often being considered to have etiological significance in the causation of psychiatric illness.

Kalra, Bhui, and Bhugra[22] studied the sacred Sikh text *Guru Granth Sahib*, searching for etiological references to mental illness. There are references to a host of supernatural causal factors in the case of depression (*dukh*), including forgetting God: "These verses warn that an individual's mind can be afflicted with terrible diseases like depression if one forgets the beloved even for a moment."[22] Karmic factors, too, are mentioned as possessing causal significance, as is excessive attachment to materialistic things. Numerous examples are also cited of the role of life events and of-this-world stressors in causing *dukh*, including the loss of loved ones, taunts, hypocrisy, loss of wealth, and drinking alcohol. One of the problems with this paper, however, is that the authors use *dukh* to refer to both suffering and depression (in the psychiatric sense) as though the two were synonymous. This sort of conflation of terms impedes more than it facilitates the emergence of a clear understanding of Sikh conceptualizations of depression.

Somatic Idioms of Distress

A significant literature documents that fact that mental illness, especially depression, is likely to be manifested in many non-European peoples in the form of somatic symptoms. This fact is relevant to any discussion of explanatory models of mental illness, as it behooves the clinician to have a critical awareness of the socially constructed nature of the very term "mental," and to appreciate that a Cartesian mind–body dichotomy underpins much of Western medical discourse.[23] Chinese populations have attracted academic attention with regards to the issue of somatization.[24-26] There has been a tendency within the Western psychiatric discourse on somatization to view the psychologization of mental distress as a superior idiom of distress than somatization,[27] but recent scholarship is challenging that assumption. Ryder and colleagues,[28] for example, observed more somatic symptomatology in Chinese as opposed to Euro-Canadian outpatients, but there were no differences in the two groups with respect to individuals' ability to identify or describe emotions. Because this research refutes the assumption that non-Europeans' somatizing tendencies are underpinned by alexithymic dispositions, the authors conclude that the study supports a nonpathological interpretation of observed differences. The authors also allude to the fact that somatization of mental illness could be more common than previously believed; indeed, they even suggest that the psychologization of mental illness may itself be a culturally specific, Western tendency.

NBEMs in Specific Psychiatric Conditions

Cinnerella and Loewenthal[29] conducted semistructured interviews with 52 women in the United Kingdom from different ethnoreligious groups (white Christian, Black Christian, Muslim, Jewish, Hindu) to ascertain variations in conceptualizations of depression and schizophrenia. Religious explanations of causality were much more likely to be invoked for depression than schizophrenia in all groups, and there was a correspondingly higher rate of use of prayer for depression. These findings held especially true with Muslim patients. Prayer was also considered to be of some help in reducing suffering in schizophrenia. This study discovered some interesting intergroup variation in religious coping: White Christians were much more likely to pray for others who were recognized as experiencing distress. All groups saw some potential merit in approaching a religious leader such as a rabbi or priest in depression, and Muslims were much more likely to express the view that help should come from a direct personal approach to God. Muslims were more likely to attribute depression to a lack of faith. The observation from this study that the Black Christian group was particularly likely to be negative about obtaining help from mental health professionals was noteworthy, as similar findings were reported by Schnittker,[30] who also found that African American women were particularly reluctant to embrace Western biomedical conceptualizations of mental illness. This was expressed in a reluctance to take psychiatric medications in contrast to a relative willingness to make a spiritual connection with God.

Bhui and colleagues[31] built on this study by interviewing 116 individuals from six different cultural groups—Bangladeshi, Caribbean, Indian, Irish, white British, and Pakistani—to show the diverse nature of religious coping strategies, such as praying, listening to religious radio, talking to God, trusting in God, and so on. This study, too, revealed some interesting tendencies within each ethnoreligious group. Christians had more of a conversational and less deferential relationship with God; Muslims were most likely to use religious coping. The ambivalent and sometimes troubled and persecuted relationship with God reported by Pargament and colleagues[32] as something that can contribute to mental distress was not seen among Muslims in this sample. Religious coping was found to be relatively uncommon among British and Irish participants, although some of the Irish participants reported obtaining guidance, wisdom, and knowledge through their religion. Indians and Pakistanis were less likely to conceptualize distress as a problem. The authors cautioned against invoking such concepts as "fatalism or external locus of control"[31,p149] to explain this finding, arguing that to do so amounts to imposing a Western scientific paradigm.

The only study of explanatory models of depression among ethnic minorities in Canada was performed by Ekanayake and colleagues,[33] but it must be interpreted extremely cautiously. While none of the 10 women invoked religious or supernatural causative models for depression, the authors did not address the potential sources of bias, including selective sampling (non-English speakers were excluded) and the influence of social desirability on the participants' responses. There is no mention that the interviewers used any suitable prompt questions to elicit perceptions or beliefs about spirituality.

In McCabe and Priebe's[34] study of explanatory models among four ethnic groups in the United Kingdom—Bangladeshi, white British, West Africans, and

African-Caribbean—a significant number of participants endorsed supernatural causal explanation for schizophrenia. Significantly more Bangladeshi, West African, and African-Caribbean participants endorsed supernatural explanation than did white British, with the Bangladeshi group being most likely to do so. Supernatural explanation was not correlated with nonadherence to medication, although it was correlated with religious help-seeking behaviors. The authors suggest that these findings be interpreted with caution given the small sample size.

A longitudinal study by Huguelet and colleagues,[35] following 92 outpatients with psychosis over a three-year period, showed that spiritual explanatory models of psychosis were independent of religious denomination and were subject to change over time. The following Christian denominations were represented in the sample: Catholic, mainline Protestant, fundamentalist Protestant, and Orthodox. Other categories represented in the sample were Islam, Judaism, Buddhism, minority religious movement, and no religious denomination.

Indigenous/Folk Explanatory Models

Based on her experiences working with indigenous communities in Tanzania and Canada, Jilek[36] identified common factors such as an emphasis on magical knowledge, relevance of extrapsychic conflicts, and disease symptoms frequently being seen as phenomena of the supernatural. More recently, Okello and Musisi[37] reported the results of a descriptive qualitative study of participants in Uganda. A clinical vignette of a case of psychotic depression was presented to faith healers, community elders, traditional healers, local leaders, and health workers, who were then invited to comment about names and causes in focus groups and in-depth interviews. Several findings emerged. First, the names ascribed to the condition themselves conveyed a statement or a belief about the presumed cause, such that the condition was referred to variably as a family problem, ancestral gods, ancestral spirits, and wind spirits. The fact that family problem and ancestral gods were cited the most frequently speaks to the fact that the collective is privileged as the cause and locus of the pathology. Second, in keeping with the findings of other research undertaken in Africa,[38] this research demonstrates that multiple levels of causation can be operant simultaneously. In this respect, the authors make a distinction between indigenous beliefs in proximate versus ultimate causes, with the former answering the question "how", and the latter answering the question "why."

In Teuton and colleagues'[38] qualitative study in Uganda, two clinical case vignettes (one presenting features of schizophrenia and the other of bipolar disorder) were presented to 20 Ugandan healers, some of whom possessed indigenous beliefs and others religious (Christian or Islamic). The methodology involved transcribing detailed interviews with the healers to ascertain their responses and their explanatory models of the case vignettes. All healers considered the individuals presented in the case vignettes as deviating from the norm in some respect, but the indigenous healers tended to attribute the problem to communications from deceased ancestors, whereas the religious healers were inclined to an explanation involving possession by evil spirits. The religious healers were also much more likely to entertain the possibility that external life stressors, much as in Western psychology, could have been of causal significance. The authors of this study, like Okello and Musisi,[37] comment on the fact that multiple explanatory beliefs can be held simultaneously. In this case, many of the religious healers simultaneously embraced religious explanations and Western psychopathological concepts—including schizophrenia and psychosis.

In their study of depressed Chinese patients in Boston, Yeung and Kam[39] found that 93% of participants considered psychological factors to be of causal importance, 45% endorsed magico-religious supernatural factors, 17% endorsed medical factors, and 14% endorsed traditional beliefs. The authors discuss the combined influence of Confucianism and Taoism on Chinese culture and Chinese sense of self, factors that in turn, influence the manner in which all illnesses are understood and expressed. In keeping with the Taoist yin-yang theory, signs and symptoms of illness are conceptualized as being due to either an excess or deficiency of yin or yang, or of one of the five fundamental elements (wood, metal, earth, wind, and fire). The treatment modality in any given case is chosen accordingly, because its aim is to restore balance to the system. Such conceptualizations of illness and its treatments are integral to the philosophy of Traditional Chinese Medicine (TCM) as well. Yeung and colleagues[12] make the very astute observation that traditional Chinese concepts may be entirely compatible with those of modern psychiatry. The modern framing of depression, for example, in terms of chemical imbalance, and the framing of treatments in terms of "restoring balance to the system"[12,p97] very much resonate with TCM health concepts.

Notions of harmony and imbalance can also be found in the Indian system of Ayurveda. Analogously to TCM, Ayurveda and the cosmological system from which it draws, posits the existence of five elements in the universe: ether, air, fire, water, and earth. The five elements are held to exist within organic as well as inorganic matter, and those elements are coded into three forces within living systems—*kapha*, *pitta*, and *vata*. These three forces, called *doshas*, are themselves composed of two or more of the elements: *Kapha* is composed of water and earth, *vata* of space and air, and *pitta* of fire. A harmonious balance between the three *doshas* is associated with health, and imbalance with disease.[40] *Unmada*, a Sanskrit term loosely translated as "insanity,"[41] is conceptualized within the Ayurvedic tradition as arising from either an excess of one of the *doshas* or excitation of all three of them.[42]

Explanatory Models of Mental Illness and Stigma

The possibility of a correlation between certain conceptualizations or explanatory models of mental illness and stigma (or some other negative social consequence for the sufferer) warrants further empirical investigation. In the contemporary psychiatric literature there is a suggestion that the promulgation of biological explanatory models may reduce stigma,[43] although that contention is not unanimously endorsed.[44] Ando and colleagues[45] reviewed the literature (19 studies in all) pertaining to stigma and mental illness in Japanese society between 2001 and 2013 and found significant stigmatization of individuals with mental illness. Stigma was measured by attitudes toward individuals suffering from mental illness, especially attitudes about social distance. There was greater stigma toward people with schizophrenia than depression, and the authors comment that mental illness in Japan is often attributed to personality weakness. The authors refrain from suggesting a causal relationship between stigma and the "weak personality" theory of mental illness (and in fact the study's design does not permit such conclusions about causality to be made), but the documented association does raise the question of the relationship between stigma and explanatory models of mental illness. Analyzing data regarding the illness beliefs of depressed Chinese immigrants in Boston, Chen and colleagues[46] observe that as this population adopts biomedical explanatory models for depressive symptoms, stigma against those symptoms may in fact increase. Later in this chapter, when we discuss the case of Meredith, there will be further discussion of this issue.

Gaps in the Literature

The above discussion attests to the fact that there is a growing literature on NBEMs, but the academic literature on explanatory models may fail to address the complexity that often characterizes real-world clinical encounters pertaining to DEMs. Real-world encounters often require a nuanced approach and skill in navigating what can at times present as thorny clinical dilemmas. There is a dearth of literature that provides pragmatic guidance to psychiatrists, psychiatric trainees, and other mental health professionals with respect to elucidating and working with patients who possess non-biomedical understandings of mental illness. The purpose of the rest of this chapter is to address that gap. Though theoretical issues will be discussed where relevant, practical and clinical issues will make up the main focus of the chapter.

WORKING WITH DEMS: THEORETICAL AND CONCEPTUAL CONSIDERATIONS

The fact that secular and biomedically based explanatory models tend to be privileged by psychiatrists and other mental health professionals over traditional, religious, indigenous, and folk models is understandable, given psychiatry's situation within a biomedical framework. However, as is the case with other medical specialties that place a greater emphasis on shared decision-making and provider–patient negotiation (e.g., primary care, pediatrics), the often-unacknowledged power differentials that result from this dynamic pose a challenge for practitioners unaccustomed to thinking in these terms. The first author of this chapter has a special interest in working with Canadian indigenous communities, a postcolonial context in which the issue of asymmetrical power relationships between mental health professionals and patients assumes particular salience. Providers must be cognizant of the role of power in each aspect of the clinical encounter, not least in the differential value that is accorded to modern biomedical versus traditional or local explanatory models of illness. Indeed, biomedical explanatory models in psychiatry tend to leave little room for other conceptualizations of distress. David Bohm's concept of *dialogue*, with its central feature of an "open mind to alternatives,"[47] is eminently relevant to the task of working with NBEMs. In what follows, we will say a little more about that concept and about Bohm.

David Bohm (1917–1992) was one of the preeminent theoretical physicists of the 20th century but also made important contributions to areas beyond physics. Especially in the latter stages of his career, Bohm became increasingly interested in social and humanitarian issues, as well as the concept of communication. In *Thought as a System*,[48] Bohm acknowledged the influence of North American Native culture on his own thinking; in fact, he maintained a fascination and admiration for indigenous culture and worldviews throughout his life.[49] The convention among North American Native people of meeting in a large circle impressed Bohm for the depth of communication and mutual understanding that it could produce. In his 1996 book *On Dialogue*,[47] he envisaged a communication process conducive to the creative emergence of new levels of understanding. Sitting in a circle establishes and reinforces a dynamic of equality because no one is a leader or has an especially authoritative role. Bohm's dialogue emphasizes a dynamic of equality between participants; each party listens actively and attentively to the other with an attitude that attempts to minimize prejudice, opinion, and judgment.

As the remainder of this chapter will demonstrate, in our work with patients who subscribe to diverse explanatory models of mental illness, we have tried to draw on Bohm's principles of dialogue. As a framework for communication, Bohm's dialogue can help psychiatrists and other mental health clinicians to cultivate a healthy self-reflexive awareness of our own biases, assumptions, and prejudices. It can help us to suspend our assumptions about the authority we normally give to biomedical explanatory models of mental illness, and the lack of authority we might accord to other explanatory models. Bohm's dialogue offers us a paradigm for communication that can help us remain open to our patients' diverse explanatory models, allowing new dimensions and depths of understanding to emerge. Yet, in advocating for the inclusion of NBEMs within the explanatory landscape, the intention is not to pit biological and nonbiological models against each other; in fact, Bohm[48] was conscious of the sorts of dichotomizing tendencies that could arise in ordinary communication, in which participants are prone to assume polarized positions. He saw such tendencies as impeding constructive communication, and his dialogue is intended to avoid such polarization.

WORKING WITH DEMS: PRACTICAL CONSIDERATIONS

We return to the case vignette presented at the beginning of the chapter. The psychiatrist established in the initial evaluation that the patient had a strong religious affiliation. That fact attuned the psychiatrist to the possibility that the patient and his family might be invoking a non-Western explanatory paradigm (at least in part) with respect to conceptualizing and making sense of Manny's difficulties. This case also illustrates the importance of taking a nonjudgmental approach, in line with Bohm's process of dialogue.

Manny was reticent to share his explanatory model, but a gentle, curious approach and the involvement of his significant other helped make him more comfortable. The following excerpted dialogue illustrates how a respectful, nonjudgmental attitude toward and affirmation of the client's explanatory model can help to establish and maintain rapport, in turn increasing patients' willingness to engage with mental health professionals and comply with biomedical treatments where indicated. Our approach here is entirely consistent with Yeung and colleagues' concept of "treatment negotiation."[12,p97] This is the step that follows the clinician's exploration of the patient's illness beliefs and disclosure to the patient of the diagnosis. Treatment negotiation "empowers the patient and shows that the clinician respects the patient's point of view; in a practical sense, it may facilitate engaging the patient into treatment."[12,p97]

DOCTOR: *Could I ask you to share with me your own understanding of what's going on here?*

MANNY: *Bad spirits.*

DOCTOR: *Okay, could you please tell me more about that? I am interested in understanding that a little more.*

MANNY: *In our culture we believe this is caused by bad spirits.* [Appearing somewhat sheepish and embarrassed]

DOCTOR: *Thank you for sharing that. I want you to know that I am interested in and have a great deal of respect for your understandings of this problem, but it is not something that I know very much about. From that perspective, would you mind sharing with me what sorts of remedies you might have previously pursued or which you might be intending to pursue in the future?*

MANNY: *We believe that it will get better with holy water. We already visited [another major Canadian city] where a church father was doing a holy water ceremony. Unfortunately, it was too busy so we were not able to be given holy water.*

DOCTOR: *Thank you for explaining that. I hope you get another chance to go to a holy water ceremony. Do you know when and where the next one is going to take place?*

MANNY'S WIFE: *The priest will be coming again to . . . We don't know when, but we will try to go to it.*

DOCTOR: *Thank you for explaining that. I am very much interested in having a greater understanding of how you understand your husband's illness from the perspective of your own cultural and religious background. From a Western (medical) point of view, I want to share with you that this problem is called "psychosis" or "schizophrenia," and it often gets better with medication. Is that something that you'd be interested in trying?*

Manny did agree to take risperidone and in fact did so more or less regularly for 6 months. Apart from minor setbacks, his psychotic symptoms remained in remission during that time. It was only during a visit to Ethiopia, where he underwent a holy water ceremony, that he stopped taking it. After that, he stayed free of psychosis for 6 months (while off medications). At that point, unfortunately, psychotic symptoms resurfaced, whereupon he resumed medication at the suggestion of the psychiatrist. Throughout the course of treatment in the local mental health center, the psychiatrist took Bohm's approach, providing gentle, affirmative, and nonjudgmental inquiry into Manny's explanatory model and associated help-seeking behavior. This assisted in the forging and maintenance of a strong therapeutic alliance, which in turn was a key factor in the patient agreeing to a retrial of medication following the relapse. At no point was the patient made to feel that his willingness to take medication required him to relinquish his explanatory model. One year later, Manny is free of psychosis and compliant with a small dose of risperidone. The psychiatrists at the mental health center continue periodically to inquire about cultural explanatory models. A recent conversation unfolded as follows:

DOCTOR: *I am glad that you are remaining well. Why do you believe that that is the case?*

MANNY'S WIFE: *The medications help, but he had holy water in Ethiopia. That was very powerful.*

DOCTOR: *Yes, I think it may well have been. I know that Christianity in Ethiopia is very deep and has a long history.*

MANNY: *Many religious people in Ethiopia live in the forest away from society because they do not want to see anything bad.*

MANNY'S WIFE: *Monastics. There are many places where people go to get healed. Places like Lalibela and Aksum are for tourists, but there are many other places.*

DOCTOR: *Do people go to heal from mental illness as well?*

MANNY'S WIFE: *Yes, you need to believe. You need to have faith.*

DOCTOR: *It sounds like your religious beliefs have helped you a lot.*

MANNY'S WIFE: *Yes, but I think the medications have helped a lot as well, maybe 80%.*

The psychiatrist's inquiry into Manny's explanatory model of illness within his family context continued over a protracted period, and it was an area that was gently and respectfully explored and revisited often. The approach taken resembled the spiral characteristics of a conversation more than it did the than linear characteristics of a checklist; the conversation often went over areas that had previously been explored, but in ever greater detail and depth. Such an approach led to a progressive deepening of rapport, as well as disclosure on the part of Manny and his wife about the details of their beliefs and their help-seeking behavior. The psychiatrist realized that the approach taken by the patient and his wife to his symptoms and their treatment was inextricably tied to their lives and worldviews. It was a privilege for the psychiatrist—based on many illuminating conversations—to expand his knowledge and understanding of the Christian Ethiopian culture within which Manny's illness beliefs and help-seeking were embedded. The psychiatrist had a strong hunch that a dynamic of reciprocity was at work in Manny's ringing endorsement of the role of medication in his healing. Such an endorsement would have been unlikely to occur if the psychiatrist himself had not respected Manny's illness beliefs and cultural background.

CASE 2: MEREDITH

Meredith is a 60-year-old Euro-Canadian woman with a mild learning disability and chronic treatment-resistant schizoaffective disorder, who is prescribed clozapine and lithium. Especially at times of stress or after sleep deprivation, Meredith is prone to experiencing transient exacerbations of auditory hallucinations, the content of which is threatening and derogatory. Meredith herself does not have a strong religious belief or affiliation, but her older brother is a devout Christian who advised Meredith that her voices are caused by satanic possession. Meredith was extremely upset about being told this, but she agreed with the psychiatrist's suggestion to have a family meeting with her brother.

DOCTOR: *Thank you for meeting with us. If you feel comfortable sharing, I would be interested to know more about the way in which you make sense of/explain Meredith's illness from the perspective of your own religious background.*

MEREDITH'S BROTHER: *I told Meredith that this voice she hears is Satan's voice.*

DOCTOR: *I have a great deal of respect for your religious beliefs, but my own belief is that the voices are not caused by Satan. What I can say is that Meredith does have a diagnosis which in medicine and psychiatry we call schizoaffective disorder. It is a disorder often thought to be associated with an imbalance of certain brain chemicals, including one called dopamine. This disorder often responds to medication. Would you agree that Meredith has been doing a lot better since she has been on her current medication?*

MEREDITH'S BROTHER: *Yes, I would most definitely agree with that.*

DOCTOR: *We also know that stress (and that includes sleep deprivation) can cause some occasional worsening of symptoms. One potentially simple solution would be to prescribe a small dose of sleeping medication to see if that helps. How does that idea sound to you?*

MEREDITH: *I would be willing to try that.*

MEREDITH'S BROTHER: *I think it would be worth trying that to see if it helps Meredith.*

This case brings attention to the potential that NBEMs have to bring harm to patients, an issue that is arguably understated in the literature on explanatory models of mental illness as well as various neuropsychiatric conditions. Jilek-All's[50] discussion of epilepsy from a historical as well as cross-cultural perspective presents a sobering reminder of how Christian conceptualizations of epilepsy as the manifestation of demonic possession, and indigenous African conceptualizations of epilepsy as a contagious entity caused by various supernatural forces, have resulted in dire social consequences for sufferers. Literature such as this, together with cases like that of Meredith, should caution clinicians against the undue idealization or romanticization of NBEMs. How should we respond to such criticism and identify a principle that can provide pragmatic guidance in such situations? While a detailed discussion is beyond the space constraints of this chapter, the next section briefly addresses this question.

In Meredith's case, the psychiatrist's assertion of a biomedical explanatory model over a religious one would appear to play into the hands of those who criticize postmodern philosophy as engendering an undisciplined "anything goes" brand of conceptual relativism. As this chapter has attempted to argue, there are negative ethical implications of the promulgation of exclusively biomedically oriented explanatory models for mental illness. We welcome the postmodern imperative[1] to challenge the authority of such totalizing models.

But postmodern philosophy itself is not without its critics. One of the points of criticism is that postmodern philosophy is anti-foundationalist,[51] meaning that it perpetuates a relativistic position in which there is a lack of an independent or predetermined way of judging the merits of any given view, position, or claim. The emerging "post-postmodern"[52] critique also brings attention to the self-refuting paradoxes that postmodern claims run into when asserting that pluralistic discourses are superior to monolithic ones. What grounds do we really have for asserting that anything is better or worse than any other thing? A comprehensive discussion of such apparent conceptual impasses, and of their nature, potential significance, and solutions, is beyond the scope of this chapter; what we can say is that such paradoxes potentially serve as important reminders of the complexity that attends clinical work with DEMs and the dilemmas that arise therein. Second, there is likely not to be just one solution to the sorts of dilemmas that will inevitably arise in clinical practice.

In Meredith's case, the privileging of the ethical consideration of nonmaleficence became an important guiding clinical principle for the psychiatrist. That is, the psychiatrist's holding up of a biomedical explanatory model served, in a sense, to *rescue* Meredith from the harmful impact that her family's (brother's) explanatory model was having on her.

This case represents an example of how a patient can be assisted by the psychiatrist's judicious navigation between several potential explanatory models. The ethical principle of nonmaleficence should undergird most clinical decisions, but in this case, it was the dominating principle informing the psychiatrist's approach to a difficult clinical situation. The psychiatrist's endorsement of a biomedical explanatory model was enough for the brother to support a medication intervention, regardless of his own religious beliefs about illness causation. This is in keeping with observations made in India by Johnson and colleagues[53] of patients continuing to embrace non-biomedical explanatory models, while nonetheless remaining adherence to treatment with medications. Meredith's brother's endorsement of medication, in combination with the psychiatrist's gentle reinforcement of a medical explanation for her symptoms, resulted in significant dissipation of Meredith's distress. This resolution occurred perhaps in part because the brother's original comment had caused a conflict in her that the family meeting helped to resolve.

SUMMARY

The worldview reflected by mainstream biomedical psychiatry is itself subject to cultural influences. That is, psychiatry reflects the values of post-Enlightenment rationalism, and the biomedical psychiatric framework is privileged over other forms of knowledge pertaining to health and illness. But such privileging —especially in an increasingly diverse society— merits examination. Mental health clinicians are well versed in biomedically based conceptualizations of health and disease, but they are likely to benefit in their clinical work from an openness to traditional, religious, indigenous, and folk explanatory models. This willingness to acknowledge or even embrace alternative conceptualizations of distress is an expression of cultural humility.

In the real-world clinical setting, patients or their families are often reticent to share the details of their NBEMs and/or the help-seeking behaviors with which these are intimately related due to concerns about negative judgment from the psychiatrist, something that itself reflects a power asymmetry. The NBEMs may therefore not be readily accessible to the psychiatrist; elucidating them requires skill and care. The psychiatrist should engage in a careful, nonjudgmental, and respectful inquiry regarding NBEMs. They may draw on David Bohm's principles of dialogue with great profit. The expectation that illness models lend themselves to being adequately explored in one sitting, based on a linear checklist type of inquiry, should probably be jettisoned. Instead a spiral model of exploration is ideal, based on a conversational or dialogic approach, that is able to revisit, in progressively greater depth, areas that have been previously explored.

In becoming cognizant of the hierarchy that frames biomedical and non-biomedical explanatory models, clinicians should avoid generating an inverse hierarchy. In other words, there are certain clinical scenarios (e.g., Case 2) in which an NBEM can lead to unnecessary torment and suffering. Clinicians should not romanticize NBEMs and should use their best clinical judgment when deciding whether to more forcefully promote a biomedical explanation in the service of relieving the patient's suffering and reducing stigma. Both cases illustrate the fact that clinicians should routinely explore DEMs within patients' systemic and familial contexts—but, of course, the patient's explanatory models will not always be identical to those of other family members.

CONCLUSION AND DISCUSSION

Through the presentation of two cases, this chapter has demonstrated that different explanatory models of mental illness, instead of vying for dominance, can coexist. Such explanatory pluralism is predicated on an ethical imperative to democratize the playing field and to allow space for non-biomedical explanations, be they religious, folk, spiritual, or indigenous, to sit side by side with biomedical and/or psychological ones, in understanding complex and subjective phenomena. Of interest is the fact that such multilevel conceptualizations of illness are often seen in indigenous/traditional health systems,[54] as well as other non-Western health systems.[53]

An approach to dialogue that is truly faithful to the description of it as set out by David Bohm would reject any notion of authority or hierarchy. Of course there is authority, hierarchy, and an undeniable power asymmetry in any psychiatrist–patient encounter, but that fact should not prevent psychiatrists from adopting dialogue as a communicative ideal or aspiration for the sort of communication that might be possible when discussing explanatory models of mental illness and associated help-seeking behaviors. Bohm speaks to that point in a section of *On Dialogue*[47] titled "Limited Dialogue," in which he recognizes that while there may be situations or variables that impede the development of dialogue in pure form, it may still be possible to carry out limited dialogue. Doing so, Bohm advises, will still be of "considerable value."[47,p49] The subject matter of this chapter attests to Bohm's point that the principles of dialogue can be profitably used during a psychiatrist–patient encounter, despite the power asymmetry that necessarily underlies that relationship. Bohm's concept of dialogue is very useful in managing to hold theoretical as well as pragmatic considerations within a single conciliatory embrace. We have seen how this applies to the example of DEMs, but the potential usefulness of dialogue to the psychiatrist–patient encounter does not stop there.

Contemporary psychiatry faces the challenge of meeting the needs of an increasingly diverse society and globalized world. Biomedical frameworks are powerful, but they represent just one way of understanding phenomena as complex as the mind and behavior, and so it behooves us to have humility about the edges of our understanding. A scenario in which diverse explanatory models coexist in a state of harmonious rapprochement is preferred to that which accords biomedical explanatory models ontologic superiority. We have alluded to the asymmetry that defines the relationship between biomedical explanatory models and NBEMs. Although an explicit critique of the former is something that has fallen outside the scope of the present chapter, it is worth noting that biomedical models of causality of the major mental illnesses are no longer endorsed as unequivocally as they might have been in previous decades. An example of that is the putative causal link between serotonin deficiency and depression, a link that is increasingly being questioned.[55] Such developments can contribute to a flattening of the conventional hierarchy of explanatory models. We hope that this chapter has shown how clinicians can identify and work with a diverse range of explanatory models.

REFERENCES

1. Bracken P, Thomas P. Postpsychiatry: Mental health in a postmodern world. Oxford, UK: Oxford University Press. 2005.
2. Ally Y, Laher S. South African Muslim faith healers' perceptions of mental illness: Understanding, aetiology and treatment. Journal of Religion and Health. 2008;47:45–56.
3. Dein S. Psychogenic death: Individual effects of sorcery and taboo violation. Mental Health, Religion and Culture. 2003;6:195–202.
4. Landrine H, Klonoff EA. Culture and health-related schemas: A review and proposal for interdisciplinary integration. Health Psychology. 1992;11(4):267–276.
5. Patel V. Explanatory models of mental illness in sub-Saharan Africa. Social Science Medicine. 1995;40:1291–1298.
6. Bhui KS, Bhugra D. Explanatory models for mental distress: Implications for clinical practice and research. British Journal of Psychiatry. 2002;181:6–7.
7. Dinos S, Ascoli M, Owiti JA, Bhui K. Assessing explanatory models and health beliefs: An essential but overlooked competency for clinicians. Advances in Psychiatric Treatment. 2017;23:106–114.
8. James CC, Carpenter KA, Peltzer K, Weaver S. Valuing psychiatric patients' stories: Belief in and use of the supernatural in the Jamaican psychiatric setting. Transcultural Psychiatry. 2014;51(2):247–263.
9. Kleinman A, Eisenberg L, Good B. Culture, illness and care: Clinical lessons from anthropologic and cross-cultural research. Annals of Internal Medicine. 1978;88(2):251–258.
10. Kleinman A. Patients and healers in the context of culture. Berkeley: University of California Press; 1980.
11. Weiss M. Explanatory Model Interview Catalogue (EMIC): Framework for comparative study of illness. Transcultural Psychiatry. 1997;34(2):235–263.
12. Yeung A., Trinh NH, Chang, TE, Fava M. The Engagement Interview Protocol (EIP): Improving the acceptance of mental health treatment among Chinese immigrants. International Journal of Culture and Mental Health. 2011;4(2):91–105.
13. American Psychiatric Association. DSM-5 Cultural Formulation Interview. Accessed July 30, 2017, from http://www.dsm5.org/proposedrevision/Documents/DSM5%20 Draft%20CFI.pdf
14. Aggarwal NK, Lewis-Fernandes R. An introduction to the Cultural Formulation Interview. Focus: The Journal of Lifelong Learning in Psychiatry. 2015;13(4) [online].
15. Malony HN. Religion and mental health from the Protestant perspective. In Koenig HG, ed. Handbook of Religion and Mental Health. San Diego, CA: Academic Press; 1998:203–211.
16. Hartog K, Gow KM. Religious attributions pertaining to the causes and cures of mental illness. Mental Health, Religion and Culture. 2005;8(4):263–276.
17. Wikler M. The Torah view of mental illness: Sin or sickness? Journal of Jewish Communal Service. 1977;53(4):339–344.

18. Al-Issa I. Mental Illness in the Islamic World. Madison, CT: International Universities Press; 2000.
19. Al-Mateen CS, Afzal A. The Muslim child, adolescent, and family. Child & Adolescent Psychiatric Clinics of North America. 2004;13:183–200.
20. Farooqi YN. Understanding Islamic perspective of mental health and psychotherapy. Journal of Psychology in Africa. 2006;1:101–111.
21. Padayachee P. Hindu psychologists' perceptions of mental illness. Unpublished Master of Arts thesis. University of Witwatersrand, South Africa, 2011.
22. Kalra G, Bhui K, Bhugra D. Does Guru Granth Sahib describe depression? Indian Journal of Psychiatry. 2013;55(2):195–200.
23. Benning TB. Should psychiatrists resurrect the body? Advances in Mind Body Medicine. 2016;30(1):32–38.
24. Tseng W. The nature of somatic complaints among patients: The Chinese case. Comprehensive Psychiatry. 1975;16(3):237–245.
25. Cheung FM, Lau BW, Wong SW. Paths to psychiatric care in Hong Kong. Culture, Medicine, & Psychiatry. 1984;8(3):207–228.
26. Zaroff CM, Davis JM, Chio PH, Madhavan D. Somatic presentations of distress in China. Australia and New Zealand Journal of Psychiatry. 2012;46(11):1053–1057.
27. Leff J. Psychiatry around the globe. London: Gaskell; 1981.
28. Ryder AG, Yang J, Zhu X, Yao S, Yi J, Heine SJ, Bagby RM. The cultural shaping of depression: Somatic symptoms in China, psychological symptoms in North America? Journal of Abnormal Psychology. 2008;117(2):300–313.
29. Cinnirella M, Loewenthal KM. Religious and ethnic group influences on beliefs about mental illness: A qualitative interview study. British Journal of Medical Psychology. 1999;72:505–524.
30. Schnittker J. Misgivings of medicine? African Americans' skepticism of psychiatric medication. Journal of Health and Social Behavior. 2003;44(4):506–524.
31. Bhui K, King M, Dein S, O'Connor W. Ethnicity and religious coping with mental distress. Journal of Mental Health. 2008;17(2):141–151.
32. Pargament KI, Koenig HG, Perez LM. The many methods of religious coping: development and initial validation of the RCOPE. Journal of Clinical Psychology. 2000;56:519–543.
33. Ekanayake S, Ahmad F, McKenzie K. Qualitative cross-sectional study of the perceived causes of depression in South Asian origin women in Toronto. BMJ Open. 2012;2:e000641.
34. McCabe R, Priebe S. Explanatory models of illness in schizophrenia: Comparison of four ethnic groups. British Journal of Psychiatry. 2004;185:25–30.
35. Huguelet P, Mohr S, Gilliéron C, Brandt PY. Religious explanatory models in patients with psychosis: A three-year follow-up study. Psychopathology. 2010;43(4):230–239.
36. Jilek-Aall L. The Western psychiatrist and his non-Western clientele: Transcultural experiences of relevance to psychotherapy with Canadian Indian patients. Canadian Psychiatric Association Journal. 1976;21(6):353–359.
37. Okello ES, Musisi S. Depression and a clan illness (eByekika): An indigenous model of psychotic depression among the Baganda of Uganda. World Cultural Psychiatry Research Review. 2006;1(2):60–73.
38. Teuton J, Bentall R, Dowrick C. Conceptualizing psychosis in Uganda: The perspective of indigenous and religious healers. Transcultural Psychiatry. 2007;44(1):79–114.

39. Yeung AS, Kam R. Illness beliefs of depressed Asian Americans in primary care. In Georgiopoulos AM, Rosenbaum JF, eds. Perspectives in Cross-Cultural Psychiatry. Philadelphia: Lippincott Williams & Wilkins; 2005:21–36.

40. Patwardhan B, Warude D, Pushpangadan P, Bhatt N. Ayurveda and Traditional Chinese Medicine: A comparative overview. Evidence-Based Complementary and Alternative Medicine. 2005;2(4):465–473.

41. Bhugra D. Psychiatry in ancient Indian texts: A review. History of Psychiatry. 1992;3(10):167–186.

42. Obeyesekere G. Ayurveda and mental illness. Comparative Studies in Society and History. 1970;12(3):292–296.

43. Angermeyer MC, Matschinger H. Causal beliefs and attitudes to people with schizophrenia. British Journal of Psychiatry. 2005;186(4):331–334.

44. Benning TB, O'Leary M, Avevor EA, Avevor ED. Biology and stigma [letter]. British Journal of Psychiatry. 2005;188(1):89.

45. Ando S, Yamaguch S, Aoki Y, Thornicroft G. Review of mental-health related stigma in Japan. Psychiatry and Clinical Neurosciences. 2013;67:471–482.

46. Chen JA, Hung GC, Parkin S, Fava M, Yeung AS. Illness beliefs of Chinese American immigrants with major depressive disorder in a primary care setting. Asian Journal of Psychiatry. 2015;13:16–22.

47. Bohm D. On Dialogue. London: Routledge; 1996.

48. Bohm D. Thought as a System. London: Routledge; 1994.

49. Peat D. Infinite Potential: The Life and Times of David Bohm. New York: Basic Books; 1997.

50. Jilek-All L. Morbus Sacer in Africa: Some religious aspects of epilepsy in traditional cultures. Epilepsia. 1999;40(3):382–386.

51. Jalloh CM. Fichte: Foundationalism, anti-foundationalism, and the new nihilism. Journal of Philosophy. 1991;8(10):542–543.

52. Benning TB. Binarism in psychiatry and its discontents. Unpublished Doctoral Thesis. California Institute of Integral Studies, San Francisco. 2018.

53. Johnson S, Sathyaseelan M, Charles H, Jeyaseelan V, Jacob KS. Insight, psychopathology, explanatory models and outcome of schizophrenia in India: A prospective 5-year cohort study. BMC Psychiatry. 2012;12:159.

54. Benning TB. Western and Indigenous conceptualizations of self, depression, and its healing. International Journal of Psychosocial Rehabilitation. 2013;17(2):129–137.

55. Cowen PJ, Browning M. What has serotonin to do with depression? World Psychiatry. 2015;14(2):158–160.

9

Religion and Spirituality in Psychiatric Care

An Experiential Seminar Model Addressing Barriers to Discussing Religion and Spirituality

SIOBHAN M. O'NEILL, JIAYING DING, AND GOWRI G. ARAGAM ■

CASE

A third-year resident in psychiatry, Dr. A, described meeting her first patient, Ms. B, in outpatient clinic:

Ms. B was a middle-aged Indian female with schizophrenia who had three older, high-achieving siblings. They cared for her immensely. Ms. B had restarted antipsychotic medication a few months earlier during a hospitalization. She was currently free of positive symptoms. She held a demanding job and was reengaging in her personal life. But despite these positive notations in her chart, when she walked in, I immediately saw sorrow in her eyes. As she sat down and shared her story, I realized that while she was no longer burdened by voices or paranoid delusions, she was tired and plagued by questions of how to bring meaning to her life.

I proceeded with the intake as I would any other, making sure to inquire about Ms. B's past medical history, social history, substance use patterns, and family history. She had been hospitalized a few times in the past decade, each time due to an exacerbation of delusions and hallucinations. She had tried several medications but was frustrated by their side effects. She had no history of suicide attempts. I asked her, "Do you have a sense of what triggered past episodes?" Ms. B said her family thought it was due to her preoccupation with God and the meaning of life after death. She told me she'd been drawn to the temple and to religious scripture and prayer. However, each time she'd allowed herself to delve into the meaning of her experience, her family said she'd quickly escalate to hearing the voice of God and putting herself in dangerous situations to "understand the truth." Her family told her this was a "delusion," but Ms. B wasn't convinced: She felt her experiences were

*meaningful, and she was heartbroken she'd been prohibited by her former doctors
and family from engaging in religion.*

*Listening to Ms. B made clear to me there was something beyond words in her ex-
perience. I started to feel nervous: Fully exploring the patient's religious and spiritual experience seemed unsafe. Where was the line between pathologic religiosity
and healthy curiosity? Would I "tip her over the edge" if I engaged in conversation
about religion during our sessions, landing her back in the hospital, or potentially
worse? Or was there some benefit to giving her the space to express herself in this
contained environment? These questions raced through my head as I sat with her,
and I found myself checking my own anxiety.*

*Ms. B's former resident doctor had suggested that she might benefit from
working with someone who could understand her spiritual concerns. I couldn't help
but notice the similarity in our skin tone, wondering if this had led others to assume
that I may be able to relate to Ms. B in a way her other doctors had not. My anxiety
increased. Trying to understand where this anxiety was coming from, I realized
I had no strategy, no experience integrating religion and spirituality into a clinical
formulation. This was not something that had been formally taught to me.*

INTRODUCTION

Psychiatrists will inevitably encounter patients with religious and spiritual experiences
in the course of clinical work. Was Dr. A's experience with her patient unusual? The
answer is no. In *American Grace*, Putnam and Campbell write that people in the
United States have high rates of religious belonging, behaving, and believing.[1,p7] In
their 2006–2007 national surveys, "83% report belonging to a religion; 40% report
attending religious services nearly every week or more; 59% pray at least weekly; a
third report reading scripture with this same frequency . . . 44% said a prayer before
each meal.[1,p7-8] These statistics are not stable, but dynamic. The United States is a
highly fluid environment where religions compete, adapt, and evolve, where religiosity is a preference rather than a fixed characteristic.[1,p4] There are radical changes,
including young people reacting against trends of the previous generation, and polarization of religion with politics.[1,p1-37]

But even as organized religion changes, religiosity and spirituality remain prominent features of American life. In 2012 and 2015, the Pew Research Center reported on the "Nones," adults with no religious affiliation. This growing segment
represented roughly 20% of the general population, and 32% of all 18- to 29-year-
olds in the general population in 2012.[2] Sixty-eight percent of the religiously unaffil-
iated say they believe in God; 58% say they often feel a deep connection with nature
and the earth; 37% classify themselves as "spiritual" but not "religious"; and 21%
say they pray every day.[2,p9-10] Numbering 56 million adults by 2015, this group was
more numerous than either Catholics or mainline Protestants in the 2015 survey.[3]
While these mainstream surveys cannot capture every nuance and orientation, they
do support that asking patients about their religious and spiritual practices is likely
to reveal a significant dimension of their lives. For patients for whom these practices
are important, asking can help improve physician–patient alliance.

Psychiatrist and medical historian Samuel Thielman notes that "physicians who have treated mental disorders, and the sufferers of mental disorders, have inevitably had to face the problem of how the spiritual and religious dimensions of human experience relate to madness in all its various manifestations."[4,p18] Matching the findings in *American Grace* and by the Pew Research Center about religion and spirituality in the general life of the U.S. public, Best and colleagues' 2015 review of 54 studies supports that many patients are interested in discussing religion and spirituality in the context of their medical care.[5] Psychiatric illnesses inevitably raise questions about meaning. And patients want to talk.

So how do you ask patients if religion/spirituality is important to them? What is religion and spirituality, and how do we understand it in relation to patient care?

How religious/spiritual needs are best addressed in medical and psychiatric care is an ongoing dialogue in the literature. The history of psychiatry has partly been defined in opposition to spirituality and religion, and psychiatrists have tended to pathologize religiosity in patients. Both patients and psychiatrists who wish to include discussion of religious and spiritual experience have met resistance in the clinical realm. However, studies and research on this issue now broadly support the position that integration of religion and spirituality in medical care is beneficial for patients.[6] Furthermore, clinician-researchers have developed interviewing tools that help medical teams assess the religious/spiritual dimensions of patients' life experience in relation to their treatment. This will be discussed later in "Clinical Tools."

However, despite research findings and the development of tools for integrating religious/spiritual assessment into medical care, discomfort, lack of training, and experience remain obstacles for many physicians. The clinical vignette illustrates a case in psychiatry. When a patient presents, whether or not he or she explicitly brings religious and spiritual concerns, the questions facing psychiatrists are: What is in the patient's best interest? What is the benefit or harm of exploring this aspect of the patient's experience at this moment in treatment? Am I supposed to be talking about this with patients? If so, how do I go about it?

These are the questions we address in this chapter. We provide a synthesis of current research and historical trends, discuss a training seminar for residents to discuss the issue, and summarize the growth in training methods in residency programs. We aim to support growth, training, and comfort discussing religion and spirituality in a clinical setting.

We posit that religion and spirituality are complex realms of human experience that we must explore if we are to understand our patients' concepts of their inner lives, how they create meaning and cope with uncertainty, how they find connection to themselves and to something beyond themselves, and how they heal, whether or not cure is possible. This is brought vividly to life by Ms. B, who recovered from her psychotic episode, but was left with sadness and internal conflict about her spirituality, and trying to find meaning in her experience. It is not the psychiatrist's role to determine whether religious or spiritual experience is harmful or beneficial (we recognize it can be both) but rather to create and hold an interpersonal space where this aspect of the patient's life may emerge and be fully included, not compartmentalized. What's best for the patient? Include all dimensions of experience. The central challenge remains: Many doctors are not comfortable addressing religion and spirituality with patients.

In training residents, summarizing different religious belief systems and various cultures' spiritual practices and traditions can lead us to believe we know something useful when we may not. Therefore, in this chapter we offer an orientation of exploration, an experiential model for training residents that values a non-knowing stance and fosters inquiry. This is our unique contribution to this field.

THE PROBLEM OF DEFINING RELIGION AND SPIRITUALITY

There are many definitions of religion and spirituality. Grappling with how to define these broad, complex terms is a recurrent theme in the literature, especially for medicine as a scientific practice. Koenig and colleagues note the importance of establishing clear, distinct definitions for the purposes of research, because if a construct is not defined, it cannot be accurately measured.[6,p36] In this light, they attempt to synthesize the definitions of many studies.

Most researchers agree that religion "involves beliefs, practices, and rituals related to the sacred."[6] An extended definition of religion is

> a multidimensional construct that includes beliefs, behaviors, rituals, and ceremonies that may be held or practiced in private or public settings, but are in some way derived from established traditions that developed over time within a community. Religion is also an organized system of beliefs, practices, and symbols designed (a) to facilitate closeness to the transcendent, and (b) to foster an understanding of one's relationship and responsibility to others living together in a community.[7]

Defining spirituality is more difficult because it is a broad concept that has changed over time. Currently, U.S. culture includes the definition of spirituality distinct from religion. Several national surveys on religion and civic life have included the categories "spiritual but not religious" and "no religious affiliation," which can include a range of people from those who do not identify with a religion to those who are atheist.[8] Traditions such as Buddhism, Hinduism, Islam, and Sikhism, present in the United States in smaller numbers, further broaden the scope of religious practice and what identifying with a specific tradition means.[1] Putnam and Campbell note that America's dynamic changes in immigration and politics have guaranteed a rich and pluralistic history that produces multiple interpretations to what people practice, how people relate, and what people think.[1,p1-37] Agreeing with Putnam and Campbell about the plurality of choice, and aligning with an understanding of Americans as individuals, Koenig and colleagues observe that "spirituality is increasingly viewed as a broader concept each individual defines for himself or herself."[6]

---

1. Putnam and Campbell write on page 31 in *American Grace* that although these traditions are different in other countries, once these traditions enter the United States, they take on some of the congregational structures of U.S. mainstream traditions. For example, Islamic mosques implemented Sunday school, and became membership groups instead of places people stop in to pray in transit in daily life.

In research, the words "religion" and "spirituality" are frequently combined using the abbreviation "R/S." However, there are inconsistencies in how this abbreviation is defined between research articles, and attempts to consider each term separately. We will not resolve these difficulties, but we wish to acknowledge them. Clinical experience rarely conforms to the constraints of research. Our goal as clinicians is to be aware of the plurality of experience and definitions, and to be open to patients' experience and how their experience informs our care.

CLINICAL TOOLS

Clinical interviewing tools have been developed to incorporate religion and spirituality assessment in medical care. Many instruments are reported in the literature. Of those, several have been validated.[9,10] Generally these tools refer to "spiritual" assessment, omitting "religion" and "religious," although they typically include questions about participation in organized religion as well as about spiritual experience.[11] The word "spiritual" is used more often in the medical literature, and only sometimes along with "religion" or "religious." We have chosen to use both terms together in most instances.

The most widely used tools are the FICA,[12] SPIRITual,[13] and HOPE[11] assessments. These tools provide prompts for starting a conversation with patients. The FICA and HOPE acronyms are paraphrased as:

Faith—Do you have faith or beliefs? Or, what gives your life meaning?

Importance—How important is your faith; how does it influence your life?

Community—Are you part of a faith community? Who are the people most important to you?

Address—How would you like this addressed in your medical care?[14]

H—sources of Hope, strength, comfort, meaning, peace, love, and connection.

O—the role of Organized religion in the patient's life.

P—Personal spirituality and practices.

E—Effects on medical care.[11]

George Vaillant provides a way to think about religion and spirituality in the context of clinical care using biological and psychological language. In *Spiritual Evolution: A Scientific Defense of Faith*, Vaillant posits that religious dogma resides in the neocortex, whereas spirituality is generated by the emotional brain.[15] He views religion as "the best means that humanity has found for bringing the positive emotions into conscious reflection."[15,p17] He argues that positive emotions are the common denominator of all major faiths and all human beings.[15,p3] He describes spirituality as "the amalgam of the positive emotions that bind us to other human beings and to our experience of 'God' as we may understand Her/Him. Love, hope, joy, forgiveness, compassion, faith, awe, and gratitude."[15,p5] He further states, "Positive emotions cannot be distinguished from what people understand as spirituality."[15,p15] Spirituality is the amalgam of positive emotions; religion is the means for bringing them into conscious reflection.

Vaillant's definitions are broad but may feel more intuitive for the clinician because he offers a framework for listening to patients. He uses a concept familiar to psychiatrists—positive emotions. While in research we may want to distinguish positive emotions from spirituality, in clinical work asking about the latter can help elucidate the former and vice versa. When a patient speaks of or expresses these emotions, these may be cues we can follow, and in the process, help our patients access an important dimension of their experience, regardless how this experience is labeled.

One of our physician colleagues, who attends Unitarian Universalist services, built on Vaillant's definition by reflecting that there is more to spirituality than positive emotions. All religions and traditions of faith are distinguished by their respective stories. When speaking about spirituality, most people eventually tell personal stories of meaningful experiences and relationships. These stories often have moral implications, which are more or less explicit. Spiritual experience, then, in addition to being an experience of positive emotions, is linked to the experience of meaning and to our conscience that acts as a guide to the rightness or wrongness of our behavior. In the words of a contemporary Unitarian Universalist minister: "It is looking out at the world from a particular perspective, and using that perspective to consider the meaning of our existence."[16]

The tension between research definitions and clinical experience can be productive. Religion is not something that exists purely as a conceptual category. Asking whether religion/spirituality is important to our patients is trying to look out at the world from their perspective. In later vignettes, Dr. A begins to explore "if spirituality is finding connection and making meaning" in aligning with her patients' experiences.

TAKING A RELIGIOUS AND SPIRITUAL HISTORY IS FREQUENTLY NEGLECTED IN CLINICAL PRACTICE

Dr. A reflects on an encounter with a young man on the psychiatric inpatient unit early in her residency training. She enquired into the man's spiritual experience and was criticized by the treatment team for doing so:

I thought back to the first time I had talked with a patient about his experience with psychiatric illness. The patient had been psychotic and was starting to improve. He tried to explain his suffering, of feeling robbed of his sense of self after starting an antipsychotic medication. He was not angry or disorganized; he was just sad. Noticing this during morning rounds, I asked him to say more. He spoke in detail about feeling isolated from himself and from his connection to a higher power. I distinctly remember feeling I'd gained a more nuanced understanding of his value system, his way of finding meaning in his existence, and his subsequent opposition to taking medication. However, I was later criticized by the treatment team for allowing him to take up precious time during rounds to "talk about unrelated topics." In reflecting on this experience more than a year later, I realized that I'd started residency more open to listening and asking about spirituality but had not been encouraged to do so in my role as a physician. Later in my training, I no longer considered discussion of spirituality to be within my purview as a psychiatrist, and that furthermore, such discussion was potentially even a poor or ineffective use of time. Someone else would do that.

Despite the availability of clinical tools, and the general literature consensus that physicians should ask patients about religion and spirituality, studies show that few physicians routinely do. In a review of 61 studies, physicians reported that lack of time and inadequate training were the most significant barriers.[17] Fears about difference and about being alienated or judged may contribute to patients' reluctance. Puchalski observes that patients need permission, some signal from physicians that these topics are appropriate and welcome.[12] As physicians, our feelings of uncertainty and vulnerability, the presence of countertransference reactions, and fears of being different or appearing ignorant may contribute to our reluctance to broach the topic with our patients. As illustrated by Dr. A's account, there also seems to be a lingering bias or unspoken taboo in our field against speaking about religion and spirituality with patients. Dr. A was left with the sense that a psychiatrist's role precludes asking questions about religion or spirituality. A brief review of the historical relationship of psychiatry and religion offers insight.

HISTORICAL ROOTS TO TODAY'S RELATIONSHIP BETWEEN RELIGION AND PSYCHIATRY

Ferngren describes in *Medicine and Religion* that through most of history, religion and medicine have been interrelated. In prehistoric and tribal cultures, shamans or religious leaders were the healers. In medieval Europe, all matters were seen through a religious worldview, including physical ailments.[18] Today, in developed countries, medicine and religion are separate domains, although there is less separation in developing countries.[6,p15-34] Numerous articles and books explore the history of the relationship between religion and medicine. The realms have often been described as opposed to one another, but contemporary historians of science and medicine such as John Brooke, Ronald Numbers, and David Lindberg view this conflict model of the relationship as simplistic.[18,p4] In fact, medicine and religion/spirituality share complex and intertwined histories. Tensions have existed historically, more intense in some eras than others. But this reflects an ongoing dialogue between medicine and religion/spirituality. There is a centuries-long tradition of exploring the relationship between religion/spirituality and mental disorders, and that tradition has been in continual evolution.[4] In the late 19th century, medicine was openly anti-religion when psychiatry was emerging as a distinct specialty seeking credibility as a scientific field. Psychiatry aligned with science through opposition to spirituality and religion.

Freud's many critiques of religious belief and practice furthered the bias of psychiatry against religion.[19] And though not all early psychiatrists agreed with Freud's views of religion, his ideas have significantly influenced the field's development. Writing in 1998 on the theoretical issues in research on religion and mental health, Levin and Chatters state, "It is important first to recognize that psychiatry and the mental health field continue to embody an active prejudice (of long standing) against issues of a religious nature."[20,p45] They support the view that the bias stems both from Freud and from the larger tensions between religion and science. The DSM-III-R[21] (1987) illustrates this bias: It was criticized by researchers for its frequent but unsubstantiated use of religious examples to illustrate psychopathology.[4] The DSM-IV-R[22] (1995) included revisions that acknowledge the importance of religion and spirituality and omitted potentially offensive references to religion.[4] The DSM-IV included for the first time the diagnostic category "religious or spiritual problem," under the heading "Other Conditions Which May be the Focus of Clinical Attention."[22] Turner and colleagues said that this change, among several, "contributes significantly to the greater cultural sensitivity incorporated into the DSM-IV."[23] Further, "the new category could help to promote a new relationship between psychiatry and the fields of religion and spirituality that will benefit both mental health professionals and those who seek their assistance."[23]

Modern-day ethical concerns that physicians could impose their religious views on patients contribute to the current tensions between medicine and religion/spirituality. Ethicist Stephen Post compares this more recent historical trend to the separation of church and state in our country proposed by Thomas Jefferson, saying there exists "a Jeffersonian wall of separation between the spheres of allopathic practice and religion and spirituality."[24,p21-22] He explains that while this separation may protect vulnerable patients from proselytizing doctors on the one hand, it "has also blinded some clinicians to the importance of spiritual and religious concerns in the patient."[24]

Our interest in this chapter is not to try to resolve the historical tensions but to acknowledge them, and to reside within them with an attitude of curiosity—the same stance we hold in psychotherapy.

THE PENDULUM SWINGS BACK

The pendulum is swinging back in the direction of integration for medicine and religion/spirituality. This is evidenced by the rapidly expanding body of research pioneered by nursing and palliative care since 1990. Another example is the treatment of addiction since the founding of Alcoholics Anonymous in 1935. According to Dermatis and Galanter, the spirituality and religiosity characteristics supported by AA, such as feeling God's presence daily and believing in a higher power as a universal spirit, were predictive of positive outcomes for people in recovery from substance use disorders.[25]

The most authoritative synthesis for integration is found in *The Handbook of Religion and Health* by Koenig and colleagues, a seminal research text on religion, spirituality, and health that reviews evidence for the connection between religion and health. The 2012 second edition reviews 2,100 quantitative research papers on religion and health published between 2000 and 2010. The 2001 first edition reviews research prior to 2000. The handbook's editor, Koenig, reviews the handbook and several other publications to highlight eight reasons for clinicians to ask about patients' religion/spirituality experience (paraphrased):

1. Many medical and psychiatric patients are religious or spiritual, and the majority have unmet spiritual needs related to medical or psychiatric illness. Unmet spiritual needs can adversely affect health.
2. Religion/spirituality influences the patient's coping; poor coping can adversely affect outcomes.
3. Religious/spiritual beliefs affect patients' medical decision-making, may conflict with medical treatments, and can influence compliance.

4. Physicians' own religious and spiritual beliefs often influence the medical decisions they make and affect the type of care they offer to patients.

5. Religion/spirituality is associated with both mental and physical health and likely affects medical outcomes.

6. Religion/spirituality influences the kind of support and care that patients receive once they return home and thus impacts adherence to treatment and follow-up.

7. Research shows that failure to address patients' spiritual needs increases health care costs.

8. Accreditation standards set by the Joint Commission and by Medicare (in the United States) require that providers of health care show respect for patients' cultural and personal values, beliefs, and preferences (including religious or spiritual beliefs).[7]

The Joint Commission also requires a spiritual assessment of patients.[26]

DR. A CONTINUES HER WORK WITH MS. B.

I decided that in order to truly understand my patient, I had to understand what gave meaning to her life. I decided to delve right in by asking her.

Over the next few sessions, Ms. B told me that she continued to download religious music and to buy books about all different religions. What struck me was her tone of voice. She stated these things like she expected to be punished. Initially, these "confessions" made my heart race. Was she becoming psychotic? Or was her exploration of religion within the scope of normal human curiosity and experience? I grounded myself as a new clinician in the more objective measurements of her functioning. She was not hearing voices. There were no ideas of reference. She continued to go to work and finish her assignments on time. She saw her family on the weekends, made her own meals, and showered daily. With that in mind, I got a hold of my fear. She was still clinically stable, and I reassured her I was interested in what brought meaning to her life: The space we'd create together was not to punish her for listening to a song or reading about religion but rather to explore what she experienced from these activities. She was holding significant internal conflict: She had been told that the thing that brought her the most peace was also what made her the sickest.

I appreciated that it was not my role to discourage Ms. B from religious and spiritual exploration, but to foster a trusting relationship in treatment so that she could discuss these experiences. My hope was to communicate an open, nonjudgmental stance.

Ms. B said she felt good and connected to people around her when she listened to religious music or read religious texts. She also understood that she'd been hospitalized when her "curiosity spiraled out of control." Over time, by allowing her to explore what she gained from religious exploration, we were able to better distinguish between her need to connect with a higher power from the perseverative thought processes that would predominate during times of high stress or isolation.

I understood my role was to treat my patient's psychosis and also to help ease her internal conflict. I became more comfortable in my ability to assess for clinical decompensation and risk and more able to welcome my patient's search for a greater purpose in life, in this case through religious means.

A SEMINAR FOR RESIDENTS: ORIENTATION AND GOALS

Dr. A's descriptions of her work with Ms. B illustrate several of the themes we have discussed:

1. Psychiatrists are faced with the problem of how the religious and spiritual dimensions of experience relate to mental illness.
2. Many patients want to talk about their religious and spiritual experience.
3. Many psychiatrists and other physicians feel unprepared or find it uncomfortable to engage patients in a conversation about their religious and spiritual experience.
4. There is a lingering bias in our field against including discussion of religion and spirituality in the clinical realm.
5. Psychiatrists can develop the capacity and flexibility as clinicians to address their patient's religious and spiritual experiences in the service of the treatment.
6. Including this exploration can strengthen the treatment alliance, supporting the patient's coping with and understanding of his or her illness and strengthening the patient's overall adherence and response to treatment.

Gaining comfort and experience working with the religious and spiritual experience of patients is the goal of the 2-hour seminar I, Dr. O'Neill, teach to third-year psychiatry residents in their "Sociocultural Psychiatry Course" at the Harvard Medical School MGH/McLean Psychiatry Residency Program. Through teaching psychiatry residents for 15 years and trying many formats, I gradually developed the seminar outlined below. Although remediating a knowledge gap might be crucial in working with a patient from a particular background, I found that, given the limited time available, there was limited utility in teaching content from the endlessly complex and diverse range of religious beliefs and practices. Similarly, there is limited utility for us clinicians to know all of the research about integrating religion and spirituality into clinical care if we cannot examine and work through our own resistance to doing so.

We work best with patients when we are grounded in experiential practice and knowledge of ourselves. Therefore, the seminar is experiential. I demonstrate a conversation about religious and spiritual experience. We also consider what gets in the way of this conversation. Residents want to increase their comfort and decrease their anxiety about talking with patients. We accomplish this by doing together what we encourage the residents to do with their patients: We talk about our own religious and spiritual histories. Following a brief introduction, the learning is completely experiential. This is a conscious shift away from the medical cultural norm of "knowing information" toward getting to know another human being.

We have discussed the evidence, which supports asking patients about their spirituality. Why a seminar on how to talk with patients about religion and spirituality? Despite the availability of multiple clinical screening tools, the vast majority of physicians still do not engage their patients in this discussion. The difficulty seems to be lack of training, discomfort, anxiety, and unspoken bias. The seminar addresses these barriers:

1. Demonstrating method: Start with the concrete. What do we ask patients? Having direction decreases anxiety.

2. Practicing/working toward mastery: Practicing a conversation in a contained setting with peers prepares us to facilitate the same conversation with patients. The lived, direct experience offers powerful learning. This is about doing instead of talking about doing. Residents see and hear me share my spiritual biography. They share theirs, listen to their peers, and ask one another questions. By practicing, residents are more likely to experience a sense of competence. We are more comfortable and less anxious when we feel competent.

3. Self-exploration: For psychiatrists, self-exploration is vital. We are the instrument; self-exploration helps us tune our instrument. We notice our own experience and let it inform our interaction with the patient. We can notice our own discomfort, name it, and nonetheless accomplish the task we would rather avoid.

4. Confronting bias: As we have noted, there is some bias against talking about religion and spirituality in psychiatry. We work toward overcoming this bias by bringing the conversation into the open and giving residents practice in a safe setting.

5. Normalizing the process: We must constantly practice in order to ask people complex questions about their private, inner lives. Our discomfort is conveyed to our patients and may unwittingly discourage their openness. We become accustomed to asking sensitive questions by asking them again and again. The seminar offers normalization through repetition. By the end of the two-hour seminar, we have heard 12 to 15 spiritual histories, each told in a unique manner.

6. Reducing anxiety and shame: Experiencing anxiety and shame when trying something new or unfamiliar is normal. Experiencing anxiety discussing deeply personal aspects of one's or another's experience is also normal. One antidote to shame is openness about that which is shameful. When I am open about my own feelings of anxiety, anxiety is normalized and shame is reduced. Ideally the resident comes away with the sense, "Okay, I can do this. I can notice this makes me a little uncomfortable, but I've done this before. I have a sense of the terrain . . . I can relax with my patient into this conversation, into the unknown, because the process is not a total unknown."

7. Cultivating curiosity: The seminar supports residents in moving toward curiosity when they approach challenging conversations. The stance is "What is this, and does it relate to me personally? Even if it does not, how might it relate to the patient in front of me?" It is difficult to feel curious when we are anxious, which is why we address anxiety.

Over the years I have worked with residents using this format, their feedback has been overwhelmingly positive—both the formal feedback given to the training program and the informal feedback offered to me after class or weeks later in the clinic hallway. The feedback is not only that the seminar is useful for practice, but that it feels like a meaningful experience.

Though there is usually some discomfort at the beginning, by the end of our time together, the group finds a way to be comfortable enough with one another in conversation about religion and spirituality. They voice surprise in discovering they have worked with one another closely in an intense training environment for two to three years, yet sometimes do not know details about the deeper aspects of each other's lives. They note the universality of spiritual experience or questioning. Occasionally, someone declines to share, but in general almost everyone has a lot to say. They curiously ask questions they have never asked one another before. A number of residents have said this seminar is a powerful experience unlike previous learning experiences. They note the high level of engagement among the participants and greatly appreciate getting to know one another better.

Overview of the Seminar

I begin by offering working definitions of religion and spirituality and briefly outline the relevance to patient care in psychiatry. Next, I set the frame and delineate the goals and working agreement for the remainder of the seminar. Then I share my own spiritual history as a model before inviting residents to share their histories. The emphasis is on inviting a conversation. I make clear that although there is the invitation to share, this is not a requirement for participation in the seminar; listening with curiosity is a form of engagement. Residents take turns telling their histories. They ask one another questions. Usually the conversation naturally evolves toward a discussion of religious and spiritual issues in the care of their patients. If not, I ask. At the end, we discuss how they felt about this seminar, what they learned, and what surprised them. Below, I discuss the main components in greater detail.

The frame and working agreements are fundamental. Knowing what to expect helps participants feel contained and safe. Establishing and maintaining a secure frame increases the possibility of true connection. The frame includes the time boundary (e.g., we will meet for the next two hours, we will end on time), the physical space (e.g., the chairs are set up in a circle, ideally without a table in the middle, in a private room with the door closed), the designated leader, and the participants (physicians in the residency class). The working agreement promotes an attitude of respect and full attention. It supports openness and trust. I let participants know that all are invited, not required to share. I ask all participants to agree to the following:

1. Maintain confidentiality (what is said in the group stays in the group).
2. Put away electronic devices.
3. Listen to one another respectfully.
4. Be as fully present as possible.
5. Stay for duration of the seminar.

The explicit request to maintain confidentiality helps establish trust.

Regarding electronic devices, I let participants know that they will not need their laptops to take notes, and they do not need their phones; we are focusing on experience. Turkle, an MIT sociologist who studies the effect of digital devices on conversation, observes that "even a silent phone inhibits conversations that matter.

The very sight of a phone on the landscape leaves us feeling less connected to each other, less invested in each other."[27,p4] If spirituality is about finding connection and making meaning, we want to model the circumstances that make this possible. Removing devices decreases distractions and implies we will be entirely present to one another. I reinforce the message that this seminar conversation is important. Occasionally some residents say they would like to use their electronic devices to take notes, perhaps as an anxiety reducer in the situation. I reassure and reiterate the request, explaining that we are focusing on being present. Devices interfere with our presence.

I then invite the group to share their spiritual histories. I ask, "What was your religious and spiritual upbringing, if any? How has that affected your experience of life and view of the world? How have your beliefs and practices changed over time? What influenced and informed these changes? What are your current beliefs and practices, if any? How do your beliefs influence and inform your reactions when patients raise religious and spiritual issues? How do you feel, sharing this aspect of your life here in this setting? How is it to listen to others?"

The first time I used this format, I asked for a volunteer to begin. No one said a word. I have a significant tolerance for silence, but I quickly appreciated that participants felt too exposed to begin. So instead, I began by sharing my history. After I shared my history, participants readily volunteered to share theirs. I now begin as a matter of course. I model the desired behavior. This imparts information and encourages imitative behavior, two therapeutic factors in experiential learning groups.[28,p8–12,17–18] I illustrate what is meant by spiritual history, and I demonstrate how one person talks about her journey, inviting participants to try something similar. My beginning breaks the ice and relieves the pressure on participants. I am surprised every year by the anxiety I feel before I share my journey. I am reminded that this is likely what participants are feeling. In part, I am feeling the anxiety of the group, and I'm reminded that this may also be what our patients feel. I often comment on my anxiety to the group to normalize anxiety they may be feeling. This discomfort is important and comes with the territory; almost always, it subsides. As the group members experience each other's engagement and interest, their anxiety subsides and curiosity and surprise emerge.

What I share:

My parents met teaching public high school soon after they left Catholic religious orders: My father had been a Jesuit for 12 years, and my mother a Franciscan nun for 16. They loved their religious communities and in many ways sought to reestablish a spiritual community in family life. The nuns and the Jesuits were a significant presence in our lives, both those who were still living in community and those, like my parents, who had left their orders.

My sisters and I were raised deeply Catholic, with rituals and traditions following the church calendar. We went to Mass on Sundays and holy days. We celebrated the feast days of the saints, said the rosary, kept vigils, fasted, and offered up our suffering for hungry children and peace in the world. This was well suited to my personality—introspective and contemplative. At 13, my mother introduced me to yoga by giving me a book for Christmas. Yoga also suited my contemplative nature.

I realized from a very early age that what mattered most was my relationship to self, others, and the larger mystery that connects us all. My decision to study medicine was surely influenced by my spiritual orientation—it was a calling.

I met my husband during residency training. I was drawn to him immediately. I learned he was living with Jesuits in Chinatown, and that he practiced yoga; clearly, we would suit each other. At that time, he was considering entering the Jesuit order himself. His plans changed. We were married by two Jesuit priests, one a close friend of my husband's and the other an old friend of my father's.

We went to Mass for a time and then gradually stopped. I deepened my yoga practice. After our sons were born, we began to think more about religious education for our children. We went back to the Catholic church but found ourselves challenged by its stance toward women and homosexuals. We grieved the widespread abuse of children and the failure of the church leadership to respond. We concluded we would not raise our children Catholic.

We joined a Buddhist sangha. For my husband, this was a return to the practices of his young adulthood. For me, though new, joining the sangha felt like a natural progression and complement to my yoga practice. I also recognized in Buddhism some of the elements that I found grounding in Catholicism, particularly the idea that any moment in life can be a spiritual practice.

Through friends in our sangha we found our way to the Unitarian Universalist church in our community. Here we found a spiritual home for our whole family. Today, we continue to practice and study Buddhist meditation. I am pursuing studies in the integration of yoga, meditation, and psychological work.

My spiritual history has had a profound influence on my professional development and practice. I had a mentor in residency who supported my interest in religion and spirituality and encouraged me toward a training program in spiritual psychology. She then invited me to develop a curriculum to teach residents about the importance of discussing religion and spirituality with patients, and how to approach this discussion.

My ongoing spiritual practices have supported my development as a person and as a clinician. Though I typically do not discuss my own views with patients, I communicate my interest in spirituality by inviting patients to talk about their experience of religion and spirituality, how their experience informs and supports their growth and wellness, as well as the ways their experience has contributed to their woundedness. I often encounter my practice of psychotherapy as a spiritual endeavor.

When I finish speaking, I reiterate that the history I've just recounted to participants is one version of my experience. My history continues to evolve. Each person will have something different to say and his or her own way of doing so. I ask, "Would someone else like to share?" It usually takes only a few seconds for someone to say, "I guess I will."

Participants take turns in no specific order. Sometimes, others ask questions for clarification or to know more, generating discussion. The overarching tone is respectful inquiry and curiosity. Rarely, there are one or two people who say little or nothing at all. Participants often reiterate the invitation with encouragement. For example, one resident might say to another, "I notice you have been quiet. If you would like to speak, I am interested in what you have to say." Each resident spends between one and five minutes speaking.

When all participants who wish to share have done so, I thank the group members for their willingness to be present and to share their experience with one another. I ask how this felt. There are usually quite a few reactions.

We then move into a discussion of their work with patients. I ask if anyone would like to share material from their cases in which themes of religion and spirituality seemed present. Residents share psychotherapy cases and also present patients they met in the acute psychiatric service, and in consultations on the medical and surgical floors. We turn our attention to not only what the patients said, but how they spoke—reluctantly or openly, with affect or detachment. We discuss how we as clinicians might ask patients about their lives in such a way that welcomes the patient's full experience.

Dr. A Reflects on Her Experience of the Seminar

I sat in a circle with my peers, and I felt exposed. My anxiety rose as my turn approached. We had been asked to share our experience with religion and spirituality during our upbringing, as well as our current beliefs and practice. This self-reflection made me aware of the inconsistency in my internal life during residency. Although I come from an incredibly religious family, one that used religion as a strong identity criterion, I didn't practice any of the rituals I'd been taught by my father all those years ago. I talked about and wanted to reengage in the meditation I'd learned as a teenager battling anxiety in high school, but even that had gone by the wayside. I wondered if I'd only been enamored with the idea of meditation as a calming and centering force. I looked around, wondering if my classmates would consider me a fraud. I was curious about their responses. None of them were Hindu, so did we share the same definition of spirituality?

As each took their turn, I appreciated we represented a continuum of experiences. Some spoke of spirituality not necessarily in terms of specific religion or practice, but rather how they chose to relate to others. They spoke of how they integrate the experiences of their lives to create meaning and a way forward. Some, surprisingly, had a lot to say. Others shared very little. Each talked about their families and up-bringing, the ways that religion, community, and family bonds were communicated to them. Though I found the nuances of our individual experiences as varied as one might expect from residents of different countries, it was clear that each person in the room had spent time contemplating these questions, whatever conclusions they reached.

Education and Training on Religion and Spirituality: Psychiatry Residencies in Context

The growing evidence supporting integration of religion and spirituality in medicine has prompted significant developments in education and training. In 1990, few psychiatry residency programs in the United States reported training residents in these topics.[29] By 2006, 32 psychiatry residency programs in the United States had received grants from the National Institute for Healthcare Research and the John Templeton Foundation to develop curricula on spirituality in medicine.[30]

The developments in medical education extend well beyond psychiatry. In 1992, only three of 125 medical schools in the United States offered courses in spirituality and medicine; by 2001, that number had risen to 72.[31] By 2000, Puchalski, who developed the FICA questionnaire as a spiritual assessment tool, had traveled all over the country and trained 4,000 practicing physicians and other health care professionals in spiritual assessment.[32]

Curricular development in psychiatric residencies grew in part in response to requirements by the American Council on Graduate Medical Education (ACGME). In 1994, the ACGME mandated that residents in psychiatry receive instruction about religious and spiritual influences on human development across the lifespan, and about the religious and spiritual aspects of culture, important for understanding patients from diverse backgrounds. In 1995, the American Psychiatric Association Practice Guidelines were updated with the recommendation that evaluations be "sensitive to the patient's . . . religious/spiritual beliefs."[33] The ACGME (item IV.A.5.b.2) continues to require that residents in psychiatry "demonstrate competence in their knowledge of . . . religious/spiritual . . . factors that significantly influence physical and psychological development throughout the life cycle."[34,p13]

Many curricula for psychiatric and family medicine residents have been described in the literature.[31,35-39] Most employ a combination of pedagogical approaches including lectures, small-group experiential learning, panel discussions, case conferences, and self-reflection. McCarthy and Peteet,[35] Grabovac and colleagues,[36] and McGovern and colleagues[37] have each highlighted the importance of addressing transference, countertransference, and ethical issues that may arise in the context of addressing these topics. Blass supports developing and refining clinical skills; he concludes, "Most clinical challenges emerging during psychiatric care of religious patients are better solved using refined clinical skills than by expecting the psychiatrist to retain exhaustive knowledge of each religion. . . . Psychiatric training programs should emphasize the goals and the methods of inquiring about the religious life of patients."[38,p30]

There are few reports in the literature on training outcomes. Anandarajah and colleagues completed an in-depth, qualitative evaluation of the longitudinal effects of a "Multifaceted Residency Spiritual Care Curriculum" (24 hours of instruction over three years) in a family medicine residency.[39] They compared participants to nonparticipants, measuring outcomes at the end of residency. They reevaluated participants eight years after graduation and concluded that "a longitudinal, multifaceted residency spiritual care curriculum can have lasting positive effects on physicians' spiritual care skills and their professional/personal formation."[39,p859] They found the most effective teaching formats were "structured spiritual self-care workshop/retreat, rounding with clinical chaplains, and patient-centered spiritual assessment skills training."[39,p869]

McGovern and colleagues found that the majority of participants in a curriculum that spanned three years of psychiatry presidency said the curriculum improved their clinical expertise and awareness regarding spiritual issues. Most considered the curriculum a helpful and meaningful experience, but responses were mixed regarding their perceived ability to take a spiritual history.[37] McCarthy and Peteet describe a required 12-hour course for PGY-4 psychiatry residents and feedback from participants. They found that "residents, no matter what their initial biases, have become more comfortable with, and more interested in addressing, patient's religious/ spiritual concerns."[35] They conclude that the "most successful sessions are actually those that help residents articulate what they themselves bring to their encounters with . . . patients."[35] They underscore the need to balance formal presentations with time for participants to reflect on their own concerns and to process differences that inevitably arise among participants. These reports support the importance of experiential learning and personal reflection.

The Harvard McLean/MGH Psychiatry residency program introduced a 10-hour curriculum in religion and spirituality in 2003. We employed a variety of teaching modalities, including review of the literature, lectures, panel discussions with clergy, small-group conversations, case conference, and experiential learning within the context of a year-long PGY-3 sociocultural psychiatry course. Due to increasing curricular demands in other areas, that time was gradually reduced. Five years ago we adopted the current format of a one-time, two-hour seminar, which emphasizes experiential learning and personal reflection.

Dr. A. Reflects on Subsequent Patient Interactions, Practicing What She Learned in the Seminar

I was asked to evaluate "suicidal ideation" in a man hospitalized for end-stage cancer. He told me he was in distress but would never commit suicide. He explained that suicide was against his belief system and that he was at peace with his illness. I asked, "Would you consider yourself a religious person? It sounds like faith brings you strength." With these questions, the patient opened up about his daily prayers, his strong belief in fate and karma, and his daily communication with close family and friends. These were the elements of his life that sustained him and calmed him, even in the face of death. It was an inspiring conversation that informed the psychiatric safety assessment and framed the treatment plan upon discharge. Ongoing contact with his priest would provide solace during his last weeks. I may never have gotten this full assessment if I had not asked him questions about where his strength comes from, and whether he was religious.

In the child and adolescent outpatient clinic, I met a young girl who had experienced sexual abuse that her parents were unaware of. She felt significant shame and guilt about the abuse and initially had difficulty sharing the extent of its effect on her. An important part of my assessment was exploring her understanding and internalization of the values and morals instilled by her parents. The strong religious fabric of her family life that consisted of weekly church, prayer, and Bible study seemed to compound her guilt and shame and at the same time to provide a valuable resource for coping and a sense of safety. The patient's confusion about this apparent contradiction, as well as the guilt and shame, contributed to her depression and anxiety symptoms. I would not have understood this without an exploration of her family and religious context.

CONCLUSION

Religion and spirituality are important dimensions of human experience that many patients would like to discuss with their physicians. Data show that patients benefit when physicians engage in this discussion, but few physicians routinely do. Lack of time, experience, and training are the main barriers. Trying to do something one does not feel competent to do leads to anxiety and avoidance. There is also a longstanding bias in psychiatry against religion and spirituality. These barriers and this bias are addressed in the experiential seminar for psychiatry residents that we described.

Physicians cannot be well versed in the myriad religious traditions and spiritual practices in the world. However, cultivating a curious stance and a willingness to confront one's own discomfort with asking patients about their particular beliefs, customs, and views provides deeply personal and relevant insights into our patients' inner lives. Our invitation and welcome can help our patients to feel seen and understood, the basis of any strong therapeutic alliance.

The exploration of spirituality also has the potential to increase the meaning physicians find in their work with patients. When we ask our patients about their spiritual lives, surprising, rich, painful, and inspiring conversations may be in store for us. Like discussions with patients about other realms of life, discussion about spirituality with patients may also cause us to reflect on our own spiritual experience or absence thereof, whether or not we have any formal practices. Such discussion is therefore an opportunity for our own personal growth and exploration. This enrichment in turn benefits the patient because the better we know ourselves, the more aware we are of our own emotions, reactions, and biases, and the more effective we are in our work with patients. Including the spiritual dimension of patients' lives and understanding their religious beliefs and practices increases our potential to be of greater service to our patients, to grow ourselves, to provide better care, and to achieve better outcomes.

ACKNOWLEDGMENT

The authors thank Drs. Karsten Kueppenbender and Robert Weber for their critical review and suggestions and Gloria J. Korsman, Research Librarian at Andover-Harvard Theological Library, for her help with literature searches and referencing.

REFERENCES

1. Putnam R, Campbell DE. *American Grace: How Religion Divides and Unites Us.* New York: Simon & Schuster; 2012.
2. Pew Research Center: The Pew Forum on Religion and Public Life. "Nones" on the rise: One in five adults have no religious affiliation. http://www.pewforum.org/files/2012/10/NonesOnTheRise-full.pdf. Published October 9, 2012. Accessed February 9, 2018.
3. Pew Research Center: Religion and Public Life. America's changing religious landscape.   http://www.pewforum.org/2015/05/12/americas-changing-religious-landscape/. Published May 12, 2015. Accessed February 9, 2018.
4. Thielman SB. Reflections on the role of religion in the history of psychiatry. In: Koenig HG, ed. *Handbook of Religion and Mental Health.* San Diego, CA: Academic Press; 1998:3–20.

5. Best M, Butow P, Olver I. Do patients want doctors to talk about spirituality? A systematic literature review. *Patient Educ Couns*. 2015;98(11):1320–1328.

6. Koenig HG, King DE, Carson VB. *Handbook of Religion and Health*. 2nd ed. New York: Oxford University Press; 2012.

7. Koenig HG. Religion, spirituality, and health: The research and clinical implications. *ISRN Psychiatry*. 2012;2012:278730.

8. Fuller RC. *Spiritual, But Not Religious: Understanding Unchurched America*. New York: Oxford University Press; 2001.

9. Borneman T, Ferrell B, Puchalski CM. Evaluation of the FICA Tool for Spiritual Assessment. *J Pain Symptom Manage*. 2010;40(2):163–173.

10. Moreira-Almeida A, Koenig HG, Lucchetti G. Clinical implications of spirituality to mental health: Review of evidence and practical guidelines. *Rev Bras Psiquiatr*. 2014;36(2):176–182.

11. Anandarajah G, Hight E. Spirituality and medical practice: Using HOPE questions as a practical tool for spiritual assessment. *Am Fam Physician*. 2001;63(1):81–89.

12. Puchalski CM, Romer AL. Taking a spiritual history allows clinicians to understand patients more fully. *J Palliat Med*. 2000;3(1):129–137.

13. Maugans TA. The SPIRITual history. *Arch Fam Med*. 1996;5(1):11–16.

14. Puchalski CM. FICA Spiritual History Tool. https://smhs.gwu.edu/gwish/clinical/fica/spiritual-history-tool. Accessed November 29, 2017.

15. Vaillant GE. *Spiritual Evolution: A Scientific Defense of Faith*. 1st ed. New York: Broadway Books; 2008.

16. Kanter DC. Faith for the Unbeliever. *UU World*. https://www.uuworld.org/articles/faith-unbeliever. Published November 1, 2017. Accessed November 18, 2017.

17. Best M, Butow P, Olver I. Doctors discussing religion and spirituality: A systematic literature review. *Palliat Med*. 2016;30(4):327–337.

18. Ferngren GB. *Medicine and Religion: A Historical Introduction*. Baltimore, MD: Johns Hopkins University Press; 2014.

19. Freud S, Erikson EH, Strachey J, Freud A. *The Standard Edition of the Complete Psychological Works of Sigmund Freud*. London: Hogarth Press; 1953.

20. Levin JS, Chatters LM. Research on religion and mental health: An overview of empirical findings and theoretical issues. In: Koenig HG, ed. *Handbook of Religion and Mental Health*. San Diego, CA: Academic Press; 1998:33–50.

21. American Psychiatric Association. *Diagnostic and Statistical Manual of Mental Disorders: DSM-III-R*. 3rd rev. ed. Washington, DC: American Psychiatric Press; 1987.

22. American Psychiatric Association. *Diagnostic and Statistical Manual of Mental Disorders: DSM-IV-TR*. 4th text rev. ed. Washington, DC: American Psychiatric Association; 2000.

23. Turner RP, Lukoff D, Barnhouse RT, Lu FG. Religious or spiritual problem. A culturally sensitive diagnostic category in the DSM-IV. *J Nerv Ment Dis*. 1995;183(7):435–444.

24. Post SG. Ethics, religion, and mental health. In: Koenig HG, ed. *Handbook of Religion and Mental Health*. San Diego, CA: Academic Press; 1998:21–29.

25. Dermatis H, Galanter M. The role of twelve-step-related spirituality in addiction recovery. *J Relig Health*. 2016;55(2):510–521.

26. Hodge DR. A template for spiritual assessment: A review of the JCAHO requirements and guidelines for implementation. *Soc Work*. 2006;51(4):317–326.

27. Turkle S. *Reclaiming Conversation: The Power of Talk in a Digital Age*. New York: Penguin Press; 2015.

28. Yalom ID, Leszcz M. The therapeutic factors. In: *The Theory and Practice of Group Psychotherapy*. 5th ed. New York: Basic Books; 2008:1–18.

29. Sansome RA, Khatain K, Rodenhauser P. The role of religion in psychiatric education: A national survey. *Acad Psychiatry*. 1990;14:34–38.

30. The GW Institute for Spirituality and Health website. http://www.smhs.gwu.edu/gwish/education/awards. Accessed February 14, 2018.

31. Puchalski C, Larson DB, Lu F. Spirituality in psychiatry residency training programs. *Int Rev Psychiatry*. 2001;13:131–138.

32. Puchalski C, Romer AL. Taking a spiritual history allows clinicians to understand patients more fully. *J Palliat Med*. 2000;3(1):129–137.

33. American Psychiatric Association. Practice guidelines for the psychiatric evaluation of adults. *Am J Psychiatry*. 1995; 152(11 suppl):63–80.

34. Accreditation Council for Graduate Medical Education. ACGME Program Requirements for Graduate Medical Education in Psychiatry. https://www.acgme.org/Portals/0/PFAssets/ProgramRequirements/400_psychiatry_2017-07-01.pdf. Published February 9, 2015. Updated February 6, 2017. Accessed February 10, 2018.

35. McCarthy M, Peteet J. Teaching residents about religion and spirituality. *Harv Rev Psychiatry*. 2003;11(4):225–228.

36. Grabovac A, Clark N, McKenna M. Pilot study and evaluation of postgraduate course on "The Interface Between Spirituality, Religion and Psychiatry." *Acad Psychiatry*. 2008;32(4):332–337.

37. McGovern TF, McMahon T, Nelson J, Bundoc-Baronia R, Giles C, Schmidt V. A descriptive study of a spirituality curriculum for general psychiatry residents. *Acad Psychiatry*. 2017;41(4):471–476.

38. Blass DM. A pragmatic approach to teaching psychiatry residents the assessment and treatment of religious patients. *Acad Psychiatry*. 2007;31(1):25–31.

39. Anandarajah G, Roseman J, Lee D, Dhandhania N. A 10-year longitudinal study of effects of a multifaceted residency spiritual care curriculum: Clinical ability, professional formation, end of life, and culture. *J Pain Symptom Manage*. 2016;52(6):859–872.

10

Gender and Sexuality

Shame and Safety in the Psychiatric Encounter

ANDREW CRUZ, JULIANNE TORRENCE,
AND CHRISTOPHER M. PALMER ■

Guilt—a feeling of violating one's ethical or cultural standards—is an emotion that serves a purpose. It causes us pause and prompts us to ask ourselves, "Is this a good decision?" It is a potentially powerful filter through which we can reflect upon decisions made to determine if the result is worth the cost. Guilt is intended to be not a burden that must be carried at all times, but rather a guidepost to help us chose our behaviors.

Shame, however, is a belief system: "I do bad things; therefore I am bad. I failed at this, so I am a failure." But who determines what is bad? Society, certainly. But what other factors contribute to a person's belief about what is inherently good or bad? Upbringing, culture, religion, education, geography, even biology shape our personalities and how we react and respond to our worlds. How do we, as clinicians, navigate this minefield of complexity?

Shame is often an inherent aspect in the very decision for someone to seek psychiatric or psychological treatment.[1,2] To reach a level of mental suffering that requires the help of another is often humiliating. Many loved ones and friends will offer advice such as "Just get over it," "Stop worrying so much," and "Snap out of it," implying that this type of suffering should be easy to overcome. Such advice further implies that those who can't manage these symptoms on their own are somehow stupid or weak. That intrinsic shame does not even factor in those feelings that emerge from the issue for which the patient is seeking treatment in the first place. Depression, anxiety, grief, relationship challenges, historical diagnoses, and difficulties successfully navigating through each day are, by their very nature, issues that can trigger shame. But what about issues that are already labeled as shameful? Discussing sexuality and behaviors that may feel taboo or deviant likely adds to an already shaming experience and can make therapy torturous for some patients.

However, the psychiatric encounter, with its intrinsic personal questions and emotional complexity, presents a unique opportunity to safely broach and explore diverse aspects of our patients' worlds, including taboo or deviant topics such as sexuality. As clinicians, we learn early in our training to meet the patient where they are, to find a way to connect. But what do you do when someone presents in your office with a situation with which you have no experience? Or no knowledge? Or have strong beliefs about? Or are uncomfortable with? What about when the patient is from, or embedded in, a culture with which you are either unfamiliar or have your own history? If we are already working to incorporate into our new doctor–patient relationship an understanding of our patient's possible shame or hesitancy to come to therapy, how do we simultaneously adjust our belief systems, our values, and our own shame to meet the patient where they are, particularly with such potentially volatile and difficult topics?

Most people have strong feelings and beliefs about sexuality and sexual behaviors, often accompanied by judgments of right or wrong. These feelings arise from entrenched values and mores in our society and are well described in the clinical literature.[3,4] To be a truly effective clinician, therefore, we must first be clearly and specifically aware of our own morals, values, beliefs, prejudices, biases, likes, dislikes, triggers, and influences around many situations and circumstances, including those involving sexuality. This is not always easy, but taking an honest and comprehensive self-assessment is the least we can do for our patients. Sound supervision around this exploration is a cornerstone to true self-awareness.

Sexuality and sexual behaviors are normal, healthy parts of human development and life. They can, at times, also be signs and symptoms of psychopathology. Distinguishing what constitutes normal, healthy sexual expression from psychopathology can be clinically challenging, and, unfortunately, there is little science to guide clinicians. As such, clinicians often must rely on what they themselves know and believe to determine which sexual behaviors may be symptomatic of a psychiatric illness and which are nonnormative but healthy consensual acts. Familiarity, therefore, with a wide range of sexual behaviors, beliefs, practices, cultures, and resources is paramount. Some sexual behaviors may indicate stand-alone psychiatric diagnoses. Many are, or can be, symptoms of a more complex psychiatric picture. Still others are "just sex," as we will explore in our cases. In addition, it is not unusual for these scenarios to overlap and change meaning with time and circumstance. The more informed a clinician is around topics of sexuality, the better he or she can distinguish what constitutes pathological versus nonpathological sexual behaviors. Several of these concepts are summarized in Table 10.2 and will be explored in more detail throughout the chapter.

Exploring issues of sexuality in the context of the psychiatric relationship will expose biases on the part of both the provider and the patient; acknowledging these biases can enhance open and honest communication between the parties. An informed understanding of both the provider's and the patient's ideas about sexuality can be the key to providing truly compassionate and competent mental health care. To illustrate the varied and complicated spectrum of human sexual behavior, we will present four clinical cases with subsequent discussion. As the cases evolve throughout the chapter, make note of the feelings, thoughts, hypotheses, diagnoses, reactions, and responses you experience, as well as how those emotions and beliefs influence your potential treatment decisions.

Resources are available to clinicians as they begin to develop their own acceptable level of comfort and style. For instance, the Centers for Disease Control and Prevention offer clear guidelines and prompts for how to comfortably incorporate

Table 10.1 TAKING A SEXUAL HISTORY

Statement/Question	Follow-up
I am going to ask you a few questions about your sexual health and sexual practices. I understand that these questions are very personal, but they are important for your health. Just so you know, I ask these questions to all my adult patients regardless of age, gender, sexual orientation, or marital status. Are you currently sexually active?	If no, ask, "Have you ever been sexually active?"
In recent months, how many sex partners have you had?	If the answer is more than zero, ask, "Are you sex partners men, women, or both?"
I'm going to be more explicit here about the kind of sex you've had over the last 12 months to better understand if you are at risk for STDs.	What kind of sexual contact do you have or have you had? Genital (penis in the vagina)? Anal (penis in the anus)? Oral (mouth on penis, vagina, or anus)?
Do you and your partner(s) use any protection against STDs?	If not, could you tell me the reason? If so, what kind of protection do you use? How often do you use this protection?
What other things about your sexual health and sexual practices should we discuss to help ensure your good health?	
What other concerns or question regarding your sexual health or sexual practices would you like to discuss?	

Adapted from Centers for Disease Control and Prevention. *A Guide to Taking a Sexual History*. CDC publication 99-8445 (pamphlet).

a thorough sexual history into a clinical interview[5] (Table 10.1). In addition, new techniques for proclivity-specific interviewing frameworks are being explored and vetted.[6,7] Although such guidelines are helpful as a baseline, clinicians will develop their own style and methods for discussing sex in clinical relationships, which must include creating a safe environment, using nonpejorative language, avoiding judgment, using open-ended questions, and being overall culturally sensitive and aware.

CASE 1

A 45-year-old male presents to a mental health clinic. When asked about what brought him in for evaluation, he says, "My depression." He elaborates that he has felt down most of his life but his hopelessness has increased during the past six months after an extramarital affair. He now finds it difficult to get out of bed in the morning, has stopped going to the gym, and is having difficulty attending his children's sporting events. He fears that he will lose his job because it has become increasingly difficult to handle the same workload that was manageable before. His wife has been supportive, but the patient does not feel worthy of her support; even more, he feels guilty for her support after his affair. The patient becomes tearful; he begrudgingly confesses that his affair was with a man. He has been attracted to men since his teenage years but has never had a relationship or sex with a male before this affair. "I'm desperate. I hate what I am and what I have done. Help me."

The patient described in this case discloses an extramarital affair in addition to presenting with symptomatology of major depression. The clinician's treatment of the patient will be preceded and influenced by a personal judgment made as the patient shares his situation. The clinician's reaction to infidelity likely depends on several factors: the clinician's personal experiences with infidelity, comfort with discussing sexuality, familiarity dealing with similar situations, and the amiability of the patient, among others. Many clinicians would assume that because this man is married to a woman and has children, he is heterosexual. When it is revealed that he is having an affair with a man, one can imagine that clinicians' reactions would be quite varied. Some may feel a sense of sadness for him—perhaps societal, religious, and cultural pressure forced him into a life that was no longer sustainable? Some may feel anger—with a family and wife at home, this patient's actions were selfish and irresponsible. Some, lacking experience with sexual minorities, may feel befuddled—a heterosexual man cannot have sex with another man without substances or an underlying pathology playing a role. Then there is, of course, the question of how the clinician would react if the gender of the patient's lover were changed. In a world free of biases, the reaction would ideally be the same regardless of the gender or sexual orientation of the patient. While that may seem impossible in the silent bias-riddled thoughts of the clinician, the way the clinician outwardly empathizes, advises, and treats all patients should be equal regardless of the sexuality dynamic. Undoubtedly, the ability of a clinician to treat patients from sexual minorities and majorities equally depends on his or her familiarity with the topic.

In your clinical practice, you will undoubtedly encounter some of the 3.5% of Americans who identify as lesbian, gay, or bisexual, in addition to the 0.3% who identify as transgender.[8] Sexual minorities experience increased rates of substance abuse, sexually transmitted infections, anxiety, and depression compared to the general population.[9] These amplified risks must be understood as a consequence of the increased bullying, isolation, shame, and guilt these patients experience and not as a direct biological consequence of their sexual orientation. These increased risks are also important clinically because of their potentially lethal implications. Risk factors for suicide, including mood and anxiety disorders, are increased in sexual minority populations.[10] Furthermore, meta-analyses have revealed a twofold excess of suicide attempts in LGBT populations.[11] Of note, even within the sexual minority communities that have an overall elevated risk of suicide, the transgender community has much higher risks. Their mental health risks, often described academically as the same, do, in fact, differ from their homosexual counterparts.

Even the astute clinician is easily tempted to focus on this patient's underlying mood disorder without truly addressing his underlying struggle with his sexuality. Omitting the patient's struggle with sexuality is a mistake. Sexual minority patients often perceive health care environments as inhospitable.[8] Their perception is shaped by the fact that they have spent their lives, closeted or not, in a largely heteronormative climate. Becoming accustomed to waiting rooms with male-female relationships depicted in posters and interview questions aimed at heterosexual relationships and sex have made an entire generation of sexual minority patients feel "less than." Health care institutions, hoping to address an obvious and troublesome health disparity, have instituted a variety of diversity training programs.[12] However, growing evidence shows that diversity training does not sufficiently address the problem.[12]

Compounding this problematic clinical scenario is the simple fact that clinicians feel uncomfortable speaking to their patients about sex.[13] As health care providers, we find it difficult to speak about subjects that we have been raised to find taboo or off limits. Yet, sexuality is a common thread that runs through all humans, has vital clinical implications, and influences human behavior in such an immense way that it cannot be ignored. As we explore ways in which that information can be pertinent to the clinical encounter, the most obvious but easily, and often purposefully, forgotten missing piece is obtaining the sexual history. Clinicians must ask patients in an open and nonjudgmental way about sexual behaviors and sexuality, particularly in the mental health field. Clinicians must not become voyeurs with their questions, but must use the sexual history to make the correct diagnosis and to provide proper treatment.

Furthermore, the sexual history can elucidate areas of sensitivity that can build rapport and enhance the clinician–patient relationship.[14] Learning to speak comfortably with our patients, including using preferred nomenclature and language, has a positive impact on the clinical relationship.[15] An example is the correct use of pronouns when working with transgender patients, as this is a basic and essential foundation of understanding between the clinician and the patient. It tells patients that they are not "others" and that the words they use to identify themselves mean enough that the clinician cares to ask about them and use them properly. Countless other situations exist in the realm of information obtained from the sexual history. Patients are often more open than clinicians may think, and only by encountering these situations and exploring them with patients can the clinician reach a place of comfort for both patient and clinician.

In the case of this patient, who presents with an episode of major depression in the setting of a same-sex affair, it is important for his treatment to delineate how his symptoms relate to his underlying mood disorder and how they similarly or differently relate to the underlying struggle with sexuality. Guilt can be a cardinal symptom of depression, though in the case of patients struggling with their sexuality, guilt and its appropriateness can be difficult to distinguish. As sexual minorities become increasingly accepted in the 21st century, it can be difficult to remember that not long ago they were ostracized, pathologized, and discriminated against. The patient's guilt or concrete feeling—that he has performed or indeed IS an offense—could be the result of a lifetime of repressed sexuality in a world that was vastly different in his formative years. Thinking about how depression often cognitively highlights negative thoughts, feelings, and emotions in patients can be helpful. The guilt this patient feels is likely multifactorial and related to a chronic feeling that is exacerbated by his current depression. These two manifestations of guilt are intimately connected and must both be addressed.

Deciding clinically how to advise the patient to proceed in this situation is controversial and will differ on a patient-by-patient basis. The patient's sexuality is still somewhat of a mystery, to the clinician and perhaps even to the patient. The framework that people are always "becoming,"[16] regardless of sexuality, can be helpful for clinicians and patients. In this case, there is no urgency to identify a sexual orientation for the patient; the focus instead must be on crisis control and stabilization. The multitude of worries the patient almost certainly has—Should he tell his wife? What is his sexuality? What will his kids think?—will be addressed over time; for now, talking through and processing his experience is the priority. The clinician must set aside preconceived notions of sexuality and, in each encounter with the patient, empathize with and learn from the patient's story. It can be helpful to step back from the certainty of clear answers and explore the similarities to all patients—each patient is looking for answers and seeking help from you.

CASE 2

A 47-year-old gay man with a history of alcohol use disorder who meets criteria for major depression presents for psychiatric care. When the clinician inquires about potentially risky behaviors, he reports that he has been "meeting up" with and having sex with different men several times a week. When asked how he meets these men, he reports using "hookup" apps on a daily basis. He reports around 700 lifetime partners. When asked if alcohol is involved, he reports that it is only involved rarely and this behavior is "normal."

"Hookup" apps have become increasingly popular in the last decade.[17] They represent a novel and, in some ways, revolutionary approach to looking for sex. These are mobile phone apps in which people of all gender and sexual identities can meet each other for everything from small talk, to dates, to sexual encounters, to full-fledged relationships. The apps are structured so that people can scroll through a hundred other people in a matter of minutes. Interestingly, people often reveal personal characteristics about themselves that, in the past, would gradually be revealed after numerous dates. It is not uncommon, for instance, for people in the public forum of the app to write about their sexual preferences, substance use habits, occupations, religious affiliations, hopes, and dreams. In a world that has become increasingly driven by instant gratification, the implications of these apps are enormous.

This case presents numerous challenges. This patient meets criteria for a mood disorder that must be addressed, but the context in which that disorder presents is equally important. Understanding the importance of hetero- and homonormative behaviors as they apply to pathology and diagnosis is challenging and often results in many assumptions and biases by clinicians.[6,18-20] The first concern, from a clinical perspective, is always safety. The patient has a history of a substance use disorder; screening for current pathology in that regard is part of a well-developed clinical interview that assesses for safety. What must also be taken into consideration is that substance use discrepancies between sexual minorities and their heterosexual counterparts are profound. In a large systematic review, the odds of recent and lifetime illicit substance abuse were over three times higher for sexual minority youth relative to heterosexuals.[21] Also of note, among sexual minority populations substance use starts at earlier ages than among their heterosexual counterparts. There is also a gender difference, with substance use being higher in men.[22] The reasons for these discrepancies are not entirely clear, but are most likely multifactorial.[22] The increased substance use may represent a combination of increased availability of substances, an attempt to cope with stressors and fear, and a mechanism for finding a community. When asking a patient with a history of substance use about current use, the clinician must be thoughtful to ensure that he or she is not missing a potential contributing factor to the patient's depression and behavior. This patient's current depression and increased sexual behavior are clinical clues—much as an uncontrolled glucose would be in a previously controlled diabetic—that either the disease itself has progressed or that there are disease-modifying behaviors contributing to this change. A comprehensive substance use screening will help to determine which of the aforementioned is primarily contributing to this patient's presentation.

An equally important aspect of this patient's presentation that must be addressed is his sexual behavior. It is important to understand that clinicians who treat sexual minority patients can have significantly different sexual orientations, gender identities, religious affiliations, and cultural backgrounds from the patients who seek their guidance. For those not familiar with sexual minority culture, particularly gay culture, hearing a patient tell you that he has had 700 lifetime partners can be shocking. Patients are intensely aware and observant of how clinicians react to such disclosures. A balanced, controlled, nonjudgmental reaction is what they hope for and what clinicians, despite their own background, must convey.

Hypersexuality is a minefield of potential incorrect diagnoses if the clinician is not careful.[23] As one of the few times that clinicians ask about sex is during psychiatric review of symptoms when concerned for mania, a clinician could attribute this patient's hypersexuality to part of a bipolar spectrum disorder. A thorough review of systems will help determine if the patient does, in fact, show signs of bipolar affective disorder. Another clinician may attribute this patient's hypersexuality to borderline personality disorder, noting that many with this diagnosis use sexual behavior to help fill a void or escape from chronic feelings of emptiness or identity confusion.[24]

One disorder that did not make the most recent *Diagnostic and Statistical Manual of Mental Disorders* (DSM-5)[25] is hypersexual disorder.[26] This disorder roughly constitutes a set of symptoms colloquially known as "sex addiction." Questions about the impact that the patient's sexual behavior is having on his life will help determine if this is, in fact, an addiction. This patient's apparent lack of concern by referring to his behavior as "normal" argues against the diagnosis of hypersexual disorder. Sex is also a common strategy for distraction from or numbing of depression, anxiety, and other mood symptoms.[27,28]

Men who have sex with men do have a higher prevalence of lifetime sex partners. The patient is a gay male. The homosexual culture has a different mindset about casual sex; hence, he may see his sexual encounters as a normal and enjoyable part of life.[29] In this context, the patient's answer that this behavior is "normal" could be as equally valid an explanation as the aforementioned diagnoses. Promiscuity does not, in and of itself, necessarily imply pathology. Regardless of its etiology, initially the patient must be assessed as with any other patient. A normal part of any clinical encounter is counseling about risky behaviors in a nonjudgmental and evidence-based way. There are very real risks to having a large number of sexual partners. Among men who have sex with men, there has been an upward trend in condomless anal sex with both casual partners and main partners, as well as condom-less anal sex with partners of unknown or discordant HIV status; there is some evidence attributing this to viewing pornography containing condom-less sex.[30] The availability of preexposure prophylaxis (PrEP) will likely reduce these risks in the future, but access is not yet widely available, and knowledge of the treatment is limited. The clinician must ask the patient about sexual practices, condom use, and HIV status of his partners. These questions and the clinical advice that follows should be similar to the questions and advice with which you would counsel any sexually active patient.

Herein lies one of the most important aspects of caring for sexual minority patients: They are minority in some ways but, like all patients, they are of course human as well. Their care has differences, yes—but it must be fundamentally the same as the care offered to all patients—humane.

Another topic of discussion is the number of partners and the implications of those numbers. While data on dating apps and their effect on sexual behaviors are emerging, there can be little doubt that apps are making an impact on sexual behavior. Men who have sex with men report having, on average, three dating app accounts, opening these apps eight times a day, and spending 1.5 hours on them.[31] Given the fast pace of the American worker and the numerous social duties that people have, these statistics are extraordinary. Furthermore, the most-cited reason for having such an app is to facilitate sex. This patient must be interviewed about his motivations for using the app he mentioned and about what he is seeking in his partners. He can be counseled about the health risks, but judgments based on the number of partners may threaten the clinical relationship. While judgmental statements must be avoided, it is worth exploring what the patient believes other people think about his behavior and whether or not that matters to him. Having a conversation, for instance, about how to deal with people who think negatively about his actions will benefit him in the future and help him to think through his responses. The normality of these behaviors is hotly debated, and clinicians will have differing opinions.

What is most important to realize, however, is that there is a novel phenomenon evolving. Sex has become digitized and accelerated, making it more available than ever before. Research will be required about the true effect of smartphone innovations on sexual behavior; for now, however, clinicians and their patients are best served by education in a nonjudgmental interview, as well as exploring the implications of present behaviors on emotions and future goals. It would be important to ask this patient if he does want a long-term relationship eventually, and how his present behaviors would work in that context. What would his future partner's reaction be? Also, exploring the emotions the patient feels before and after the encounters will be important clinical information. Have there been times when the encounters felt dangerous or did not go according to plan? What were his emotions then? These questions and their answers can serve to elucidate the patient's diagnosis while simultaneously building a clinical relationship and validating his experience.

CASE 3

A concerned mother brings in her 15-year-old son for evaluation. By history, he meets criteria for major depression. As you begin to explore his symptomatology, he endorses extreme guilt around daily masturbation while viewing pornography. He was raised in a religious household and believes that he cannot share his struggle with his parents or friends. His mother is aware of his pornography use and believes that it is the primary reason for the patient's symptoms.

Sexual behaviors, even those considered normal by the health care community, become complicated in the setting of cultural and religious influences.[32,33] In the case of masturbation, there is potential for embarrassment, as well as a general sense of discomfort and lack of knowledge from clinicians, regarding this normal part of sexual development. Masturbatory behavior is a common concern for parents and children and has implications across several clinical fields, particularly mental health. While a wide range of statistics exists, some 90% to 94% of males and 50% to 60% of females report masturbating during their childhood.[34] Despite the commonness of the behavior, it is still a difficult subject for patients and clinicians to talk about, even within the confidentiality of the clinical relationship. Clinicians need to explore such issues when presented with cases in which the patient is struggling. Often that requires asking patients directly. Knowledge of the research about pornography and masturbation is essential for the clinician to feel comfortable counseling the distressed patient in this case.

Masturbation, commonly accepted as normal adolescent behavior, can be contrasted with the more controversial and divisive act of viewing pornography. Although they often accompany each other, the mental health literature has not reached as widely an accepted consensus about adolescent pornography usage as it has for masturbation. Studies have shown both negative and positive consequences from viewing internet pornography. Among the potentially damaging consequences are an increased number of partners and substance use at last sexual encounter.[35] Concerns about erectile dysfunction, inability to reach orgasm, and other sexual dysfunction associated with porn usage have not been confirmed with evidence in studies and may have been misguided.[36,37] More encouraging outcomes have shown that young adults view pornography consumption as helpful by increasing their sexual knowledge and general quality of life.[38] It is important to understand though, that in the context of the present case, the benefits and drawbacks of masturbation are of little importance; the adolescent's guilt and how that is contributing to his mood is the primary concern.

When clinicians encounters a patient, regardless of age, who is struggling with a sexual behavior, their duty, as with any clinical problem, is to assist in healing. Understanding cultural and religious contexts, while simultaneously setting them aside and educating the patient, is an appropriate and beneficial technique. In other words, reassuring the patient about which behaviors are in the realm of "normal" based on statistics and the available literature is the duty of the clinician, not debating religious or cultural norms.

In the case of this patient, speaking with the mother is important to understand where her concerns originate. Her concern may come from seeing the change in mood and personality in her son and, looking for answers, she associates these symptoms with his masturbation and pornography usage. If that is the case, education and reassurance to the mother would prove helpful. A more difficult situation is when the mother's ideology and personal truth is at odds with clinical truth. In that case, depending on the rigidity of the belief system, educating the parent may not be as beneficial; however, educating the teenager can help him with his self-hate. The importance of reassuring the patient cannot be overstated. Studies have shown that religiosity is a strong predictor of perceived pornography addiction, even when controlling for the actual level of pornography usage.[39] This is concerning for several reasons, but most importantly, teenagers could feel distressing guilt and perceive a personal addiction, separate from a clinical measurement of their behavior. In this patient, the overwhelming guilt could have been the catalyst for his current major depressive episode. While medications can be helpful, it is unlikely that his subsequent depression would resolve in the setting of continued inappropriate and misguided guilt. Understanding the inseparable interplay of the sexual behavior and the patient's underlying mood disorder is the key to addressing his suffering.

CASE 4

Mary is a 35-year-old white woman with a history of borderline personality disorder (BPD) referred to therapy by her primary care physician due to difficulties in her marriage.

Self-aware clinicians will pause here to reflect on what feelings, thoughts, and assumptions are provoked from just this piece of the clinical picture. For instance, does Mary's or the clinician's race, gender, or socioeconomic status influence assumptions about Mary? What about marital status or sexual orientation? Do clinicians' family dynamics, culture, or religion impact their thoughts and feelings about marriage, and, therefore, the patient? What about the BPD? A clinician's biases and experience working with BPD will influence the interaction and influence the framework through which to best explore and understand Mary.

Many clinicians develop strong emotions—negative or positive—when working with BPD patients;[40–42] a successful clinician will determine how best to manage these intense feelings, while at the same time considering how these intense emotions will influence treatment decisions. Clinically, Mary's history of BPD will influence the approach that the clinician takes in exploring and understanding her relationships and sexuality. That is not to say that all of Mary's marital and life issues are a direct product of her BPD; rather, in therapy, those issues need to be viewed within the context of a BPD history and the clinician's response to it. Astute clinicians will acknowledge that they may have already made assumptions, and possibly judgments, about Mary just from this small amount of information from the referring clinician. Does this self-awareness help or hinder a clinician's ability to formulate an accurate clinical assessment? To fully assess and address issues within the marriage—the presenting problem here—the clinician must ask about numerous aspects of the relationship and marital life, including the sexual relationship. But will the assumptions and judgments already made about Mary color the exploration of issues around sexuality and sexual behaviors?

The referral goes on to note that Mary has reported a possible history of sexual abuse but has no specific memories of abuse.

This is another issue that can produce strong emotions in clinicians. Many will make assumptions about how this might influence her marriage, sexuality, and her diagnosis of BPD.

When Mary walks into the office, she is casually dressed and well groomed. She seems to have difficulty making and maintaining eye contact, has an almost rigid posture, and holds her hands together on her lap as she takes her seat. The clinician asks Mary what brings her to the office today. Mary is guarded with her answers, offering little or no specific information other than, "I am having trouble communicating in my marriage." Trying to engage Mary in further conversation, the clinician reviews her history as presented in the referral; Mary confirms with one-word answers, showing no change in affect or body language as she responds. When asked about the possibility of her having been sexually abused, Mary replies, "I think I might have been. I'm not really sure why, but I think I might have been. I am not really sure, though." Mary never makes eye contact with the clinician as she speaks. Mary's guarded responses and approach make further exploration difficult. The session comes to an end, and Mary makes another appointment for next week.

Before the next session, a clinician should formulate a plan for working with Mary—how to lessen her guardedness and engage her in difficult conversations about her potential abuse history, as well as her marital issues.

In the second session, recognizing that being in therapy might be difficult and shameful for Mary, the clinician asks Mary what she would like to talk about. Still guarded, Mary slowly reports that she finds she has difficulty making friends and maintaining relationships. She speaks about childhood relationships, as well as her parent and sibling connections. Mary reports that she and her husband have known each other for "a long time" through mutual friends at a club to which they both belong, and that they have been married for 2 years, the longest romantic relationship Mary has ever had.

Curious to see if Mary believes that her BPD plays a role in her history of relationship issues and her current marital stressors, the clinician asks Mary if she has ever considered that. Mary looks a bit amused as she answers, "Um . . . that is what being a borderline is, so, umm, yeah." Mary then laughs and makes eye contact with the clinician. The clinician is relieved that Mary is more insightful than assumed and that they have finally made a connection, but the session has come to an end. The clinician smiles back and says, "At our next session, we will really get to work to get to the bottom of your relationship issues with your husband."

When Mary comes for her third session, the clinician is ready with a plan to actively explore her specific marital issues that bring her to treatment, hoping that it will lead to an opportunity to ask about her possible sexual abuse and her current sexual behaviors. As is often the case, the patient shatters the best-laid plans. Mary comes into the session with a sense of determination and says, "I know you want to look at my BPD. And you probably want to have me talk about my sexual abuse, but I came here to talk about communication with my husband!" Mary goes on to tell the clinician that she has been in therapy before and feels that she has already explored and understands those issues. "I have to learn to communicate with my husband better. He asked me to do something, and I did it, and I liked it, but now I feel guilty, and I am scared, and I think he is going to like her more."

Mary appears and presents very differently today. Is this about her BPD? Did her husband ask her to do something that triggered memories of sexual abuse? Was her initial guarded and flat presentation about depression?

Before the clinician can articulate the next question, Mary says, "Look, I don't have time to not talk about this, so I am just gonna tell you—my husband and I are in 'the Lifestyle.' He is my Dom and I am his submissive. He and I negotiated and agreed to add a play partner to our D/s relationship. We did, and now I am feeling insecure and worried that he will like her better than me. I need help talking to him about this without him thinking I am crazy, or overreacting, or moody, or screwed up. Whatever else is wrong with me, I don't think that my feelings right now about this are wrong or crazy or unrealistic. I just want somebody who will help me talk about that." Mary has grown tearful, sitting silently shaking after her confession.

The typical clinician might not know what a D/s relationship is, or what BDSM is, so confusion and insecurity can be common feelings. BDSM is actually a collection of abbreviations that are adopted to best suggest a participant's preferences. BD describes bondage and discipline; DS represents dominance and submission; SM describes sadism and masochism or slave and master power exchanges.[43] Even for those with awareness of this lifestyle, all clinicians must take stock and assess how they feel about someone who engages in such behaviors. Sexual sadism and masochism disorders, along with exhibitionistic disorder and voyeuristic disorder, are all in DSM-5.[25] Do these BDSM behaviors automatically equate, then, to pathology? Does BDSM imply active abuse, or can the dynamic and consensual power exchange ever be a healthy one? And what if a BDSM participant has a psychiatric diagnosis such as Mary's BPD? Does a client's possible sexual abuse history play a role in her involvement in the practice of BDSM? Should it? Could she be consciously or unconsciously reenacting her possible sexual abuse? If so, is that automatically unhealthy, or could it possibly be part of a healing process? Does it automatically pathologize the practice of BDSM if one or more partners is a victim of domestic or sexual abuse? In this case, should the possibility of sexual abuse even factor into the exploration of the BDSM aspects of Mary's presenting marital issues? How does a clinician differentiate pathology from potentially healthy thinking and behavior in such a complex clinical presentation?

Although this case study is rich with clinical opportunity, let's focus on the shame that is inherent in several aspects of Mary's presentation. Right or wrong, many clinicians have negative perceptions of people with BPD, often using the pejorative term "a borderline," rather than a person with BPD. With the mere mention of a BPD diagnosis, assumptions are made, and the lens through which a patient is viewed is tinted. Most people with BPD are aware of other's responses, reactions, and beliefs about them due to this diagnosis.[42,44]

It is the overlying belief of people who engage in the BDSM lifestyle that most clinicians have negative attitudes toward them, that they lack knowledge of sexual subcultures, and that they are often not adequately aware of their own values and beliefs around these subcultures.[20] Furthermore, they are acutely aware that many of the practices in which they engage are diagnosable pathologies in DSM-5.

Imagine, then, the courage it must take for Mary to enter the therapist's office carrying the shame of a troubled marriage and the baggage of a BPD diagnosis, and wanting to talk about her "deviant" sexual practices that she fears the clinician will not understand or may disapprove of. Whatever beliefs and assumptions the clinician has, appreciating Mary's bravery in coming to treatment will be an important tool in developing a therapeutic alliance.

To do this, clinicians cannot simply ignore or stop feeling emotions and reactions; in doing so, their response would be disingenuous and therefore unhelpful. Instead, good clinicians must be aware of and acknowledge their emotions and reactions, but also be aware of their own limitations around their knowledge base. It can be helpful to have at least some knowledge of BDSM practices and power exchanges to be able to properly assess and treat people who participate in these activities. Relationship issues that fall into these dynamics, such as ownership, objectification, pick-up play, punishment and reward, service and obedience, the differences between a top and a Dom, as well as a bottom and a submissive, switching (top/bottom), and play partnerships, can all be helpful. Many patients will not be willing to teach the therapist about BDSM for fear of rejection or revulsion.[15,20,45]

Acknowledging these limitations is important when the clinician's scope of knowledge and familiarity interfere with the therapeutic connection. Clinicians are human, too, and our emotions, histories, beliefs and values are as real as our patients'. We do no one a service—in fact we do a disservice to patients—if we are unwilling to acknowledge our own limitations. But rather than plowing on with generic treatment planning, good clinicians will try to understand the specific issues and look for resources that are available to learn about and get support on these topics. When this is not possible, or when the clinician's own beliefs and values prohibit this process, a referral to a colleague who might be a more appropriate fit for the patient may be the best course of action.

In Mary's case, this assessment needs to be applied to sex—kinky sex in particular. Mary identifies that she is part of the BDSM lifestyle living as a submissive to a Dominant. You may believe that you do not know anyone who engages in these practices, either in your clinical work, as colleagues, as friends, or as neighbors. And yet, research shows that 1% to 25% of the North American population is or has been involved in BDSM activities,[46,47] with even higher percentages reporting interest in them. A commonly accepted general belief is that 10% of American adults are involved or interested in BDSM activities.[48,49] Pop culture appears to be increasing the acceptance of alternative sexual practices, as evidenced by the dramatic popularity of *50 Shades of Grey* and the subsequent increase in sales of men's restraints and blindfolds.[50]

If that isn't enough incentive for clinicians to gain even basic knowledge about alternative sexualities, perhaps the American Psychological Association's acknowledgment of the burgeoning population of people whose sexual identities, beliefs, and practices vary from the "norm" will. As a result of this acknowledgment, the association altered its definition of sexual orientation in its code of ethics to include a person's sense of identity based on those attractions, related behaviors, and membership in a community of others who share those attractions. With this new definition, BDSM is considered a sexual minority group; as such, BDSM and other alternative sexual lifestyles are now included in the association's ethical requirement to obtain adequate training, experience, consultation, and supervision to develop competency in this area.[51–53]

In the context of using this definition of sexual orientation, it is important to note that the DSM-5 and the International Classification of Diseases, Tenth Revision, Clinical Modification (ICD-10-CM)[54] billing codes define many of these nonnormative practices as deviant and unusual—fetishism, masochism, sadism, frotteurism, exhibitionism, pedophilia, transvestism, and voyeurism specifically.[25] But by whose definition are they deviant or unusual? Clarifying the ambiguity of these labels has clinical, theoretical, practical, and legal ramifications. A literature search of studies that might clarify this ambiguity resulted in the discovery of only 17 studies published between 1995 and 2012, most of which focused on college-age participants and did not include sufficient statistical analysis.[55] When left with no clarification on how deviance is assigned to such activities, clinicians are left to make that determination through their own lens of knowledge and beliefs.

To attempt to clarify this ambiguity, Joyal and colleagues conducted a study to more clearly define which sexual fantasies—the basis for a paraphilic classification—are rare, unusual, common, or typical. Participants rated 55 sexual fantasies derived from established norms and popular internet and pornographic download histories. Two sexual fantasies were labeled rare (2.3% or fewer of the respondents endorsing them), nine were statistically unusual (15.9% or fewer of the respondents endorsing them), and five were identified as typical (84.1% or more of the respondents endorsing them). For the remaining 39 sexual fantasies, 23 were considered common in men and 11 in women. The most notable result in this common category is that both men and women have statistically significant interest in domination and submission fantasies—including being sexually dominated, being tied up for sexual pleasure, being spanked or whipped, and being forced to have sex,[55] all of which are included under the BDSM umbrella. As the determination of pathology is defined by unusual or deviant sexual fantasies, care clearly must be taken in assigning pathology when the majority of the 55 identified sexual fantasies have not been statistically identified to be unusual. As for deviance, its association with such sexual fantasies is pejorative in and of itself, and is subjective in nature. Table 10.2 lists several of the notable sexual fantasies from which the participants chose, in descending order of interest for both men and women.

It is encouraging, both for BDSM practitioners seeking treatment and for clinicians who are willing to treat them, that despite the popular opinion that all BDSM practices are stereotypically perceived by both lay and clinical people as "bad," Kelsey and colleagues showed that the majority of clinicians polled did not universally equate unconventional sexual activities with individual psychopathology or dysfunctional relationships. In their study, 68% of responding clinicians endorsed that people can engage in BDSM without experiencing emotional problems, and 70% of those polled agreed that BDSM activities should not be targeted for reduction in therapy without the patient specifically identifying this as a desired goal for treatment. Furthermore, they conclude that BDSM practices should not be considered as a central therapeutic issue if they are only peripherally related to the client's presenting concern.[20] Wismeijer and van Assen dispelled the notion that engaging in BDSM practices was associated with psychopathology by showing that BDSM practitioners are, as a whole, less neurotic, more extroverted, more open to new experiences, more conscientious, and less sensitive to rejection; and have higher subjective well-being—all suggesting favorable psychological characteristics compared to the control group.[56]

But what of the reverse situation? Mary came to treatment specifically because of activities within her BDSM dynamic. If BDSM is the client's primary concern, what is our obligation as therapists to also factor in the client's history of pathological diagnoses and possible sexual abuse? Are they mutually exclusive or intricately linked? In Mary's case, the possibilities are endless.

One must explore Mary's involvement in BDSM to fully understand her current dilemma. An astute clinician will do so in such a way as to simultaneously discern if there is a connection to either her BPD diagnosis or her possible past sexual abuse history. Hypersexuality can certainly be part of a BPD presentation.[24] Desperate means to engage in and maintain relationships can also be a piece of that clinical puzzle, with remorse and self-doubt equally so. Are clients with BPD more vulnerable to coercion in an effort to be accepted? Mary's insecurities about her appeal to her husband can certainly be attributed to her BPD. At the same time, being a submissive in a D/s relationship is also a very vulnerable position; in submission, insecurities can either be heightened or erased, depending on the Dominant and the dynamic. Is the

Table 10.2 PREVALENCE AND DIVERSITY OF FEMALE AND MALE SEXUAL FANTASIES IN THE GENERAL POPULATION

Women's Sexual Fantasies	% Women	Men's Sexual Fantasies	% Men
I like to feel romantic emotions during a sexual relationship.	99.2	I like to feel romantic emotions during a sexual relationship.	88.3
I have fantasized about having sex in an unusual place (e.g., in the office; public toilets).	81.7	I have fantasized about having sex with two women.	84.5
I have fantasized about having sex with someone that I know who is not my spouse [...].	66.3	I have fantasized about having sex in an unusual place (e.g., in the office; public toilets).	82.3
I have fantasized about being dominated sexually.	64.6	I have fantasized about having anal sex.	64.2
I have fantasized about making love openly in a public place.	57.3	I have fantasized about watching someone undress without him or her knowing.	63.4
I have fantasized about having sex with more than three people, both men and women.	56.5	I have fantasized about dominating someone sexually.	59.6
I have fantasized about being tied up by someone in order to obtain sexual pleasure.	52.1	I have fantasized about being dominated sexually.	53.3
I have fantasized about dominating someone sexually.	46.7	I have fantasized about tying someone up in order to obtain sexual pleasure.	48.4
I have fantasized about tying someone up in order to obtain sexual pleasure.	41.7	I have fantasized about being tied up by someone in order to obtain sexual pleasure.	46.2
I have fantasized that my partner ejaculates on me.	41.3	I have fantasized about having sex with two men.	45.2
I have fantasized about having homosexual (or gay) sex.	36.9	I have fantasized about spanking or whipping someone to obtain sexual pleasure.	43.5

(*continued*)

Table 10.2 CONTINUED

Women's Sexual Fantasies	% Women	Men's Sexual Fantasies	% Men
I have fantasized about being spanked or whipped to obtain sexual pleasure.	36.3	I have fantasized about being forced to have sex.	30.7
I have fantasized about being forced to have sex.	28.9	I have fantasized about being spanked or whipped to obtain sexual pleasure.	28.5
I have fantasized about having sex with a fetish or non-sexual object.	26.3	I have fantasized about having sex with a fetish or non-sexual object.	27.8
I have fantasized about spanking or whipping someone to obtain sexual pleasure.	23.8	I have fantasized about forcing someone to have sex.	22
I have fantasized about forcing someone to have sex.	10.8	I have fantasized about my sexual partner urinating on me.	10

Adapted from: Joyal CC, Cossette A, Lapierre V. What exactly is an unusual sexual fantasy? *J Sex Med*. 2015;12(2):328–340.

vulnerable nature of being submissive exacerbating Mary's insecurities that may or may not stem from her BPD? These are all questions that must be explored, carefully, to truly understand Mary's marital issues.

The potential of past sexual abuse adds another complicated clinical dynamic in this case. Mary is uncertain at best if she is the victim of abuse, but that possibility is very real. Is Mary's interest in submitting to another a result of, or in protest to, her having been abused? Does giving her consent to be taken sexually somehow reduce or ameliorate her residual feelings of being taken sexually against her will in previous abuse? And if her sexual history plays a role in her becoming involved in BDSM, does that necessitate a pathological context or an empowering one? Is Mary aware of the possible connection?

Richters and colleagues concluded that BDSM practice is a variety of sexual interest that is not, in and of itself, a symptom of sexual abuse or sexual pathology, noting that the prevalence of a sexual abuse history is similar between populations of BDSM practitioners and nonpractitioners.[46] However, sexual and domestic abuse histories do exist in the BDSM culture. How a BDSM practitioner reconciles this history to current desires is a complicated and difficult matter. Clinicians who are comfortable with and knowledgeable about sexual subcultures, including BDSM practices, can play an integral role in helping to explore this connection.

But what about Mary?

The best way to comprehensively assess Mary's situation and the myriad potential interpretations is to talk with her and assess all of these complicated areas and considerations. Tackling difficult topics is best accomplished with open-ended, nonjudgmental questions and responses. Given patients' reluctance to disclose many aspects of sexual behaviors for fear of rejection or disapproval, clinicians often need to advance these conversations by initiating questions about specific sexual practices, demonstrating awareness of these practices and an openness to hearing honest answers. This can be accomplished only when clinicians increase their knowledge of sexual subcultures, while becoming aware of their own values and beliefs regarding them.

Finally, clinicians must not allow their clinical assessment to be influenced and biased by prejudice and stereotypes. Consistent and thoughtful supervision throughout a clinician's development and career is an important aspect in accomplishing this goal.

CONCLUSION

The cases presented in this chapter illustrate some of the challenging and complex ways that sexuality and sexual behaviors can intersect with the psychiatric encounter, influencing diagnostic formulations, treatment, rapport, and the therapeutic relationship. We hope this chapter has provided a framework for approaching and formulating such situations.

REFERENCES

1. Love M, Farber BA. Let's not talk about sex. *J Clin Psychol.* 2017;73(11):1489–1498.
2. Zaslav MR. Shame-related states of mind in psychotherapy. *J Psychother Prac Res.* 1998;7(2):154–166.
3. Ho T, Fernández M. Patients' sexual health: Do we care enough? *J Ren Care.* 2006;32(4):183–186.
4. Herson L, Hart KA, Gordon MJ, Rintala DH. Identifying and overcoming barriers to providing sexuality information in the clinical setting. *Rehabil Nurs.* 1999;24(4):148–151.
5. Centers for Disease Control and Prevention. *A Guide to Taking a Sexual History.* CDC publication 99-8445 (pamphlet).
6. Sprott RA, Randall A, Davison K, Cannon N, Witherspoon RG. Alternative or nontraditional sexualities and therapy: A case report. *J Clin Psychol.* 2017;73(8):929–937.
7. Kolmes K. An introduction to BDSM for psychotherapists. Retrieved from: http://www.societyforpsychotherapy.org/an-introduction-to-bdsm-for-psychotherapists
8. Hafeez H, Zeshan M, Tahir MA, Jahan N, Naveed S. Health care disparities among lesbian, gay, bisexual, and transgender youth: A literature review. *Cureus.* 2017;9(4):e1184.
9. Gonzales G, Henning-Smith C. Health disparities by sexual orientation: Results and implications from the behavioral risk factor surveillance system. *J Community Health.* 2017;42(6):1163–1172.
10. Mullaney C. Reshaping time: Recommendations for suicide prevention in LBGT populations. *J Homosex.* 2016;63(3):461–465.
11. King M, Semlyen J, Tai SS, et al. A systematic review of mental disorder, suicide, and deliberate self-harm in lesbian, gay and bisexual people. *BMC Psychiatry.* 2008;8(1):70.

12. Dean MA, Victor E, Guidry-Grimes L. Inhospitable healthcare spaces: Why diversity training on LGBTQIA issues is not enough. *J Bioeth Inq*, 2016;13(4): 557–570.

13. Dyer K, Nair RD. Why don't healthcare professionals talk about sex? A systematic review of recent qualitative studies conducted in the United Kingdom. *J Sex Med.* 2013;10(11):2658–2670.

14. Gay and Lesbian Medical Association (GMLA). *Healthy People 2010: A Companion Document for LGBT Health.* San Francisco: GMLA; 2001 Apr. Retrieved from: http:// www.glma.org/_data/n_0001/resources/live/HealthyCompanionDoc3.pdf

15. Rehor JE. Sensual, erotic, and sexual behaviors of women from the "kink" community. *Arch Sex Behav.* 2015;44(4):825–836.

16. Klein K, Holtby A, Cook K, Travers R. Complicating the coming out narrative: Becoming oneself in a heterosexist and cissexist world. *J Homosex.* 2014;62(3):297–326.

17. Beymer MR, Weiss RE, Bolan RK, et al. Sex on demand: Geosocial networking phone apps and risk of sexually transmitted infections among a cross-sectional sample of men who have sex with men in Los Angeles county. *Sex Trans Infect.* 2014;90(7):567–572.

18. Kort J. *Gay Affirmative Therapy for the Straight Clinician: The Essential Guide.* New York: W.W. Norton & Co.; 2008.

19. Nichols M. Psychotherapeutic issues with "kinky" clients: Clinical problems, yours and theirs. *J Homosex.* 2006;50(2-3):281–300.

20. Kelsey K, Stiles BL, Spiller L, Diekhoff GM. Assessment of therapists' attitudes towards BDSM. *Psych Sex.* 2013;4(3):255–267.

21. Marshal MP, Friedman MS, Stall R, et al. Sexual orientation and adolescent substance use: A meta-analysis and methodological review. *Addiction.* 2008;103(4):546–556.

22. Demant D, Hides L, Kavanagh DJ, et al. Differences in substance use between sexual orientations in a multi-country sample: Findings from the Global Drug Survey 2015. *J Public Health (Oxf).* 2017;39(3):532–541.

23. Montgomery-Graham S. Conceptualization and assessment of hypersexual disorder: A systematic review of the literature. *Sex Med Rev.* 2017;5(2):146–162.

24. Sansone RA, Sansone LA. Sexual behavior in borderline personality: A review. *Innov Clin Neurosci.* 2011;8(2):14–18.

25. American Psychiatric Association. *Diagnostic and Statistical Manual of Mental Disorders.* 5th ed. Washington, DC: APA; 2013.

26. Karila L, Wéry A, Weinstein A, et al. Sexual addiction or hypersexual disorder: Different terms for the same problem? A review of the literature. *Curr Pharm Des.* 2014;20(25):4012–4020.

27. Chatzittofis A, Arver S, Öberg K, et al. HPA axis dysregulation in men with hypersexual disorder. *Psychoneuroendocrinology.* 2016;63:247–253.

28. Kalra G. The depressive façade in a case of compulsive sex behavior with frottage. *Indian J Psychiatry.* 2013;55(2):183–185.

29. Zablotska IB, Grulich AE, Wit JD, Prestage G. Casual sexual encounters among gay men: Familiarity, trust and unprotected anal intercourse. *AIDS Behav.* 2010;15(3):607–612.

30. Schrimshaw EW, Antebi-Gruszka N, Downing MJ. Viewing of internet-based sexually explicit media as a risk factor for condomless anal sex among men who have sex with men in four U.S. cities. *PLoS One.* 2016;11(4):e0154439.

31. Macapagal K, Coventry R, Puckett JA, et al. Geosocial networking app use among men who have sex with men in serious romantic relationships. *Arch Sex Behav.* 2016;45(6):1513–1524.

32. Heinemann J, Atallah S, Rosenbaum T. The impact of culture and ethnicity on sexuality and sexual function. *Curr Sex Health Rep.* 2016;8(3):144–150.

33. Hogan RM. Influences of culture on sexuality. *Nurs Clin North Am.* 1982;17(3):365–376.

34. Strachan E, Staples B. Masturbation. *Pediatrics in Review.* 2012;33(4):190–191.

35. Braun-Courville DK, Rojas M. Exposure to sexually explicit web sites and adolescent sexual attitudes and behaviors. *J Adolesc Health.* 2009;45(2):156–162.

36. Landripet I, Štulhofer A. Is pornography use associated with sexual difficulties and dysfunctions among younger heterosexual men? *J Sex Med.* 2015;12(5):1136–1139.

37. Prause N, Pfaus J. Viewing sexual stimuli associated with greater sexual responsiveness, not erectile dysfunction. *J Sex Med.* 2015;3(2):90–98.

38. Kvalem IL, Træen B, Lewin B, Štulhofer A. Self-perceived effects of internet pornography use, genital appearance satisfaction, and sexual self-esteem among young Scandinavian adults. *Cyberpsych J Psychosocial Res Cyberspace.* 2014;8(4), Article 4.

39. Grubbs JB, Wilt JA, Exline JJ, et al. Moral disapproval and perceived addiction to internet pornography: A longitudinal examination. *Addiction.* 2018;113(3):496–506.

40. Bourke ME, Grenyer BF. Psychotherapists' response to borderline personality disorder: A core conflictual relationship theme analysis. *Psychother Res.* 2010;20(6): 680–691.

41. Bodner E, Cohen-Fridal S, Iancu I. Staff attitudes toward patients with borderline personality disorder. *Comp Psychiatry.* 2011;52(5):548–555.

42. Aviram RB, Brodsky BS, Stanley B. Borderline personality disorder, stigma, and treatment implications. *Harv Rev Psychiatry.* 2006;14(5):249–256.

43. Connolly PH. Psychological functioning of bondage/domination/sado-masochism (BDSM) practitioners. *J Psych Human Sex.* 2006;18(1):79–120.

44. Nehls N. Borderline personality disorder: The voice of patients. *Res Nurs Health.* 1992;22(4):285–293.

45. Kleinplatz PJ, Moser C. Toward clinical guidelines for working with BDSM clients. *J Contemp Sex.* 2004;38(6):1–4.

46. Richters J, de Visser R, Rissel C, et al. Demographic and psychosocial features of participants in bondage and discipline, "sadomasochism" or dominance and submission (BDSM): Data from a national survey. *J Sex Med.* 2008;5:1660–1668.

47. Wiseman J. *SM 101: A Realistic Introduction.* San Francisco, CA: Greenery Press; 1996.

48. Kleinplatz PJ. Learning from extraordinary lovers: Lessons from the edge. *J Homosex.* 2006;50(2-3):325–348.

49. Easton D, Liszt C. *When Someone You Love Is Kinky.* Oakland, CA: Greenery Press, 2000.

50. Dray K. The *Fifty Shades of Grey* effect. *Cosmopolitan.* https://www.cosmopolitan.com/uk/love-sex/relationships/a16761/fifty-shades-of-grey-sees-400-percent-increase-in-sex-toy-sales/. Published March 27, 2018. Retrieved April 15, 2018.

51. American Psychological Association. *Ethical Principles of Psychologists and Code of Conduct.* 2010. Retrieved from http://www.apa.org/ethics/code/index.aspx

52. American Psychological Association. Guidelines for psychological practice with lesbian, gay, and bisexual clients. 2011. Retrieved from http://www.apa.org/pi/lgbt/resources.guidelines.aspx#

53. American Psychological Association. Sexual orientation & homosexuality: Answers to your questions for a better understanding. 2011. Retrieved from http://www.apa.org/topics/sexuality/orientation.aspx

54. World Health Organization. International Classification of Diseases (ICD). Retrieved November 23, 2010.

55. Joyal CC, Cossette A, Lapierre V. What exactly is an unusual sexual fantasy? *J Sex Med.* 2015;12(2):328–340.

56. Wismeijer A, van Essen M. Psychological characteristics of BDSM practitioners. *J Sex Med.* 2013;10(8):1943–1952.

11

Implicit Bias in Mental Health Care

ANDREA S. HEBERLEIN, JUSTIN A. CHEN,
AND NHI-HA T. TRINH ■

CASE

An intern, Dr. Travis Smith, is rounding on the inpatient psychiatry service with his attending, Dr. Kamala Johnson, and his senior resident, Dr. Karen Chang. The intern is white and a man, the attending is a Black woman, and the resident is an Asian American woman. He walks into the room and the patient, a 75-year-old white man with depression, turns to him and says, "Hi Doc, I'm so glad to see you." Dr. Smith introduces himself and mentions that his attending is Dr. Johnson and his senior resident is Dr. Chang. The patient takes a look at Drs. Johnson and Chang and back at the intern and says, "Right, you're the doctor, and they must be your nurses." Dr. Smith corrects him, and gestures to their name badges. Dr. Johnson and Dr. Chang try to shake the patient's hand but he just smiles at them and turns back to Dr. Smith. During the interview, the patient responds to questions from the team by addressing only Dr. Smith. The intern grew up in a small town in Alabama, and his accent reflects that. The patient's wife seems sensitive to this: She muses aloud that Dr. Smith seems really smart "for someone from the South," queries where he went to medical school, and raises an eyebrow skeptically when he notes that his degree is from the University of Alabama-Birmingham, the state's flagship school (an excellent medical school, though he doesn't point that out to her). Dr. Johnson laughs at this; she means only to put everyone at ease, as she knows Dr. Smith is highly competent, but Dr. Smith flushes. The patient's wife seems to be confused as on whom to focus.

IMPLICIT BIAS

Some behaviors can easily be linked to bias—a negative attitude about a group that then translates into negative attitudes about (and, often, discriminatory behavior toward) individuals one believes to be members of that group. We can see these effects easily in others, and occasionally have the perspective to see them in ourselves. However, one of the major lessons of psychological research of the second half of the 20th century (with some intellectual debt reaching back to Freud) is that people are far less aware of the workings of their minds than introspection might reveal. For example, in the realm of visual perception, we are not aware of the existence of blind spots on our retinae because the perceptual "filling-in" of the missing information from this spot is so seamless in our conscious perception. Notably, we also cannot *will* ourselves to not have a blind spot, nor can we prevent the filling-in of our consciously experienced world. And yet, while people might experience wonder at how much of visual perception happens outside of consciousness (and without being affected by intentions), individuals are often less ready to accept that a great deal of other mental processing also happens outside of conscious awareness.[1]

One might expect that mental health clinicians would have a particularly keen awareness of unconscious processes, since the very concept of unconsciousness was popularized by the influential psychoanalyst Sigmund Freud. Examples of unconscious reactions that play out in everyday clinical interactions include transference and countertransference—that is, unconscious redirections of feelings from patients to clinicians and vice versa that are based on prior relationships from childhood. However, many mental health clinicians may not have applied these concepts specifically to biases about patients, particularly with regard to race, religion, or gender. In this chapter, we will focus on a useful distinction between *explicit* attitudes (those that people know they hold, and which can thus be measured using questionnaires and rating scales) and *implicit* attitudes (those that people are not aware they hold). Explicit attitudes are what we typically think about when we discuss prejudice and bias; implicit attitudes are not as intuitively understood.

Two decades of research on implicit attitudes have shown that, while explicit attitudes are obviously predictive of behavior, implicit attitudes have greater predictive validity in a particular set of situations: those in which people have a motivation to not express, and/or not be aware of, a particular (usually negative) attitude. Think back to the examples above: Were the patient to be asked about his beliefs, he might well not express any negativity (toward women, Asians/Asian Americans, or Black/African American individuals); he might further be fully committed to, for example, his daughter's access to professional training, and/or genuinely be able to point to valued friendships with African Americans. In other words, he might not express any explicit prejudice; he might in fact be deeply committed to *eradicating* prejudicial treatment, both societally and in his own behavior. Why, then, did he treat the intern with more respect than the senior resident and the attending doctor? And why did his wife's estimation of the intern's competence decline when she heard his accent? What associations or habits of thought might underlie such behavior?

Thinking through these questions reveals two critical features of implicit associations: First, implicit attitudes may well lie *contrary* to one's explicitly held, conscious attitudes. The patient's behavior toward Drs. Chang and Johnson did not reveal an intention to harm them. Implicit stereotypes and bias do not necessarily correlate with hostility and often coexist with explicit egalitarian attitudes. (In fact, people sometimes struggle with the *bias* component of *implicit bias*, because we think of bias as explicit hostility, which implicit bias by definition is not.) Second, implicit associations can nonetheless be destructive in interpersonal interactions, even when they are contradicted by one's explicit attitudes and beliefs. In the case above, Drs. Smith, Johnson, and Chang may not have been impeded in their ability to interview, examine, diagnose, and formulate a treatment plan for the patient—though if the patient or his wife isn't able to trust one or more of the doctors, any of these activities might actually be compromised. However, imagine that Dr. Smith feels defensive, and this is reflected in his nonverbal behavior. Now, the patient or his wife might feel wary about sharing sensitive information; they might feel unhappy with the encounter. Further, if repeated over time, such seemingly subtle comments may gradually serve to erode Drs. Johnson's and Chang's confidence in their own abilities, given their implication, however inaccurate, that these professionals do not fit the bill of what a doctor "should" look like. Such comments may put Dr. Smith in the uncomfortable position of caretaking for his senior resident and attending, or even undermine his confidence in their level of competence. And seeing Dr. Smith's competence questioned by patients or their family members might also subtly weaken his supervisors' confidence in him.

Although the preceding case vignette illustrated implicit bias of a patient and his family member, in this chapter we will primarily focus on the implicit biases of care providers, and provide a framework for educating trainees about these common, unconscious processes and their effects on patient care. This chapter has three goals: (1) to describe implicit attitudes and associations and how they are measured; (2) to review literature on their predictive validity: What specific behaviors have been linked to implicit associations, especially as compared to explicit associations?; and (3) to suggest how one might counteract one's own unwanted implicit associations and thus minimize the potential for one's own behavior to harm others in clinical contexts.

IMPLICIT ASSOCIATIONS AND ATTITUDES

Implicit mental constructs are ones that we are not consciously aware of and cannot consciously control. Thus, in contrast to explicit attitudes and associations, implicit attitudes and associations cannot be measured with questionnaires or other self-report. A quick but important note about terms: In psychological research, *association* refers to a relationship or connection between concepts, and *attitude* refers to a positive or negative inclination toward some target. For example, I might have a positive attitude toward the concept *coffee*, as well as associations between the word, the smell, the taste, and the feeling of being energized and productive. We can think of an attitude as a mental association between a concept (like *coffee*) and either *positivity* or *negativity*—in other words, attitude is just an association with valence. All of this is relevant because the most common measure of implicit attitudes, the IAT, is known as both the Implicit Attitude Test and the Implicit Association Test: It uses the same method to measure either one. The IAT measures what Cronbach and Meehl (1955) called the "nomological net": a web of relationships and associations between stored conceptual representations.[2] IATs and related measures test this web or network using speeded response times.

Imagine that I wanted to test whether you implicitly associated coffee with productivity or with leisure. I might ask you to categorize images related to coffee (e.g., mugs, percolators) versus images related to some comparison beverage like lemonade (e.g., lemons, glasses), by pressing one key for coffee-related words and a different key (with your other hand) for lemonade-related words (Fig. 11.1). At the same time, I would ask you to categorize words related to productivity (e.g., goals, accomplishment, work) with either the same left-hand key or the same right-hand key as one of the previous categories, and to categorize words related to leisure (e.g.,

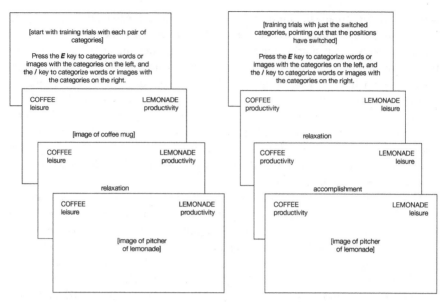

Figure 11.1 Examples of critical trials on the IAT. Participants first complete two blocks of training trials, sorting words or pictures for just one pair of categories (e.g., first sorting pictures related to coffee and to lemonade, and next sorting words related to leisure and then to productivity). Then, participants categorize randomly ordered words and pictures simultaneously, as shown in the example screenshots on the left. Next, one of the pairs switches sides (productivity and leisure, in this example), and participants practice categorizing according to these new positions. Finally, participants categorize randomly ordered words and pictures simultaneously, but with the switched pairings, as shown in the example screenshots on the right. Note that half of participants would get the pairing that is consistent ("congruent") with the stereotype first, as in the screenshots on the right, and the other half would get this pairing second and get the incongruent pairing first. This controls for any differences in timing associated with practice or learning. On average, people will respond slower when the pairings of categories are not consistent with existing mental associations. If we tend to associated coffee more strongly with productivity than with leisure, and lemonade more strongly with leisure than with productivity, then we would categorize words and pictures faster when the categories are arranged as in the example trials on the right, and slower when the categories are arranged as in the example trials on the left.

relax, hammock, nap) with the other hand and response key. Do you think you would respond more quickly when words related to coffee and to productivity required the same response (and words related to lemonade and to relaxation required the other response), or when the responses were paired in the opposite way (coffee/relaxation, lemonade/productivity)? This difference in how quickly people respond to one possible pairing of concepts (coffee/productivity) versus another (coffee/relaxation) is a powerful technique for revealing underlying conceptual associations and is the basis for the IAT. Examples are available online at https://implicit.harvard.edu/implicit/.

In the above example, your explicit associations between coffee (vs. lemonade) and productivity (vs. leisure) are likely identical to your implicit associations; few of us, even non–coffee drinkers, would respond faster to a lemonade/productivity pairing than a coffee/productivity pairing. However, explicit and implicit associations don't always line up so neatly. At times, we may not honestly report our attitudes to others. For example, explicit reporting of prejudicial attitudes (such as toward groups of individuals) is constrained by individuals not wanting to admit attitudes they believe to be inappropriate. At other times, we may not *want* to hold a given association and thus may not even admit fully to ourselves that we hold it—for instance, in the case of an accomplished female scientist discovering to her chagrin that she more easily associates male names with "science" than female names. In such cases, the IAT and other measures of implicit associations can serve as a kind of psychological mirror, revealing otherwise inaccessible aspects of our minds to ourselves—or to experimenters.

Where do implicit attitudes and associations come from? Humans tend to think categorically—it's a ubiquitous cognitive feature with obvious advantages for efficiently responding to a world with some predictable elements. However, our categories are informed by inputs outside of our control (or even our awareness, in some cases). In the case that started this chapter, it's likely that the patient would have disavowed explicit racism, and potentially also explicit sexism. His wife may well not have rated Southerners as less intelligent or less competent than Northerners on a questionnaire. The patient may not have intended to show disrespect to the two more senior doctors in the room, but his behavior and his spouse's were being informed by their implicit associations—by the complex web of conceptual associations that they each have developed through their lifetimes of interactions, exposure to cultural input, and previous medical experience. In fact, some researchers debate whether the IAT measures cultural knowledge, as opposed to personally held implicit associations. The exact nature of the relationship between explicit and implicit attitudes is also a topic of ongoing research and debate.[3–5] As noted above, the nature of implicit associations causes some to question whether negative implicit attitude should be termed *bias* at all. It is critical to remember both that implicit attitudes predict behavior *and* that people can reject their own implicit attitudes and associations.[5]

PREDICTIVE VALIDITY OF IMPLICIT MEASURES

To minimize the negative impacts of implicit bias on medical care, we must understand the mechanisms by which implicit attitudes impact interpersonal behavior. The IAT has not been found to predict overt hostility.[1] However, recent meta-analyses have found that implicit measures predict a wide range of measures (including physical actions, judgments, choices, and physiological reactions) with roughly similar validity, on average, as explicit measures do, though explicit and implicit measures vary in their correlation with each other.[4,6] The real utility of implicit measures, though, lies in their ability to predict behavior *better* than explicit measures, which has been found to occur most commonly in cases where there is societal and/or situational pressure against expressing particular attitudes. For example, implicit attitudes, as quantified by the IAT and related measures, predict both verbal and nonverbal elements of interracial interactions better than do explicit measures, especially in cases where explicit and implicit attitudes diverge—as in cases where an individual maintains an explicit egalitarian value but also holds implicit negative attitude towards an outgroup.[7-9] Implicit attitudes have also been found to diverge from explicit attitudes related to sexual orientation, age, skin color (distinct from race), body weight, religion, disability status, and mental health status.[1,6,10] Given that only explicit measures are under intentional control, such dissociations likely result from the effect of social pressures on people's explicitly reported attitudes. In an explicit test of this idea, Banse and colleagues (2001) found that people *instructed* to fake positive attitudes toward gay men could do so on a self-report questionnaire, but not on an attitude IAT.[11]

As an aside, there are other notable instances when implicit measures have diverged from explicit measures in ways that are very relevant to mental health care.[12] The IAT has been used to measure attitudes toward food in people with eating disorders,[13] attitudes toward alcohol in people with disordered alcohol use,[14] and associations between one's self and death in people at risk for suicide[15]—all situations in which individuals may well avoid explicitly reporting, or may not even themselves be aware of, their associations. Individuals could appear low in anxiety on a questionnaire when instructed to "make a good impression" (for a job context) but not on an anxiety self-concept IAT.[16] Further, IATs measuring associations between oneself and concepts relevant to eating disorders, alcohol abuse, anxiety, and depression predict clinical symptoms.[17]

Studies of the predictive validity of implicit measures, particularly for behavior relevant to interpersonal interactions, illustrate how implicit attitudes and associations can sabotage egalitarian intentions. This is true both for action and perception: White individuals' explicit (self-reported) attitudes predict their verbal behavior toward Black Americans, but implicit attitudes predict nonverbal friendliness as rated by observers.[8] When interacting with others, we are particularly sensitive to nonverbal behavior, perhaps *because* it is so difficult to control. In a study of the effects of explicit and implicit attitudes on perception, white Americans' implicit attitudes toward Black Americans predict a greater readiness to perceive anger in Black faces—but explicit attitudes toward Black Americans do not correspond to predictions of anger, and neither explicit nor implicit measures predict how likely participants are to perceive anger in white faces.[18]

An influential functional imaging study provides insight into the mechanisms relating explicit and implicit attitudes to perception of other-race faces: Cunningham and colleagues used fMRI to examine neural responses of white participants viewing Black and white faces. They found that implicit bias against Black Americans predict activity of the white participants' amygdala (a medial temporal lobe nucleus related to fear and threat processing), but only when the faces are presented subliminally (30 ms). When faces were presented for longer durations (525 ms), and thus were consciously perceived, the same white participants do not have greater amygdala activity when viewing Black faces compared to when they view white faces.[19] Beyond supporting a distinction between implicit and explicit bias, this study illustrates the *dual-process* nature of prejudice. Widespread in experimental psychology, dual-process models include an automatic/intuitive component (System 1) and an effortful/rational component (System 2).[20,21] Both contribute to behavior, including decisions and judgments, but only System 2 is under direct control. In Cunningham and colleagues' study, when white participants—all of whom expressed a motivation to respond without bias—viewed photos of Black individuals *and were consciously aware of what they were seeing*, not only do they exhibit lower amygdala activity, but they also exhibit higher activity in prefrontal regions associated with cognitive control.[19] This implies not only that people who have an expressed motivation to be unbiased nevertheless evidence implicit bias, but importantly that people can control their responses in conditions where rational, conscious processes can be brought to bear.[22] However, decades of research on dual-process mechanisms clearly show that System 1 processes—automatic, unconscious, intuitive—drive a substantial proportion of human behavior,[20] consistent with the findings reviewed above, of implicit bias affecting nonverbal behavior in detectable ways even in explicitly egalitarian individuals.

Additional research suggests mechanisms by which implicit attitudes could affect social interactions. In a recent study, white participants were assigned to an "instructor" role in pairings with either white or Black participants assigned to a "learner" role. The implicit bias of these white participants negatively predicted Black learners' performance. Explicit attitude did not, and there was no relationship between implicit bias and the performance of white learners. When videos of the instructors were coded, both instructor anxiety and lesson quality were found to mediate this effect.[23] In general, negative implicit attitudes lead to nonverbal behaviors reflecting discomfort, anxiety, or other negative affective states, which in turn are readily perceived by the targets of these implicit attitudes.[8,24-27]

IMPLICIT BIAS IN MEDICINE

Explicit bias is generally condemned in medicine,[28] but substantial evidence exists for implicit bias in physicians and nurses toward groups that are likely to comprise significant proportions of their relevant patient populations. This is likely to impact patient care in at least two main ways: First, physicians' and nurses' implicit stereotypic associations can impact treatment recommendations and information given to patients, and second, as noted above, implicit bias is reflected in nonverbal behaviors in ways that are difficult to control, yet easily detectable.[8]

The existence of implicit bias in medical professionals is well documented. For example, a study of 2,535 physicians found an implicit preference for white relative to Black patients, using the IAT;[29] the degree of bias was stronger than the explicit bias expressed within all demographic groups examined within this sample except Black physicians, who did not on average show an implicit preference in either direction. Emergency department care providers (physicians and nurses) exhibit implicit bias against American Indian children and adults relative to non-Hispanic white individuals,[30] an effect that differed by age (with older providers exhibiting lower levels of implicit bias) but not by provider type, rural versus urban location, or the percentage of American Indian children seen during a typical work shift.

The prevalence of implicit race bias cannot be dismissed in the face of documentation that nonwhite patients have been shown to receive different care than white patients: less empathy, less attentive care, differential care, and less control over treatment decisions.[28,31-33] It's notable that, at least until recently, white clinicians have tended to believe that racial or ethnic bias does not influence patient care, whereas roughly half of Black and Latino respondents *do* believe that bias affects care.[34,35] Not only has the existence of implicit bias now been well documented, but it has been shown to predict treatment differences. An influential study of 287 internal medicine and emergency medicine residents published in 2007[28] directly links differences in treatment decisions to implicit bias. In this study, physicians completed IATs, one measuring implicit race bias (against African Americans), and two others measuring implicit associations between whites versus African Americans and cooperativeness, both generally and within medical contexts. They were then given a patient case vignette describing cardiac symptoms, paired with either an African American or a white male face. All three of the IATs predicted physicians' recommendations of thrombolysis; explicit measures of race bias did not.[28] In a similar vignette-based study, Sabin and Greenwald found that implicit pro-white bias predicted differential prescription of postoperative opioid medication for white versus African American patients among pediatricians.[36] However, other vignette-based studies, while typically documenting implicit bias, have not found relationships between implicit measures and hypothetical treatment recommendations (in studies of pediatricians,[37] surgical nurses,[38] primary care and family medicine physicians' recommendations for total knee replacement,[39] and Indian Health Service physicians[40]). In at least one of these samples, the physicians were noted to typically see a high proportion of minority patients, which may have led to the lack of differential treatment recommendations.

The field of psychiatry is certainly not immune to the pernicious influence of implicit bias. A recent review of 24 years of empirical research regarding the association between race and diagnosis of psychotic disorders found a pervasive pattern in which African American/Black and Latino American/Hispanic patients were disproportionately diagnosed with psychotic disorders at rates of approximately three to four times that of their European American/white counterparts.[41] The authors of this review note that these disparities may be attributed to clinicians' unconscious bias. Specifically, some psychiatrists have argued that higher rates of psychotic disorder diagnoses correspond to long-held stereotypes of African Americans as potentially dangerous or violent.[42] In another study of racial-ethnic differences in diagnosis and treatment of psychiatric conditions across the Mental Health Research Network, a consortium of 11 private, not-for-profit U.S. health care delivery systems, non-Hispanic blacks were almost twice as likely as non-Hispanic whites to be diagnosed with schizophrenia.[43] When Black patients are prescribed psychiatric medications, there is evidence to suggest that the most appropriate choice is not always selected. A review of Texas Medicaid claims data found that even after controlling for a number of relevant sociodemographic and clinical disease severity variables, Black patients were significantly less likely than whites to receive newer second-generation antipsychotic medications such as risperidone or olanzapine as opposed to older medications such as haloperidol, which are associated with significant side effects such as acute dystonia and tardive dyskinesia, and are therefore generally less favored as first-line treatment.[44] This disparity in prescribing patterns may provide further evidence that black patients with psychosis are perceived as more potentially violent or dangerous and therefore as requiring more powerful medications.

Alongside effects on diagnosis and treatment decisions, implicit bias can have deleterious effects on communication between medical professionals and patients. In a survey of nearly 3,000 patients, primary care clinicians with higher levels of implicit bias (measured by IAT) were rated lower on four subscales of the Primary Care Assessment Survey by Black patients.[45] (Interestingly, in the same study, Latinx patients did not rate clinicians differently as a function of their implicit bias on a Latino/white IAT.) A construct known as *aversive racism* may explain this effect: Dovidio and colleagues[8,9] define *aversive racism* as the combination of low explicit racism but high implicit racism, particularly in the context of beliefs about the importance of equal access. A substantial (and growing) body of research has found that aversive racists convey mixed messages during interracial interactions. For example, a study of family medicine residents found that Black patients' satisfaction ratings were predicted by a combination of explicit and implicit bias measures in the residents in a surprising pattern. When residents had low levels of explicit bias, patients' ratings of them were negatively predicted by their implicit bias (higher implicit bias led to lower ratings; this is unsurprising). However, when residents had high levels of implicit bias, explicit bias was *positively* correlated with patient satisfaction: In other words, residents with concordant, *high* levels of explicit bias were liked *more* than residents with discordant high-implicit, low-explicit bias.[46]

Implicit bias and implicit stereotypes about compliance in Black (vs. white) patients also predicted communication patterns of physicians in an intervention focused on communication in the management of hypertension and depression.[47] Clinician verbal dominance and patient-centeredness were coded from medical visit audio recordings, using the Roter Interaction Analysis System.[48] Other dependent variables in this study included emotional tone and questions from a post-visit survey given to patients (e.g., "My doctor likes me"). Both white and Asian doctors showed, on average, moderate levels of bias on both IATs; Black doctors did not. Higher levels of implicit bias on a race attitude IAT predicted more clinical verbal dominance with both Black and white patients, and lower patient positive affect scores after Black patient visits. Black patients also believed that physicians with higher IAT-measured bias had lower respect for them and liked them less; Black patients also responded that they were less likely to recommend these doctors to others. Implicit racial stereotypes about compliance, as measured by the second IAT, predicted lower patient-centered dialogue in visits with Black patients. With both Black and white patients, implicit racial stereotypes about compliance were also associated with lower predicted probabilities of patients perceiving the clinician as involving them in decisions.[47] It's important to note that the two IATs were not highly correlated, highlighting that even in the absence of general race-based attitude difference (or bias), individuals may still hold implicit stereotypes related to race, for example regarding differential compliance.

As Murray-García and colleagues[27] note, the communication patterns between white clinicians and nonwhite patients, predicted by clinician implicit bias and stereotypes, can "set in motion parallel, self-reinforcing cycles" between clinicians and patients leading to breakdowns in (or barriers to) a collaborative, cooperative relationship—and this effect can carry over into subsequent clinician–patient relationships. Clinicians can create a self-fulfilling prophecy, in which they unintentionally confirm their own (implicit or explicit) beliefs by asking some questions and omitting others.[49-53] Self-fulfilling prophecy effects can result from both physician and patient expectations, and particularly from combinations of these: Hagiwara and colleagues[54] examined the simultaneous influence of physician bias and patients' past perceptions of discrimination and found that both of these influence the ratio of time that physicians versus patients spent talking in a clinic visit. Non-Black primary care providers' implicit bias predicted higher physician talk time relative to patient talk time; in contrast, their explicit bias did not—further evidence for the higher predictive validity of implicit measures. Black patients with higher levels of past perceived discrimination tended to talk *more*, and patients who talked more were less likely to adhere to treatment recommendations.[54] Another study by these researchers[55] used similar predictor variables to address the mechanisms underlying these effects. Analyses of videos from physician–patient encounters found that physicians' affect and level of engagement were predicted by the relationship between explicit and implicit bias, but only in the context of patients with a history of perceived discrimination. Patients' affect was predicted by their history of perceived discrimination. In other words, physicians who demonstrate the aversive racism pattern interacting with patients who were less trusting or warier are particularly likely to evidence more negative affect and lower engagement.[55]

The cultural transmission of implicit attitudes continues into medical school: A large-scale survey of medical students (the Medical Student Cognitive Habits and Growth Evaluation Study [CHANGES]) found that hearing negative comments about African American patients in the clinic (which might be considered part of the "hidden curriculum" modeled by supervising physicians) predicted an increase in implicit racial bias between the first and fourth year of medical school.[56] In another publication based on the same large survey, Phelan and colleagues[57] found that faculty role modeling of weight bias predicted an increase in both implicit and explicit bias toward overweight individuals, as did training in dealing with difficult patients. This latter (somewhat surprising) result may result from the deleterious effects of categorization; that is, thinking of overweight individuals as a category associated with "difficultness" (or thinking of difficult patients as a category unto themselves) may increase stereotyping along this dimension.[57]

Though we have focused primarily on the impacts of implicit bias and stereotypes related to race and ethnicity, which have been well documented, other forms of bias and stereotyping also affect the care that individuals receive. Implicit negative attitudes or implicit beliefs about groups defined by social class, immigration status, sexual orientation, region of origin, weight, and mental health diagnosis can all affect both nonverbal behavior and communication patterns, with deleterious effects for clinician–patient relationships and ultimately for the patient's health outcomes. Such negative attitudes and stereotypes are widespread, including within medicine. For example, the CHANGES survey of medical students found that nearly half of the 2,088 heterosexual respondents expressed at least some *explicit* bias toward gay and lesbian individuals, and 81% exhibited at least some implicit bias on an IAT.[58] The majority of all respondents in the same CHANGES survey expressed both explicit and implicit bias against overweight individuals.[59] Bias against overweight individuals was also observed in a large study of physicians (N = 2,284), who exhibited both strong explicit and implicit biases,[60] and in a study of nursing and of psychology preprofessional students, who exhibited implicit bias.[61] Stereotypes associated with overweight and obese individuals include noncompliance, lack of intelligence, and weak will,[62] behaviors associated with decreased agency. Attributing—implicitly or not—lower levels of agency to individuals is a subtle form of dehumanization with obviously deleterious effects on communication and the clinician–patient relationship.[63,64] Experiencing this form of stereotyping and dehumanization leads many overweight and obese individuals to avoid medical care, including for weight-associated health problems.[62] In general, people tend to rely on stereotypes more for outgroup members; group membership can be defined in a large number of ways, any combination of which may be relevant in a given interaction.

Members of the general public not only have implicit biases against people with mental health diagnoses (measured in an IAT comparing attitudes toward mental illness and physical illness), but also have stronger associations between mental illness and helplessness, and between mental illness and blameworthiness[65]—negative implicit attitudes that parallel explicit evaluations for negativity and helplessness. This same experiment found that negative implicit and explicit attitudes were also present in participants with mental illness diagnoses—a form of internalized prejudice. Another study exploring links between implicit and explicit bias toward patients with mental illness found that (reassuringly!) people with mental health training—including graduate students and professionals with clinical psychology or counseling psychology PhDs, social workers, and psychiatrists—displayed lower levels of implicit bias than did undergraduates, members of the public, or people in "helping professions" not directly linked to mental health (e.g., other medical professionals or people working in social services).[10] Notably, explicit and implicit attitudes toward patients with mental illness were only weakly correlated, and showed differential predictive validity: Explicit attitudes predicted more negative prognoses based on patient vignettes (and implicit attitudes did not), but implicit attitudes predicted overdiagnosis (and explicit attitudes did not). Of note, many such IATs are available at www.ImplicitMentalHealth.com, which contains both educational and research information on implicit biases relating to patients with mental illness.

Biases against individuals with mental health diagnoses are not limited to members of the public. In a 2010 mixed-methods study of 256 primary care physicians, physicians reported more negative attitudes for patients with schizophrenia with bizarre affect (SBA) as compared to schizophrenia with normal affect, depression, or eczema as control.[66] There were few differences in clinical decisions measured quantitatively or in charting, but qualitative data revealed less trust of patients with SBA as reporters, with more reliance on sources other than the patient. Physicians often alerted colleagues about SBA, thereby shaping expectations before interactions occurred. The authors concluded that the results are consistent with common stereotypes about people with serious mental illness, as vignettes did not include intentional indication of unreliable reporting or danger. One interpretation of this study is that physicians have an implicit (almost explicit?) bias that such patients with signs of mental illness are not reliable historians and thus may not be adherent to care. Thus, clinicians' implicit bias may result in disparate care for those afflicted with particular diagnoses.

In sum, a significant body of research suggests that implicit bias exerts powerful effects in medical care in general, and in mental health care in particular. Clinicians' unconscious biases contribute to disparities in both the diagnoses and treatments that certain patients receive. A first step toward eliminating disparities, then, must involve clinicians becoming aware of their implicit biases, for example by undergoing IAT, recognizing that such biases are a natural human tendency, and actively challenging themselves to think more objectively in future situations. Clinicians should also be aware that their patients are likely to struggle from the effects of implicit bias regarding many forms of mental illness in other settings, including in health care as well as society at large.

INTERVENTIONS: HOW TO DECREASE IMPLICIT BIAS

A first step in decreasing one's implicit bias is seemingly straightforward: to acknowledge the existence of implicit components of attitudes and associations. In other words, in some cases, simply being aware of implicit bias can lead one to dampen its effects on one's behavior. For example, non–African-American medical students who took a race-bias IAT during the first year of medical school showed lower levels of implicit bias in their fourth year than other students who did not have the experience alerting them to their implicit bias.[56] There is evidence that individuals who focus on reducing their *implicit* bias, specifically, are able to do so.[67] Becoming aware of one's implicit biases and stereotypes is challenging, however, because they affect behavior, by definition, without awareness, and thus are frequently invisible to those who hold them.[68] Particularly when we are motivated *not* to hold such attitudes and associations, our awareness tends to be limited to our explicit attitudes. Remember the surveys showing a disparity between what white physicians and Black and Latinx members of the public believed about disparities in health care?[34,35]

In addition, there are two key pitfalls to avoid when educating individuals about implicit bias. One potential pitfall resulting from increased awareness of one's own implicit bias is a category of what we might call ironic effects.[69] Ironic effects result when one tries not to attend to some mental content, and ironically ends up being unable to think of anything else (this is sometimes known as the white bear effect, after the illustrative exercise to *Try not to think about a white bear*—which ends up, typically, resulting in many more white bear–related thoughts than would have occurred otherwise). Suppressing stereotypes or negative attitudes can lead to one's being hypersensitive to thoughts related to the suppressed content; focusing on specific salient categories of others can paradoxically lead to increased activation of these stereotypes. Instead of suppressing, Burgess and colleagues recommend that we think about professionalism and providing excellent care to all patients, acknowledge the human tendency to categorize others,[70] and mindfully train ourselves to be aware of the potentially negative consequences of stereotyping.[71]

Paradoxically, teaching about cultural competence can inadvertently feed into both explicit and implicit stereotyping behaviors. The opposite of stereotyping is to treat each person as an individual: to acknowledge that, while there may be cultural differences that predict certain elements of a person's values, beliefs, or behavior, each individual reflects a unique combination of influences from his or her culture(s), temperament, and experiences. Individuating is cognitively demanding; the pressure to stereotype and categorize is driven by the need for cognitive efficiency.[1,49] If one learns about an unfamiliar culture and learns that members of that culture tend to share some behavior or cultural value, one might unthinkingly use that knowledge to stereotype individuals of that culture.[68] Put another way, cultural competence might lead to better categories, but learning about categories may end up reinforcing the mental habit of putting people into categories. (This is not to say that cultural competence training should be abandoned! Instead, one might imagine its best use, in this light, as enlightening about what differences in values *could* exist. Enabling us to become aware of our assumptions is useful; making new assumptions is not.) Understanding that individuation is effortful, and an important way to counteract stereotyping and improve relationships, is thus critically important.[70]

The second potential pitfall resulting from increased awareness of one's own implicit bias is that it is deeply troubling to acknowledge our implicit biases in cases when they conflict with our explicit attitudes. Confronting one's implicit bias leads to feelings of guilt and defensiveness, and thus merely making an individual aware of his or her bias, without adequate support for the feelings that this engenders, can backfire.[27] Murray-García and colleagues offer a list of questions that should inform education on implicit bias to minimize backfire effects:

> When you first see and hear the awkwardness that informs the anxiety in my dialogue, will you see it as implying ill will or bigoted intent? When you reveal to me the painful and embarrassing duplicity of my aversive racism and how it can subconsciously undermine relationship-building with patients, will you also give me a place where I won't be judged by my peers or evaluated harshly by you, my instructor? Will this be a space wherein I can deal with my self-betrayal, self-disappointment, and guilt, and find nonjudgment, and even healing and absolution, from you and my peers? Who will reassure me that I am not fatally flawed, but rather in an important stage of my racial identity development . . .? Will you show me how not to consume the energy I need to recover in dialogue, how not to consume that energy on defensiveness, avoidance, and even resentment? Will you protect the often already marginalized non-White students from the colluding, silencing, and retaliatory behaviors of their White peers, behaviors which can predictably spring from my guilt, anger, and need for mastery? Are you skilled enough to make this a constructive rather than a divisive experience for my peers and me? Is there an authority figure in the room who can help me walk out of here—maybe not on this day, but on some day—with the sense of hope, inspiration, investment, and courage it will take to sustain this lifelong path of self-discovery, self-critique, and learning you have asked and implicitly required me to embark on . . .?[27]

To summarize, a first, critical step in reducing implicit bias and stereotyping is to acknowledge the existence of one's implicit biases—conscientiously, with the aid of tools such as cultural competency training and information about the historical significance of racist attitudes, and in a supportive atmosphere that enables us to experience the range of emotional reactions that might follow this new awareness.

ACKNOWLEDGMENT

The authors would like to acknowledge Ms. Andrea Madu's contribution to the background research of this chapter.

REFERENCES

1. Banaji, M. R., & Greenwald, A. G. *Blindspot: hidden biases of good people.* New York: Delacorte Press, 2016.
2. Cronbach, L. J., & Meehl, P. E. Construct validity in psychological tests. *Psychol. Bull.* **52**, 281–302 (1955).

3. Nosek, B. A. Moderators of the relationship between implicit and explicit evaluation. *J. Exp. Psychol. Gen.* **134**, 565 (2005).

4. Hofmann, W., Gawronski, B., Gschwendner, T., et al. A meta-analysis on the correlation between the Implicit Association Test and explicit self-report measures. *Pers. Soc. Psychol. Bull.* **31**, 1369–1385 (2005).

5. Nosek, B. A., Ranganath, K. A., Smith, C. T., et al. Pervasiveness and correlates of implicit attitudes and stereotypes. *Eur. Rev. Soc. Psychol.* **18**, 36–88 (2007).

6. Greenwald, A. G., Poehlman, T. A., Uhlmann, E. L., & Banaji, M. R. Understanding and using the Implicit Association Test: III. Meta-analysis of predictive validity. *J. Pers. Soc. Psychol.* **97**, 17 (2009).

7. Dovidio, J. F., Kawakami, K., Johnson, C., et al. On the nature of prejudice: Automatic and controlled processes. *J. Exp. Soc. Psychol.* **33**, 510–540 (1997).

8. Dovidio, J. F., Kawakami, K., & Gaertner, S. L. Implicit and explicit prejudice and interracial interaction. *J. Pers. Soc. Psychol.* **82**, 62 (2002).

9. Gaertner, S. L., & Dovidio, J. F. *The aversive form of racism.* San Diego, CA: Academic Press, 1986.

10. Peris, T. S., Teachman, B. A., & Nosek, B. A. Implicit and explicit stigma of mental illness: links to clinical care. *J. Nerv. Ment. Dis.* **196**, 752–760 (2008).

11. Banse, R., Seise, J., & Zerbes, N. Implicit attitudes towards homosexuality: reliability, validity, and controllability of the IAT. *Z. Für Exp. Psychol.* **48**, 145–160 (2001).

12. Roefs, A., Huijding, J., Smulders, F. T., et al. Implicit measures of association in psychopathology research. *Psychol. Bull.* **137**, 149 (2011).

13. Vartanian, L. R., Polivy, J., & Herman, C. P. Implicit cognitions and eating disorders: their application in research and treatment. *Cogn. Behav. Pract.* **11**, 160–167 (2004).

14. Houben, K., & Wiers, R. W. Implicitly positive about alcohol? Implicit positive associations predict drinking behavior. *Addict. Behav.* **33**, 979–986 (2008).

15. Nock, M. K., & Banaji, M. R. Prediction of suicide ideation and attempts among adolescents using a brief performance-based test. *J. Consult. Clin. Psychol.* **75**, 707 (2007).

16. Egloff, B., & Schmukle, S. C. Predictive validity of an Implicit Association Test for assessing anxiety. *J. Pers. Soc. Psychol.* **83**, 1441 (2002).

17. Werntz, A. J., Steinman, S. A., Glenn, J. J., et al. Characterizing implicit mental health associations across clinical domains. *J. Behav. Ther. Exp. Psychiatry* **52**, 17–28 (2016).

18. Hugenberg, K., & Bodenhausen, G. V. Facing prejudice: implicit prejudice and the perception of facial threat. *Psychol. Sci.* **14**, 640–643 (2003).

19. Cunningham, W. A., Johnson, M. K., Raye, C. L., et al. Separable neural components in the processing of black and white faces. *Psychol. Sci.* **15**, 806–813 (2004).

20. Kahneman, D. A perspective on judgment and choice: mapping bounded rationality. *Am. Psychol.* **58**, 697 (2003).

21. Gilovich, T., Griffin, D., & Kahneman, D. *Heuristics and biases: the psychology of intuitive judgment.* Cambridge, UK: Cambridge University Press, 2002.

22. Devine, P. G. Stereotypes and prejudice: their automatic and controlled components. *J. Pers. Soc. Psychol.* **56**, 5 (1989).

23. Jacoby-Senghor, D. S., Sinclair, S., & Shelton, J. N. A lesson in bias: the relationship between implicit racial bias and performance in pedagogical contexts. *J. Exp. Soc. Psychol.* **63**, 50–55 (2016).

24. Blascovich, J., Mendes, W. B., Hunter, S. B., et al. Perceiver threat in social interactions with stigmatized others. *J. Pers. Soc. Psychol.* **80**, 253 (2001).

25. Dovidio, J. F., & Fiske, S. T. Under the radar: how unexamined biases in decision-making processes in clinical interactions can contribute to health care disparities. *Am. J. Public Health* **102**, 945–952 (2012).

26. Dovidio, J. F., Penner, L. A., Albrecht, T. L., et al. Disparities and distrust: the implications of psychological processes for understanding racial disparities in health and health care. *Soc. Sci. Med.* **67**, 478–486 (2008).

27. Murray-García, J. L., Harrell, S., García, J. A., et al. Dialogue as skill: training a health professions workforce that can talk about race and racism. *Am. J. Orthopsychiatry* **84**, 590 (2014).

28. Green, A. R., Carney, D. R., Pallin, D. J., et al. Implicit bias among physicians and its prediction of thrombolysis decisions for black and white patients. *J. Gen. Intern. Med.* **22**, 1231–1238 (2007).

29. Sabin, D. J. A., Nosek, D. B. A., Greenwald, D. A. G., & Rivara, D. F. P. Physicians' implicit and explicit attitudes about race by MD race, ethnicity, and gender. *J. Health Care Poor Underserved* **20**, 896 (2009).

30. Puumala, S. E., Burgess, K. M., Kharbanda, A. B., et al. The role of bias by emergency department providers in care for American Indian children. *Med. Care* **54**, 562 (2016).

31. Johnson, R. L., Saha, S., Arbelaez, J. J., et al. Racial and ethnic differences in patient perceptions of bias and cultural competence in health care. *J. Gen. Intern. Med.* **19**, 101–110 (2004).

32. Basáñez, T., Blanco, L., Collazo, J. L., et al. Ethnic groups' perception of physicians' attentiveness: implications for health and obesity. *Psychol. Health Med.* **18**, 37–46 (2013).

33. DeVoe, J. E., Wallace, L. S., Pandhi, N., et al. Comprehending care in a medical home: a usual source of care and patient perceptions about healthcare communication. *J. Am. Board Fam. Med.* **21**, 441–450 (2008).

34. Henry J. Kaiser Family Foundation. *Race, ethnicity and medical care: a survey of public perceptions and experiences.* (1999). Available at https://www.kff.org/disparities-policy/poll-finding/race-ethnicity-medical-care-a-survey-of/

35. Henry J. Kaiser Family Foundation. *National survey of physicians part I: doctors on disparities in medical care.* (2002). Available at https://www.kff.org/uninsured/national-survey-of-physicians-part-i-doctors/

36. Sabin, J. A., & Greenwald, A. G. The influence of implicit bias on treatment recommendations for 4 common pediatric conditions: pain, urinary tract infection, attention deficit hyperactivity disorder, and asthma. *Am. J. Public Health* **102**, 988–995 (2012).

37. Sabin, J. A., Rivara, F. P., & Greenwald, A. G. Physician implicit attitudes and stereotypes about race and quality of medical care. *Med. Care* **46**, 678–685 (2008).

38. Haider, A. H., Schneider, E. B., Sriram, N., et al. Unconscious race and social class bias among acute care surgical clinicians and clinical treatment decisions. *JAMA Surg.* **150**, 457–464 (2015).

39. Oliver, M. N., Wells, K. M., Joy-Gaba, J. A., et al. Do physicians' implicit views of African Americans affect clinical decision making? *J. Am. Board Fam. Med.* **27**, 177–188 (2014).

40. Sabin, J. A., Moore, K., Noonan, C., et al. Clinicians' implicit and explicit attitudes about weight and race and treatment approaches to overweight for American Indian children. *Child. Obes.* **11**, 456–465 (2015).

41. Schwartz, R. C., & Blankenship, D. M. Racial disparities in psychotic disorder diagnosis: a review of empirical literature. *World J. Psychiatry* **4**, 133 (2014).

42. Lawson, W. How Americans' view of Black men affects mental health care. *Psychiatric News* (2013). Available at https://psychnews.psychiatryonline.org/doi/full/10.1176/appi.pn.2013.10b22

43. Coleman, K. J., Stewart, C., Waitzfelder, B. E., et al. Racial-ethnic differences in psychiatric diagnoses and treatment across 11 health care systems in the Mental Health Research Network. *Psychiatr. Serv.* **67**, 749–757 (2016).

44. Opolka, J. L., Rascati, K. L., Brown, C. M., & Gibson, P. J. Ethnicity and prescription patterns for haloperidol, risperidone, and olanzapine. *Psychiatr. Serv.* **55**, 151–156 (2004).

45. Blair, I. V., Steiner, J. F., Hanratty, R., et al. An investigation of associations between clinicians' ethnic or racial bias and hypertension treatment, medication adherence and blood pressure control. *J. Gen. Intern. Med.* **29**, 987–995 (2014).

46. Penner, L. A., Dovidio, J. F., West, T. V., et al. Aversive racism and medical interactions with Black patients: A field study. *J. Exp. Soc. Psychol.* **46**, 436–440 (2010).

47. Cooper, L. A., Roter, D. L., Carson, K. A., et al. The associations of clinicians' implicit attitudes about race with medical visit communication and patient ratings of interpersonal care. *Am. J. Public Health* **102**, 979–987 (2012).

48. Roter, D., & Larson, S. The Roter interaction analysis system (RIAS): utility and flexibility for analysis of medical interactions. *Patient Educ. Couns.* **46**, 243–251 (2002).

49. Burgess, D. J., Fu, S. S., & Van Ryn, M. Why do providers contribute to disparities and what can be done about it? *J. Gen. Intern. Med.* **19**, 1154–1159 (2004).

50. Cooper, L. A., Roter, D. L., Johnson, R. L., et al. Patient-centered communication, ratings of care, and concordance of patient and physician race. *Ann. Intern. Med.* **139**, 907–915 (2003).

51. Ashton, C. M., Haidet, P., Paterniti, D. A., et al. Racial and ethnic disparities in the use of health services. *J. Gen. Intern. Med.* **18**, 146–152 (2003).

52. Ferguson, W. J., & Candib, L. M. Culture, language, and the doctor–patient relationship. *Family Med.* **34**, 353–361 (2002).

53. Epstein, A. M., Taylor, W. C., & Seage III, G. R. Effects of patients' socioeconomic status and physicians' training and practice on patient-doctor communication. *Am. J. Med.* **78**, 101–106 (1985).

54. Hagiwara, N., Penner, L. A., Gonzalez, R., et al. Racial attitudes, physician–patient talk time ratio, and adherence in racially discordant medical interactions. *Soc. Sci. Med.* **87**, 123–131 (2013).

55. Hagiwara, N., Dovidio, J. F., Eggly, S., & Penner, L. A. The effects of racial attitudes on affect and engagement in racially discordant medical interactions between non-Black physicians and Black patients. *Group Process Intergroup Relat.* **19**, 509–527 (2016).

56. van Ryn, M., Hardeman, R., Phelan, S. M., et al. Medical school experiences associated with change in implicit racial bias among 3547 students: a medical student CHANGES study report. *J. Gen. Intern. Med.* **30**, 1748–1756 (2015).

57. Phelan, S. M., Puhl, R. M., Burke, S. E., et al. The mixed impact of medical school on medical students' implicit and explicit weight bias. *Med. Educ.* **49**, 983–992 (2015).

58. Burke, S. E., Dovidio, J. F., Przedworski, J. M., et al. Do contact and empathy mitigate bias against gay and lesbian people among heterosexual medical students? A report from medical student CHANGES. *Acad. Med. J. Assoc. Am. Med. Coll.* **90**, 645 (2015).

59. Phelan, S. M., Dovidio, J. F., Puhl, R. M., et al. Implicit and explicit weight bias in a national sample of 4,732 medical students: the medical student CHANGES study. *Obesity* **22**, 1201–1208 (2014).

60. Sabin, J. A., Marini, M., & Nosek, B. A. Implicit and explicit anti-fat bias among a large sample of medical doctors by BMI, race/ethnicity and gender. *PloS One* **7**, e48448 (2012).

61. Waller, T., Lampman, C., & Lupfer-Johnson, G. Assessing bias against overweight individuals among nursing and psychology students: an Implicit Association Test. *J. Clin. Nurs.* **21**, 3504–3512 (2012).

62. Puhl, R., & Brownell, K. D. Bias, discrimination, and obesity. *Obesity* **9**, 788–805 (2001).

63. Haque, O. S., & Waytz, A. Dehumanization in medicine: causes, solutions, and functions. *Perspect. Psychol. Sci.* **7**, 176–186 (2012).

64. Waytz, A., Gray, K., Epley, N., & Wegner, D. M. Causes and consequences of mind perception. *Trends Cogn. Sci.* **14**, 383–388 (2010).

65. Teachman, B. A., Wilson, J. G., & Komarovskaya, I. Implicit and explicit stigma of mental illness in diagnosed and healthy samples. *J. Soc. Clin. Psychol.* **25**, 75–95 (2006).

66. Welch, L. C., Litman, H. J., Borba, C. P., et al. Does a physician's attitude toward a patient with mental illness affect clinical management of diabetes? Results from a mixed-method study. *Health Serv. Res.* **50**, 998–1020 (2015).

67. Blair, I. V., Ma, J. E., & Lenton, A. P. Imagining stereotypes away: the moderation of implicit stereotypes through mental imagery. *J. Pers. Soc. Psychol.* **81**, 828 (2001).

68. Stone, J., & Moskowitz, G. B. Non-conscious bias in medical decision making: what can be done to reduce it? *Med. Educ.* **45**, 768–776 (2011).

69. Wegner, D. M. Ironic processes of mental control. *Psychol. Rev.* **101**, 34 (1994).

70. Burgess, D., Van Ryn, M., Dovidio, J., & Saha, S. Reducing racial bias among health care providers: lessons from social-cognitive psychology. *J. Gen. Intern. Med.* **22**, 882–887 (2007).

71. Burgess, D. J., Beach, M. C., & Saha, S. Mindfulness practice: a promising approach to reducing the effects of clinician implicit bias on patients. *Patient Educ. Couns.* **100**, 372–376 (2017).

12

Responding to Patients' Provider Preferences

KIMBERLY L. REYNOLDS, KIRA KNIGHT RODRIGUEZ, LOUCRESIE RUPERT, AND MICHAELA OWUSU ■

In our increasingly diverse world, there has been a call for increased diversity in the ranks of physicians and other health care providers in all specialties. This diversity will lead to patients interacting with physicians who are of very different racial, ethnic, religious, and/or geographical backgrounds. In this chapter, we will explore the various requests that a patient may make when visiting the psychiatrist in terms of race, gender, religion, and language preferences. This chapter will differ considerably from the other chapters in this textbook: Because that each patient request has unique implications, it is imperative that each preference be explored in the unique context in which it may present during a patient encounter. Following each case, we will discuss the historical, ethical, patient-related, provider-related, and organizational factors that come into play when deciding whether to accede a patient's request (Box 12.1).

RACE-BASED PREFERENCES

Case

Dr. Cassie Knowles is a second-year resident in a prestigious psychiatry residency program. She has received pass-off from a graduating resident about one of her outpatient psychopharmacology patients, Mr. Jake Thompson. Mr. Thompson is a 37-year-old man with a diagnosis of schizophrenia. Mr. Thompson is being treated with risperidone and benztropine and is adherent to his medications. He is married and has two young children, ages 2 and 4. On her first day in the outpatient clinic, Dr. Knowles retrieves Mr. Thompson from the clinic waiting room and introduces herself as the new resident taking over from the previous doctor. Mr. Thompson smiles but appears distracted by something on his phone. Dr. Knowles begins by asking him how he is feeling.

Box 12.1

Factors to Consider in Analyzing a Patient's Provider Preference

- Relevant historical perspective
- Ethical considerations
- Patient factors
- Provider factors
- Organizational factors

"I don't mean to be rude," Mr. Thompson states, "but I am going to need a new doctor."

Dr. Knowles smiles knowingly. Her chief residents prepared her for the difficult transition that sometimes occurs when new residents take over in clinic.

"I understand that it is difficult to transition to a new physician," she states calmly.

"I don't think you understand," Mr. Thompson states, looking up from his phone for the first time. "You are not the type of physician that I need. You are Black. I need to see a white doctor."

Fearing she did not hear him correctly, Dr. Knowles asks, "Excuse me?"

Mr. Thompson reiterated, "I want to be seen by a white physician. It's nothing personal."

Taken aback, Dr. Knowles stands up from her chair and stumbles back. She mumbles, "I'll be back in a minute" and flees the room. She runs into her attending, Dr. Hopper, in the hallway.

"Done so soon?" he questions.

Dr. Knowles explains the situation to her attending, trying to keep her composure as her voice shakes. What should be Dr. Hopper's next step?

Historical Perspective

To evaluate the case for the request made by Mr. Thompson, we first must examine the history of race relations in America as a way of adding context to the request. Until relatively recently, the history of Black physicians in this country has been one of discrimination and marginalization by mainstream medical associations and hospitals. At the annual meeting of the American Medical Association (AMA) in 1870, the organization refused to seat two Black delegates. Subsequently, the organization enacted a series of policies that marginalized Black physicians and denied them access to membership in the AMA. Out of this marginalization arose a new organization, the National Medical Association, which was formed to counteract the discriminatory practices of the AMA.[1] In addition to the discrimination faced by local and national organized physician groups, many hospitals did not allow Black physicians to practice medicine on their wards, or they were relegated to segregated wards. Black physicians then opened their own medical schools and hospitals; however, many of these were closed in 1910 after the AMA commissioned the Flexner Report. Traditional medical schools in the Jim Crow era did not admit many Black physicians, and the number of Black physicians plummeted in the subsequent years.

In 2008, the AMA officially apologized for its history of discriminatory practices. However, the legacy of segregation and discrimination remains: Black physicians are persistently underrepresented in medicine and are less likely than white physicians to hold key leadership positions in medical schools and hospitals.[2]

This country's history of racial discrimination against physicians of color is a unique factor in the decision to accommodate a patient's race-based request.

Racism and Psychiatry

Many aspects of psychiatry are unavoidably racialized. There are dominant "norms" that are considered to exist in general society, and Western society more specifically; deviations from these norms often result in incorrect diagnoses. For example, there is known to be a higher rate of diagnosis of schizophrenia in Black patients.[3] It is postulated that differences in patterns of speech and mannerisms, as well as the incorrect belief that Black patients have lower rates of affective disorders, contribute to the differences in diagnosis.[3]

Ethical Considerations

PATIENT AUTONOMY

Patient autonomy is the hallmark of the practice of American medicine. We hold true to the belief that patients are the best ones to decide on their own care. This principle is reinforced throughout traditional medical education and forms the foundation of institutional review boards, informed consent, and so on. Indeed, many would argue that honoring the request for a physician of a particular race is in accordance with the ethical principle of patient autonomy. However, in the instance outlined in the above case, one must take into consideration not only the patient's autonomy but also the impact on the resident physician. Her role in this must not be understated, for it is the resident physician who must go on to care for other patients. Her mental well-being and sense of self must also be valued and taken into consideration. Furthermore, physicians are entitled to a workplace that is free from discrimination, based on Title VII of the Civil Rights Act of 1964.[4] The law has supported health care workers (mostly nurses) who sue when race-based requests are accommodated.[5]

However, patients with the mental capacity to make medical decisions have the ethical and legal right to refuse care from any physician.[4] Forcing a patient to be treated and examined by a physician he or she does not wish to engage with can amount to battery, particularly in a nonemergent situation.

JUSTICE

The ethical principle of justice is related to the fair distribution of resources within a society.[6] In this case, the resource would be health care services for the patient. When resources are limited, the principle of justice often directly conflicts with patient autonomy. Whereas a patient may request a physician of a particular race, there may not be a physician of that race available. It may also be the case that using a physician of a specific race takes that physician away from another patient who may need him or her. These factors must also be considered when the case for a physician of a particular race is examined.

NONMALEFICENCE
The ethical principle of nonmaleficence requires that we avoid intentionally harming or causing injury to a patient.[6] This may also involve choosing the "lesser of two evils" when two problematic choices are at play.

BENEFICENCE
This principle of beneficence refers to the duty of a physician to be a benefit to the patient.[6] On the surface, it may not seem as though the principle of beneficence directly relates to a patient preference of a provider. However, let us examine the following case to illustrate the relevance of this ethical principle.

Case

A.K., a 54-year-old woman with a history of hypertension and type 2 diabetes mellitus, is referred to your psychiatric office for the treatment of suspected depression. A.K. is a homemaker, and her husband works as a manager at a local manufacturing plant. You walk in the room to find a pleasant, African American female who appears her stated age, is well groomed, and has a pleasant affect. You briefly review the chart as you exchange pleasantries with the patient. You spot a note from the nurse stating that A.K. is nonadherent with her hypertension and diabetes regimens. A.K. smiles pleasantly as you begin to ask her questions but states that she was hoping she would have an African American physician, like her last psychiatrist. You begin thinking of the literature that shows that many African American patients have better outcomes when they see a racially concordant physician. Should you continue treating A.K., or should you refer her to an African American colleague?

This case differs significantly from the first case that we explored, in that while the patient is passively making a request for a physician of a different race, the physician is aware of potential benefits to the patient. Indeed, there is an abundance of literature confirming this physician's initial thoughts. Taylor and colleagues showed that African American patients were less likely to be adherent to cardiovascular disease medications, but those African American patients who had racially concordant physicians were more likely to adhere to their medications.[7] Cuffee and colleagues showed that, among inner-city African Americans, self-perceived racial discrimination was associated with lower medication adherence to hypertension medications.[8] Regarding mental health specialties specifically, Cabral and Smith conducted a meta-analysis of 81 studies of patient perceptions of therapists and showed that patients tended to perceive racially concordant therapists more positively.[9] However, they did not find an overall effect on patient outcomes.[9] In the Cabral and Smith study, African American patients were the most likely to experience improved outcomes as a function of racial/ethnic matching; racial/ethnicity matching was least beneficial for white/European Americans. Jerant and colleagues found that matching of patients and providers by race/ethnicity did not show improvements in ratings of provider communication.[10]

Despite the lack of evidence that racial concordance results in improved outcomes on an aggregate level, there is clear evidence that racial/ethnic matching benefits outcomes specifically among African American patients due to increased levels of trust, satisfaction, and understanding.[11] This firmly places the requests from Black/African American patients in an entirely different category than requests from white patients, namely because racial/ethnicity matching does not result in better outcomes for white/European patients. Furthermore, the history of racial discrimination in this country, and specifically within the medical community, must be considered when determining the decision to yield to the requests of a patient. Psychiatry is a unique specialty in which patient trust is paramount to treatment success. Any measures that improve trust should be employed, so long as employing them does not delay care or create undue stress on the patient, physician, or health care system.

Additionally, it is well documented that African American patients face significant mental health and health care disparities. The 2001 U.S. Surgeon General's Report on Mental Health supplement was unambiguous in its assertion that Black/African American patients are less likely to receive the mental health services they need, and when they do receive the services, they are poorer in quality, leading to a "greater loss to their overall health and productivity."[12] This is not simply about the patient's experiencing a connection with the psychiatrist solely for the purposes of having a pleasant experience; the overall health and well-being of African American patients can be impacted when racial concordance is taken into consideration. It is for these reasons that the requests of a Black patient should be assessed as the overall health of the patient is considered.

Organizational Factors

According to Title VII of the Civil Rights Act, all employees have a right to a workplace that does not discriminate based on race, color, religion, sex, and national origin.[13] However, health care entities also have a fiduciary duty to the patients they serve. When the rights of the patient to be autonomous conflict with the rights of the physician to work in an environment free of discrimination, whose rights ultimately win out?

Paul-Emile and colleagues have proposed a framework for deciding whether to accede to a patient's race-based requests, taking into consideration patient-level factors such as medical condition, decision-making capacity, and the reason for the request (clinically or ethnically appropriate reasons versus reasons based on bigotry or racism). Each of these considerations is explored further below. As each case will be different, organizations can be proactive in developing algorithms that take into consideration the above-named factors that allow physicians to make informed decisions regarding whether to accede to patients' requests. Medical leadership within the organization should be trained on the use of the algorithm. Organizations can also employ mock patient request scenarios that are taped, followed by debriefings, to ensure that the algorithms are being employed appropriately. Individual physicians should also undergo this training during orientation as well as periodically, with an emphasis on whom to consult when such a request arises during patient care.

Patient Factors

In psychiatry, it is important to assess the status of the patient when considering whether to honor his or her race-based requests for another physician. As suggested by Paul-Emile and colleagues, we believe that three factors should be taken into consideration whenever a patient makes a race-based request: capacity, severity of presentation, and the reason for the request.[4]

CAPACITY

Psychiatrists are uniquely suited to determine the capacity of a patient, or whether a patient has the mental ability to make his or her own decisions. If a patient is incapacitated and unable to make decisions on his or her own, then physician must walk a fine line between dismissing the patient's desires and honoring the request. If the treatment required is emergent or urgent, physicians must ultimately do what is best for the patient, as we are ethically, morally, and legally bound to treat and stabilize. If a physician who fulfills the patient's desires is present, however, it may be reasonable to transfer care, so as to protect the emotional well-being of the physician in this case, whose well-being is also important.

SEVERITY OF PRESENTATION

When handling an urgent or emergent case in a patient with decision-making capacity, the consequences of a delay in treatment must be the first consideration in deciding whether to accede to a patient's request. When in doubt, in an emergent and/or life-threatening situation, the patient should first be treated and stabilized if a transfer of care will result in delay. Additional factors to consider are the skill level of the physicians involved (i.e., who would be the best to take care of the patient).

REASON FOR THE REQUEST

The reason for the request is paramount when determining whether a patient should be transferred at a patient's request. Paul-Emile and colleagues state that requests based on bigotry against a physician from a historically marginalized group should not be accommodated. However, these authors provide an example of a patient who is a war veteran with posttraumatic stress disorder (PTSD) and is being treated by a physician who belongs to the same ethnic group as the enemy opponents. The patient may experience transference that may hinder the building of a therapeutic alliance between the physician and patient. Given the sensitive nature of the diagnosis of PTSD and the potential triggers, it may be appropriate to acquiesce to this particular patient's request.[4] On the other hand, a patient in this scenario may benefit greatly from working through his or her transference and developing a positive relationship with a provider to whom he or she may have initially had a strong negative reaction. This approach should be discussed in depth with the patient to determine if the long-term benefits of such a relationship may outweigh the potential fear and triggering. Again, minority patients, and specifically Black patients, who experience worse outcomes and poorer care overall, may not benefit from a discordant relationship reminiscent of the racial hierarchy and systemic oppression they experience on a day-to-day basis. This may do more harm than good.

Impact on Providers

In discussing the impact of racial concordance on patients, we must also consider the impact of patients' race-based requests on providers. In particular, minority and foreign-born physicians must regularly deal with discrimination at both the micro and macro levels within the institutions in which they work.[2] As these physicians navigate complex work environments with structural and interpersonal barriers to advancement compared to their white counterparts, a race-based request predicated on bigotry can be an additional hurdle these physicians must overcome. However, negating such a request may hinder the ability of the provider to form a meaningful therapeutic relationship with the patient. The countertransference Dr. Knowles will likely experience may impede the physician–patient relationship. Furthermore, the severe emotional toll that racism takes on its victims may impede her ability to function at full capacity. Care must be taken to discuss such factors with the psychiatrist to determine his or her comfort level moving forward, regardless if the request is honored or denied.

Summary

Patients who make requests for a psychiatrist based on race present a unique challenge. The decision to honor race-based requests will vary based on the historical perspective of the patient and physician involved in the scenario; ethical considerations such as autonomy, justice, and beneficence; patient factors such as whether race concordance leads to improved outcomes in this case; provider factors such as countertransference; and organizational factors.

In the case of Dr. Knowles, who is Black, and Mr. Thompson, a white patient, we recommend a thorough deconstruction of the salient elements of the case before deciding whether to allow Mr. Thompson be transferred to a white physician. Dr. Knowles represents a largely underrepresented group in medicine that has experienced significant racial bias, both in the medical profession and in society in general. In evaluating Mr. Thompson's contributing factors, we find him likely to possess the capacity to make decisions about his own care. Furthermore, his case is not severe or life-threatening at the moment. It is difficult to ascertain his reasons for requesting a white physician, but bigotry is implied in the manner in which it was asked. There are data to suggest that acceding to Mr. Thompson's concerns would result in better outcomes. Conversely, Dr. Knowles continuing with the encounter may lead to a strained physician–patient relationship, while not allowing her to perform optimally.

What should Dr. Hopper do? After a thorough review of the pertinent aspects of this case, Dr. Hopper would be wise to allow Dr. Knowles to determine her comfort with acceding to the request versus denying it. Dr. Knowles and the patient may indeed benefit from attending to the inevitable transference and countertransference that will likely play out in this scenario, but we propose that Dr. Knowles should be the one to make the decision, as she is arguably the more vulnerable individual in this scenario.

GENDER-BASED PREFERENCES

Case

A.G. is a 27-year-old female with a past medical history of polycystic ovarian syndrome and a past psychiatric history of PTSD secondary to a sexual assault by a male perpetrator approximately nine years ago. She presents today as a new referral in your 10-provider outpatient clinic to reestablish care for an exacerbation of symptoms following the ending of her marriage to an abusive male partner. On arrival to the clinic, staff inform her that today's psychopharmacology intake is scheduled with the clinic's specialist in trauma treatment, a senior cisgender male psychiatrist. The patient appears anxious and requests "any other female provider" as a replacement. While many of the office therapists are female, the only two psychiatrists are male. How should this clinic conceptualize and navigate the patient's gender preference?

Historical Perspective

In the United States, there have been several generational gender shifts in the mental health clinician workforce. Political challenges to power differentials and discrimination against women have increased national recognition of women's competence as clinicians. This has led to increases in the number of nonmale trainees in medicine, psychology, and ancillary fields. For example, the percentage of U.S. psychiatrists self-identifying as female has risen to 38% in 2015.[14] This increase is reflective of the 2017 U.S. national percentage of female-identifying physicians, at 34.6%.[15] Yet while the female psychiatrist remains underrepresented relative to the general population, there has been a gradual "feminization" of psychotherapy practice by nonphysicians. In other words, the fields of clinical psychology, counseling, and social work are increasingly female dominated.[16]

Despite increased numbers of women practicing in mental health fields, gender remains a significant structural determinant of mental health due to continued female social subordination.[17] For example, highly prevalent psychiatric illnesses such as depression and anxiety disproportionately affect women and are recognized as among the leading causes of disability worldwide.[17] Historically, psychiatry and psychology have engaged in gender-biased formulations, diagnoses, and treatments that have since been deemed discriminatory.[17] For example, the prescribing of psychotropic medications can be predicted by female gender.[17] Further, women presenting with identical complaints as men are more likely to be diagnosed with depression than men and are less likely to be diagnosed with a comorbid substance use disorders.[17]

Given the relative primacy of gender to one's experience of navigating the world, people often express a preference for the gender of their treater. In medicine, there is evidence that this occurs most commonly for intimate medical conditions such as gynecological problems. Mental health treatment requires emotional intimacy, most notably for psychotherapy, the success of which is largely dependent on the client–treater relationship.[18] While most people do not enter mental health clinics mandating characteristics of their treater, when they do, gender preference is the most common.[19] Female patients more often request mental health professionals of their own gender, regardless of whether the chief complaint is gendered. Furthermore, as stated previously, there is evidence that patients who are able to be matched with a provider of their preference have small but measurable improvements in communication with providers, a relevant necessity in psychiatric care.[10]

Research studies on preferences for provider gender indicate that it is difficult to know which patient profile will state which gender preference. In a study of adolescents choosing their pediatrician, preference for provider gender decreased with age of the participants. Boys generally had less frequent preferences than did girls, who tended to prefer female physicians. However, Kapphahn and colleagues showed that male adolescents with sexual assault histories had a shift toward female physician preference.[20] Liddon and colleagues identified through survey data that equal numbers of men and women have no gender preference for "psychological" care, at 62% and 61% respectively.[21] However, among those with a stated preference, there is a clear gender divide, with 34% of women versus 22% of men desiring a female treater. In comparison, only 5% of women versus 17% of men desired a male treater.[22]

Ethical Considerations

As with all assertions of provider preference, requests regarding gender place the ethical principles of autonomy and nonmaleficence into conflict with justice. That is, patients' rights to assert their preferences and to avoid an interaction that they anticipate may be detrimental to their well-being or, alternatively—to seek one that will promote their well-being—conflicts with the public health concern for equitable distribution of limited resources.

Patient Factors

As above, providers must first consider whether the patient has the capacity to make the gender-based request. Even if the patient is deemed capable, does the severity of the presentation warrant immediate treatment, trumping consideration of the patient's request? If the request is based on bigotry, as in the case of a male patient refusing to be treated by a woman due to bigoted views of female providers, care must be taken not to appear to side with the bigoted view. Depending on the patient's symptoms and/or diagnosis, working with a female provider may be of great benefit to the patient, either because the particular provider possesses unique expertise that relates to the patient's presentation, or because the patient may be able to address and work through these bigoted views in the context of a therapeutic alliance.

For many patients, the expression of gender preference in their provider is a proxy for desired personality traits. These patients may have unconsciously identified a series of desired characteristics that are associated with a particular gender stereotype. For example, the patient may assume that a female physician will be nurturing and deferential, or a male will be confident and dominant.[22] Helping patients to translate their request into more specific personality traits may deepen mutual understanding of the request. Furthermore, such an approach may identify bigotry and reduce gender discrimination in a society where gender expression and identity are increasingly less dichotomous or predictable.

For other patients, their preference for provider gender is an expression of their desired and feared emotions in the interpersonal process. To discuss one's inner experience with a mental health practitioner requires a high level of comfort and trust. As such, provider gender preference may serve as a proxy for comfort, implicit trust, empathic understanding, and avoidance of fear and shame. This preference may be particularly salient to individuals for whom trust and comfort has been severely ruptured in a gendered or sexual manner, and may help to explain the greater expression of provider gender preferences from women due to their position as a lower-status gender group compared to men.[21] Of note, male veterans with experiences of military sexual trauma had high rates of preferring female mental health providers at 50%, though some 25% still requested male treaters.[23] This gender preference following assault likely reflects altered preconceived notions of the interpersonal interactions. However, it remains unclear which specific assumed qualities of the exchange—comfort, trust, empathic understanding, fear, or shame—cause this alteration.

Provider Factors

An understanding by practitioners of their patients' desired and feared emotions resulting from assumed and explicit gender dynamics may help identify circumstances in which respecting a gender preference can ease the development of a trusting therapeutic relationship and consequently hasten patient healing. For some patients, however, the impact of the stated preference may be far less significant than initially perceived. For these patients, the opportunity to develop a trusting therapeutic relationship with a treater of the less-preferred gender may actually provide greater healing. For example, a woman with a history of difficult relationships with men may express a preference for a female treater but might actually achieve greater insight and progress by working with a male provider, due to the challenge it offers to her preconceived notions, and the opportunity to forge new, more positive experiences in a therapeutic relationship with a man. We recommend that such a challenge should only be pursued in discussion with the patient, and only if it would not inhibit the patient's willingness to enter into treatment.

Organizational Factors

Similar to the scenario described in the race-based preferences section, there are many laws and statutes that ensure the ability of women to work in environments that are free of discrimination based on gender, such as Title VII of the Civil Rights Act, and U.S. Code Title 42, Chapter 21.[13] While such regulations exist, because of the ubiquity of gender-based preferences as discussed above, as well as the knowledge that they may benefit patient outcomes, it is important to consider the implications of acceding to requests at the organizational level and possibly to formulate specific guidelines.

Practitioners working in individual clinics may consider speaking to clients about their gender preferences and assumptions at initial intake to determine fit. Those working in larger clinic environments should be vigilant for representative gender diversity among all specialties in their practice. Training clinics may have less flexibility to comply with preferences for treaters due to training requirements that necessitate exposure to a wide range of demographic and illness populations. As gender representation becomes more equitable, clinics with a desire to respect gender preferences for providers can do so with greater ease and flexibility. As above, we advise assisting both patients and clinic staff to understand the motivation behind the stated preference, as well as its impact on initiating a therapeutic alliance.

Summary

Let's return to the case presented at the beginning of this section. To recap, A.G. is a female patient with PTSD following the sexual assault by a male nine years ago, and the recent breakup with a partner who was also abusive, who is presenting to reestablish care. She is scheduled to see a male psychiatrist but is visibly shaken at the prospect and requests a female physician. As PTSD is characterized by a reexperiencing of the traumatic event that can take on the form of emotional distress and physical reactivity, we suggest that it would not be in the patient's immediate best interest to continue with psychiatric care at this clinic at the present moment. The heightened emotional reaction at simply the prospect of a male physician is suggestive of the severity of the illness. The clinic should offer the patient a referral to a female physician who specializes in dealing with patients with PTSD. However, once her symptoms are better controlled, she may benefit from developing a therapeutic relationship with a male provider in the long run. Working through her transference and establishing a relationship with a trusted male psychiatrist may be an important step on her path to healing.

RELIGIOUS PREFERENCES

Case

A 10-year-old girl and her parents are seen by a pediatrician, who recommends referral to psychiatry for evaluation of irritability and inattention in the child. This family has been to therapy before, but the parents state they are not very trusting of psychiatry as a whole. When the pediatrician asks for more details, they state that psychiatry has the reputation of not being friendly to those who have strong religious values. The family has a Christian background.

Patients will enter your practice with a set of theological beliefs, whether they align themselves with a particular religion, atheist/agnostic beliefs, or spirituality in general. Those beliefs will have varying effects on the concerns they present with and their responses to treatment. For some, there may be little to no effect, whereas for others, their religious/spiritual beliefs, or lack thereof, may play a significant role in how they will accept their diagnosis and respond to psychiatric treatment. It has been observed that it is not necessarily the specific type of religious beliefs/spirituality that determines its importance in treatment, but more so the commitment level of the believer.[24] Those beliefs may at times be a positive factor in treatment, and at other times may actually deter achieving treatment goals. Religious beliefs can also be protective factors or risk factors, depending on the patient and context. For example, religious beliefs are generally a protective factor in suicides, whereas an externally imposed morality system may lead to guilt over perceived wrongdoings that can exacerbate depression and anxiety.[25] Some belief systems hold the mentally ill in high regard as spiritual leaders, whereas others teach that all mental illness is a result of either demonic possession or attacks from the spiritual world. These attacks are perceived as punishment or as a test or trial to make the patient stronger. There are many belief systems that understand mental illness through a combination of spiritual and physical explanations. Followers of these beliefs may describe that while spiritual forces influence our world, there are also biological causes for symptoms of mental illness. These individuals may encourage the use of prayer in addition to seeking medical treatment.

Psychiatry and Religion

Religion in psychiatry can be approached in one of four ways:

1. The familiar and traditional approach is for the clinician to limit discussion of religious content to the psychological and psychiatric implications. For example, a mother's anger at God regarding the illness of her child may be discussed and examined through the lens of normal emotional catharsis, or perhaps considered as another expression of a persistent pattern of anger at authority figures throughout her life.
2. A second approach clarifies spiritual and psychosocial aspects of the problem and then refers the family to resources for dealing with these spiritual issues, such as a religious community or outside authority (e.g., hospital chaplain).
3. A third approach addresses the clinical problem indirectly, discussing the patient's beliefs, worldview, or philosophy of life in detail and reviewing how the family can make better use of the resources of the tradition. This approach presumes the clinician has some knowledge of the basic faith groups that can help inform meaningful dialogue.
4. The final approach is to address the clinical problem directly through a shared perspective or worldview. This is most commonly done when the therapist shares the same religious traditions and worldview of the patient and family. This approach requires careful attention to ethical issues, particularly those related to transference, therapeutic boundaries, and consent.[25]

Contrary to popular belief, there are actually some similarities between religion and psychiatry, particularly psychotherapy. The Christian Bible provides ample examples that can help illustrate some of these similarities. In therapy, "positive thinking" or "changing thoughts" is a significant component of cognitive-behavioral therapy, dialectical behavioral therapy, and other treatments. Therapies use principles such as recognizing automatic negative thoughts and irrational thoughts, and challenging, or even replacing, those thoughts with positive thoughts. The Christian Bible mentions the same principle in the form of scriptures such as Philippians

4:8: "Whatsoever things are just, whatsoever things are pure, whatsoever things are lovely, whatsoever things are of good report; if there be any virtue, and if there be any praise, think on these things."

There is also a connection between the psychotherapeutic principle of "mindfulness" and several spiritual belief systems. Mindfulness itself is derived from Eastern religious practices, namely Hinduism and Buddhism, and has been adapted to its current form by Western spiritual practitioners, mental health clinicians, and researchers. There is also a link between mindfulness as a psychotherapeutic principle—namely an attitude of nonjudgmental openness focused on moment-to-moment experience—and the Islamic principle of *khushoo* (often translated as "sincerity" or "concentration") in *Salah* (Muslim daily prayers). Muslims are encouraged to focus on speaking with God and to leave behind the distractions of worldly affairs.[26] Similarly, in the Christian religion, Matthew 6:25–27 admonishes its readers not to worry or focus on negativity, as worry will not "add a single hour to your life."

These examples illustrate the importance of psychiatrists not only familiarizing themselves with the religious beliefs of their patients, but also attempting to address psychiatric illness through the patient's individual lens, when appropriate. Let's explore some relevant cases that illustrate the fourth approach outlined above when approaching religious content in a psychiatric clinical setting.

Case

A 50-year-old Nigerian woman presents to the hospital with suicidal ideation and depression. She does not speak English. The patient was brought in by her husband. Her husband had initially taken the patient to their Pentecostal/tribal spiritual leaders, who believed she was demonically possessed. The patient continued to decline and presented with severe psychomotor retardation; it took her no less than 10 minutes to walk across a room. She became unable to care for her 10 children or herself, was not eating, and was unable to perform her activities of daily living. After admission to the psychiatric unit, the family is very resistant to any interventions, especially psychotropic medications. It is clear that this family is suspicious of psychiatry for many reasons. The resident assigned to this case happens to be Black and Pentecostal. The resident, through an interpreter, explains that she too is Pentecostal. She explains that she believes in God and miracles, but that she also believes that God led her to be a psychiatrist to help others. She further suggests God has given her the tools to use to help patients improve, and that in itself could be an answer to prayer. The resident even prays with the family. Though there is still cultural and language differences, the similarities of being Black and Pentecostal like the patient and her family significantly aid the therapeutic alliance. The family is much more open and agrees to treatment, and the patient significantly improves in time with medications.

Historical Perspective

Despite a common impression that psychiatry and religion are incompatible, mental illness has in fact long been explained in spiritual terms. Whereas some religious traditions do describe mental illnesses as resulting from negative influences from the spiritual world (e.g., demonic possession), this is not always the case. Early religions provided both spiritual and physical explanations for what would later be described as mental illnesses. Religious traditions and rituals may also provide positive coping skills for adherents, although some negative coping skills can be found in some religious practices as well. These characteristics are not specific to a particular religion, but are more often related to the commitment people have to their particular religion.

Many religions embrace positive coping skills such as seeking support from clergy or a faith community, finding spiritual meaning in stressful events, belief and faith in a higher power, prayer/meditation practice, and believing one's life is a part of a larger plan. Some negative coping skills include believing that external forces are in complete control, which can lead to abnegation of personal agency, and believing that stressors are a punishment from God or an attack from the devil or a demonic power. Religion is not "one size fits all," and individuals may express their religious beliefs in various ways.

Ethical Considerations

Just as with other patient requests for providers of particular backgrounds, multiple ethical principles must be considered when patients request a physician of a specific religion. Autonomy forms the basis of most physician–patient interactions and has an elevated role in the field of psychiatry. However, justice must also be taken into account, as we consider the lack of psychiatric providers in a particular region, which can be framed as a resource issue. Conversely, for some patients a therapeutic alliance with a provider of the same background may be of tremendous clinical benefit, particularly if there is an initial distrust in the medical establishment, or in psychiatry in general. Thus, the beneficence afforded the patient of acceding to the request may alleviate that distrust and allow for improvement in the patient's clinical status, if such a provider is available. However, care must be taken not to cause harm by making the patient wait a significant amount of time to see a psychiatrist of a particular faith. Thus, autonomy, justice, beneficence, and nonmaleficence must be considered as a whole to achieve the best outcome.

Patient Factors

Being aware of a patient's baseline religious beliefs and practices is an important part of psychiatric care. This aids in diagnosis, as what might be interpreted as hyperreligious thoughts or behaviors in one person may be culturally appropriate for another. In the Southern United States, for instance, it is cultural and normal to hear people say, "God told me ____," or, "I had a flat tire today—that was the devil's doing." A physician not familiar with the religious beliefs of a particular area or culture may mistakenly diagnose psychosis, delusions, or hyperreligiosity associated with mania. With a healthy level of curiosity, further questioning by the clinician may reveal that these individuals deny hearing an audible voice but may reference being "led by the spirit" or through scripture. In the same vein, a change from baseline religiosity may be a cause for concern. For instance, if a patient's family endorses prior spirituality but little religiosity, but now states that the patient is spending hours writing religious texts, praying, or reading about religion, this change from baseline may be a cause for concern.

The above discussion lends credence to the notion that, in certain situations, advocating for religious concordance may be in the best interest of certain patients to avoid the bias that may occur with interreligious encounters. As with the race and gender-based preferences discussed above, care must be taken to understand the patient factors that interact when the request is made. Does the patient have the capacity to make such a decision? Does the severity of the presentation and the need for rapid treatment override the patient's request in the short term? What is the reason for the request? Does it stem from the patient's wanting a therapeutic alliance with a physician who shares his or her worldview, or does the patient possess bigoted beliefs that are being transferred onto the providers? A thorough analysis of the patient-level factors can aid in decision-making when a religion-based request is made.

Provider Factors

Granting a request to provide a physician of the same or similar religious background to the patient can provide immense benefit, as in the case example. One thing to consider, however, is the countertransference of the psychiatrist. Shared spirituality can be a very intimate bond. The psychiatrist in this situation must guard against overidentification with the patient, as well as the use of the religious similarities to guide the patient's decisions. Instead, religious similarities should serve as a support while respecting the individual patient's autonomy. Below is an example of the pitfalls of this approach.

A 17-year-old female with a history of bipolar disorder that is well controlled on medications comes for a follow-up visit. She confides in you that she has just found out that she is eight weeks pregnant. You and the patient are of the same religious background—in fact, she sought you out for treatment because of this. She feels ill equipped to care for a baby in the near future and seeks your professional counsel on whether she should terminate the pregnancy. Given your shared religious beliefs, you mention to her that it is against your religion to terminate a pregnancy, and she agrees. You offer to provide her with the names and contact information of teen pregnancy support groups, as well as adoption services.

In the case, you may feel that you are connecting with the patient's spirituality, but you are actually doing the patient a disservice by not providing her with all of her options and allowing her to make the best decision for herself.

Organizational Factors

There are no overarching legal or regulatory requirements that aid in our assessment of whether a provider should accede to a patient's request for a physician of a particular religious background. The *2013 Diagnostic and Statistical Manual of Mental Disorders* (DSM-5) does not offer guidance to clinicians on religious-based requests.[27] Of note, if the patient's request represents a form of bigotry, in that a patient holds bigoted views toward adherents of a particular religion, the approach outlined in the race-based request section may be of particular benefit, and the provider can use the decision tree outlined by Paul-Emile and colleagues.[4]

On the micro-organizational level, an important factor to consider is the availability of a physician of the requested religion. In teaching environments, physicians may rotate on different clinical services, which may limit the outpatient clinical availability of a physician of a specific background. Of note, many nonprofit organizations discourage overt discussion or involvement of religious affiliations in the professional environment, so it may be difficult to identify a physician with a particular background. Physicians may not want to disclose their religious affiliations and may be hesitant to be assigned to a patient solely based on their religion. Given these factors, it may be very difficult to accommodate the religious needs of patients in most settings. Organizations can provide guidance to physicians by compiling referral lists of community physicians who do disclose their religious affiliations and are willing to work with patients of a particular religion. The clinic may offer the services of or a referral to a licensed therapist, as there are many therapy practices that advertise therapists who have a particular religious background. This may be a useful addition to a patient's care team.

Summary

This section began with the case of a 10-year-old girl and her parents referred by the pediatrician to a psychiatrist. The parents express concern that psychiatry has the reputation of not being friendly to those who have strong religious values. Recognizing the importance of the family's spiritual worldview in their decision-making, the physician recommends that the parents approach their pastor for a recommendation for a specific psychiatrist. The parents agree and are ultimately referred to a Christian psychiatrist known to their pastor. With this referral, the family expresses being more comfortable with the referral to psychiatry. The patient and family meet with the psychiatrist, who recommends additional referral to psychology for further testing. Due to the family's trust of the psychiatrist, they accept the referral and participate with the psychologist (who does not have the same belief system; this does not seem to bother the parents for a one-time consultation). The patient is eventually diagnosed with depression and attention-deficit/hyperactivity disorder, is treated with medications and therapy, and improves greatly in a short time.

In analyzing the opening case of this section, we find that the pediatrician leveraged his or her knowledge of the family's strong religious beliefs and recommended that the family talk to their religious leader. The patient's autonomy was preserved, and the outcome of the case reveals that this was indeed to the patient's benefit. No harm was done, as the patient received the care she needed and improved on the necessary therapies under the care of a provider who was able to bridge the worldviews of psychiatry and Christianity. Of course, even if a Christian provider were unavailable, the pediatrician would still be obligated to recommend referral to a psychiatrist for evaluation and treatment of the patient's symptoms, which the family may subsequently decline.

LANGUAGE PREFERENCES

Case

L.M. is a 43-year-old man with no prior psychiatric history referred to the emergency department (ED) for suicidal ideation. The patient was seen by his primary care provider earlier the same day for his annual examination. During that visit, the patient endorsed difficulties in his marriage as well as increased fatigue. When asked about suicidal ideation, the patient endorsed having a gun at home and a plan to shoot himself "if things don't work out with my wife soon." As a result, the physician sent him to the ED on a psychiatric hold. In the ED, he refuses to answer the ED physician's questions and states that he only wants to speak to physicians "who speak my language." The patient is Puerto Rican and speaks fluent English but states that someone who speaks Spanish would "understand me more." It is explained to the patient that there are currently no physicians who are Spanish-speaking in the hospital, but a live interpreter is available. The patient then becomes combative and threatens to harm the next person who comes in the room without speaking Spanish. The patient has no weapons on his person but is anxiously pacing the room. You are the on-call psychiatrist who is covering the ED that day. You do not speak Spanish. What is your next step?

There are over 320 languages spoken in the United States. The U.S. English Foundation, Inc., a research and education organization that studies language issues within the United States, reported on the amount of "linguistic diversity" in our nation, which varies widely from state to state, and even within states. The term "language diversity" or "linguistic diversity" refers to the number of languages spoken in the United States and the number of people who speak them. This country's rich melting pot history, driven by waves of immigration over the centuries, contributes to the extent of the language diversity that exists here. As a result of patterns of migration and settlement, "Each state, county and metropolitan area has its own unique linguistic composition."[28] This poses several challenges for organizations attempting to provide clinical care for increasingly diverse populations, as language discordance/barriers significantly impact effective health care delivery and safety.

Historical Perspective

Beginning in the 18th and 19th centuries, the immigration and settlement of large numbers of non–English-speaking European immigrants was a key starting point in the development of a polyglot nation with a diverse array of languages. As the country grew in size, acquiring vast territories throughout North America, a significant proportion of the nation's inhabitants spoke a language other than English. According to the 1910 census, the national population was 92 million, with 10 million immigrants reporting a mother tongue other than English or Celtic (Irish, Scotch, or Welsh).[29]

While the United States maintains a reputation of great linguistic diversity fueled by mass immigration, there is a key historical period characterized by language extinction and English dominance. This decline in linguistic diversity began during World War I, with the cessation of mass European immigration. This downward trend and plateau continued as a result of restrictive U.S. immigration quotas, global depression, World War II, and ultimately Europe's shift from being a region of mass emigration to one of immigration.[29] The percentage of foreign-born U.S. citizens fell steadily, from 14.7% in 1910 to an all-time low of 4.7% in 1970; with this decline, most immigrant native tongues were replaced by English.[28]

The recovery of linguistic diversity began during the postwar period as mass immigration resumed after 1970. The percentage of foreign-born residents rose steadily back toward its historical high, reaching 12.9% in 2010. The demographics of this new wave of immigrants was significantly different than the earlier waves. Prior to the mid-20th century, immigrants to the United States were predominantly white and from Europe; these individuals now represent only about 10% of immigrants. The remainder of U.S. immigrants today are predominately people of color and hail from numerous parts of the world, most notably from Latin America and Asia.[30] The Latino population has contributed significantly to the growing diversity of the United States, accounting for half of the national population growth since 2000; Spanish is the most widely spoken non-English language in the United States today.[30] Approximately 20% of the U.S. population, or 65 million people, speak a language other than English at home, with 8.6% being defined as having limited English proficiency (LEP).[31] LEP refers to individuals who do not speak English as their primary language and who have a limited ability to read, speak, write, or understand English.[32] Studies have found three key determinants of English language fluency among immigrants from non–English-speaking countries: age at arrival, years/level of education, and time spent in the United States. Individuals who arrived before adolescence, who are well educated, and who have lived in the United States for over a decade are more likely to speak fluent English.[29] As the population of LEP individuals grows, the availability of linguistically appropriate health care services has become a pressing issue facing the U.S. health care system.

LEP patients may ask to use their children as translators and interpreters in clinical encounters, reasoning that "they know better English than I do." *Ad hoc interpreting* is defined as having an untrained family member, friend, or clinic employee serve as an interpreter during a clinical encounter.[33] This is not illegal, but the consensus in the medical literature is that ad hoc interpreting is inadvisable on account of quality and safety. Specifically, family members should not play this role because:

- They are not trained interpreters.
- There may be a conflict of interest.
- Vital information can be withheld or omitted as family members may not understand the need to interpret everything the patient says, and may summarize information instead.
- Misinformation can lead to misdiagnosis.
- There is a strong likelihood for breach of confidentiality.
- Patients may have an incentive to withhold important relevant information (e.g., related to intimidation or abuse by a partner, or simply a reluctance to speak of taboo topics in front of a family member).

Bilingual staff members are also untrained interpreters, and their language skills may not match the needs of the patient. They are also not accountable for the interpretation that they provide.

Therefore, it is crucial that accurate information and details of a diagnosis be effectively communicated in the patient's native language, and that hospital systems provide the resources, such as telephone-based professional interpreter services, necessary to provide high-quality care.

Ethical Considerations

It is important to perform a nuanced analysis of the relevant ethical principles at play as the physician decides whether to agree to the request of the patient in the case above. Once again, the patient's autonomy in requesting a particular language must be considered yet balanced with justice (the accessibility of a provider who speaks that language). Language is a very personal and fundamental part of a patient's cultural identity, and as such may present a challenge when the patient requests a provider who speaks a particular language. This is particularly the case for psychiatry, which arguably uses language to a higher level and in a more central way for diagnosis and treatment than any other medical specialty.

There is clear evidence that patient outcomes are improved when patients are treated by providers who speak their language, particularly in minority communities.[34] Thus, both beneficence and nonmaleficence must also be considered. In general, LEP patients should be granted the opportunity to be seen by a provider who speaks their particular language if available, given that this can promote better clinical outcomes. However, given the ever-growing diversity within our borders, it is impossible that every language group will be represented among providers. As described above, every provider should have access to high-quality interpretation services for LEP patients, as well as for patients who require American Sign Language interpretation services.

Patient Factors

As in the other sections discussed earlier in this chapter, the provider must first attempt to determine the capacity of the patient to make decisions, whether the severity of the patient's presentation warrants an immediate intervention, and the reason for the request. Once these factors are considered, the provider can go on to evaluate the individual patient factors that are germane to the decision to comply with the request. Unlike the other factors we have discussed, however, including race, gender, and religion, language is fundamental to an individual's cultural identity and self-expression, due to its central role in communication. Language is the most basic format through which people express their emotions, thoughts, beliefs, and values.[35] Therefore, language-based requests may be even more important to accommodate than other requests.

In understanding variations in need for linguistic matching, it is often helpful to classify patients according to generational groups. When taking a patient's history, understanding the patient's family background can provide insight into his or her language literacy and preferences. The first generation is often defined as immigrants born outside the United States; the second generation are therefore those born in the United States to immigrant parents; the third generation are those born in the United States to native-born parents and one or more immigrant grandparents; and the fourth generation are natives with both native-born parents and native-born grandparents.[28] While exposure to a non-English language while growing up may remain quite common in the second generation, research has found a rapid drop in non-English literacy (reading and writing ability) despite a person's ability to understand or speak that foreign language in subsequent generations, such that proficiency and effective use of languages other than English may effectively die out in the third and fourth generations.

Working with immigrant populations and LEP patients brings specific clinical challenges, especially within the fields of psychiatry and mental health. Overcoming these language barriers through the use of professional interpreters continues to be a significant challenge for clinicians.[36] The underuse of professional interpreters by mental health providers who work with immigrant clients with language barriers represents a failure to meet basic professional standards of care. Language barriers affect key areas of ethics, including clinical assessment, decision-making, client confidentiality, and informed consent.[35]

Certain patient factors may also influence use of language services during clinical visits. An interpreter is required when a patient requests one or mentions that he or she prefers to speak, and is more fluent in, a language other than that of the health care provider. Unfortunately, many health care systems cannot provide enough language-concordant providers to meet the demand.[33] In 2012, Hacker and colleagues published a retrospective cohort study examining the role of language concordance or interpreter usage and healthcare utilization (hospitalization, ED visits, and glycemic control). These authors found that patients who had language concordance or the use of an interpreter were less likely to have diabetes-related ED visits.[34] This result reinforces the findings cited earlier, that patients have better outcomes when they are treated by language-concordant physicians.[34]

Provider Factors

Numerous factors can contribute to health care providers' resistance to using interpreters. For one, interpreters may be deemed too costly in terms of time and effort. Waiting for each sentence to be understood and interpreted can add significantly to the evaluation time, leading some providers to wish to take a shortcut and rely on the patient's limited English skills to obtain the most important information. Furthermore, adding another person into the clinical encounter can change patient–provider dynamics, affecting trust and loyalty, as well as raising concerns about confidentiality. Many providers have the common misconception that if the patient has adequate English proficiency, they do not require a professional interpreter. This misconception is often reinforced by patients themselves, as they attempt to demonstrate their proficiency in English.[35]

Even when the need for a professional interpreter is agreed upon by both parties, issues arise regarding the appropriate role of the interpreter in the clinical encounter. Are interpreters meant to translate word for word, or do they act as cultural brokers, conceptualizing the information about the patient's culture and experience? Despite the lack of consensus, it is generally understood that translations go beyond "just words" and require the cultural interpretation of meaning. Professional interpreters are trained in helping to clarify misunderstandings that arise due to cultural differences between provider and patient.[35] Hence, it is not only problematic to use untrained interpreters, but serious ethnical issues can arise, compromising the patient's care. Overall, in the fast-paced environment of the everyday clinical encounter, working with professional interpreters can be seen as time-consuming and labor-intensive, but language barriers can significantly affect the clinician's ability to provide ethical care. Poor communication as a result of linguistic mismatch affects important aspects of mental health care—reassurance, motivation, empathy, and rapport—and therefore needs to be avoided at all costs.

Organizational Factors

Title VI of the Civil Rights Act of 1964 requires that all organizations receiving federal funds must ensure that patients with LEP have appropriate and meaningful linguistic access to these federally funded health care programs.[37] In addition, many state and local programs also have provisions requiring language services for LEP individuals. Despite these laws and regulations, research has consistently shown that language barriers persist in clinical settings, with detrimental effects on overall safety and quality of care. Indeed, LEP patients have been found to be at increased risk of adverse health care events.[37]

Health care organizations have options available to assist with the language diversity prevalent in the U.S. population today. These include interpreters, translated written and multimedia materials, electronic sign-in machines that offer language preference selection, communication boards, and so on. Unfortunately, with the dynamic nature of patients' levels of English proficiency, the variability in interpreter availability, the limited availability of language-concordant health care providers, as well as the complexity of patient visits, challenges frequently arise for adequately responding to patients' provider language preferences.[33] Patients who do not share the same language as their health care providers receive reduced interpersonal support, fewer referrals/follow-ups, fewer preventive or public health services, and poorer quality of pain treatment, yet they utilize more resources, such as more diagnostic tests and longer hospital stays.[34] It is thus in the organization's best interest to respond to the patient's language preference and determine the best possible option to assist in effective communication. The Agency for Healthcare Research and Quality recommends providing translated materials in plain language, especially for informed consent, presurgical instructions and postsurgical care, and discharge instructions.[38]

To avoid hiring discrimination actions, health care organizations should not just seek bilingual providers, but should also develop training programs to build the language capacities of all the providers in the system. Organizations should in addition develop strategic initiatives geared toward attracting and retaining competent bilingual providers.

Summary

Of all of the provider requests, language-based requests appear, at face value, to be the most straightforward. However, the case presented here poses a unique challenge. In this case, the patient possesses decision-making capacity, but the situation appears to be severe enough (warranting presentation to the ED) that the patient's request should not be honored at this time. A trained interpreter, preferably live, should be offered in the acute setting, while an effort is made to secure a Spanish-speaking provider for the patient during the inpatient hospitalization. The interview should be conducted with security present if available given the patient's threat of violence.

CONCLUSION

In this chapter, we have reviewed various scenarios in which a patient asks to be seen by a psychiatrist of a certain race, gender, or religion, or one who speaks a specific language. Each individual case warrants an analysis of the historical factors, ethical considerations, patient-level factors, and organizational-level factors contributing to the decision about whether to accommodate a patient's request. Although one size does not fit all, this chapter provides guidelines that physicians can use when confronted with such clinical scenarios.

REFERENCES

1. Davis RM. Achieving racial harmony for the benefit of patients and communities: contrition, reconciliation, and collaboration. *JAMA*. 2008;300(3):323–325.
2. Price EG, Gozu A, Kern DE, et al. The role of cultural diversity climate in recruitment, promotion, and retention of faculty in academic medicine. *J Gen Intern Med*. 2005;20(7):565–571.
3. Jones BE, Gray BA. Problems in diagnosing schizophrenia and affective disorders among blacks. *PS*. 1986;37(1):61–65.
4. Paul-Emile K, Smith AK, Lo B, Fernández A. Dealing with racist patients. *N Engl J Med*. 2016;374(8):708–711.
5. *Chaney v Plainfield Healthcare Center*, 612 F3d 908 (7th Cir 2010). Available at http://trace.tennessee.edu/cgi/viewcontent.cgi?article=1006&context=rgsj; accessed November 15, 2017.
6. Principles of Bioethics. Available at https://depts.washington.edu/bioethx/tools/princpl.html; accessed November 7, 2017.
7. Traylor AH, Schmittdiel JA, Uratsu CS, et al. Adherence to cardiovascular disease medications: does patient–provider race/ethnicity and language concordance matter? *J Gen Intern Med*. 2010;25:1172.
8. Cuffee YL, Hargraves JL, Rosal M, et al. Reported racial discrimination, trust in physicians, and medication adherence among inner-city African Americans with hypertension. *Am J Public Health*. 2013;103(11):e55–e62.
9. Cabral RR, Smith TB. Racial/ethnic matching of clients and therapists in mental health services: a meta-analytic review of preferences, perceptions, and outcomes. *J Couns Psychol*. 2011;58:537–554.
10. Jerant A, Bertakis KD, Fenton JJ, et al. Patient-provider sex and race/ethnicity concordance: a national study of healthcare and outcomes. *Med Care*. 2011;49(11):1012–1020.

11. Cooper LA, Roter DL, Johnson RL, et al. Patient-centered communication, ratings of care, and concordance of patient and physician race. *Ann Intern Med.* 2003;139:907–915.
12. Office of the Surgeon General (US); Center for Mental Health Services (US); National Institute of Mental Health (US). *Mental Health: Culture, Race, and Ethnicity: A Supplement to Mental Health: A Report of the Surgeon General.* Rockville, MD: Substance Abuse and Mental Health Services Administration, 2001. Available from https://www.ncbi.nlm.nih.gov/books/NBK44243/
13. Title VII of the Civil Rights Act of 1964. Equal Employment Opportunity Commission. Available from http://www.eeoc.gov/laws/statutes/titlevii.cfm; accessed November 10, 2017.
14. Association of American Medical Colleges. 2016 Physician Specialty Data Report. Available from https://www.aamc.org/data/workforce/reports/457712/2016-specialty-databook.html; accessed October 30, 2017.
15. Association of American Medical Colleges. 2017 State Physician Workforce Data Report. Available from https://www.aamc.org/data/workforce/reports/442830/statedataandreports.html; accessed October 26, 2017.
16. Carey B. "Need therapy? A good man is hard to find." *New York Times.* May 21, 2011. Available from http://www.nytimes.com/2011/05/22/health/22therapists.html; accessed October 26, 2017.
17. Astbury J. Gender disparities in mental health. In: *Mental Health.* Geneva, Switzerland: WHO, 2001:73–92.
18. Wampold BE. How important are the common factors in psychotherapy? An update. *World Psychiatry.* 2015;14:270–277.
19. Landes SJ, Burton JR, King KM, Sullivan BF. Women's preference of therapist based on sex of therapist and presenting problem: an analogue study. *Couns Psychol Q.* 2013;26(3-4):330–342.
20. Kapphahn CJ, Wilson KM, Klein JD. Adolescent girls' and boys' preferences for provider gender and confidentiality in their health care. *J Adolesc Health.* 1999;25:131–142.
21. Liddon L, Kingerlee R, Barry JA. Gender differences in preferences for psychological treatment, coping strategies, and triggers to help-seeking. *Br J Clin Psychol.* 2018;57(1):42–58.
22. Greenberg RP, Zeldow PB. Sex differences in preferences for an ideal therapist. *J Pers Assess.* 1980;44(5):474–478.
23. Turchik JA, Rafie S, Rosen CS, et al. Perceived barriers to care and provider gender preferences among veteran men who have experienced military sexual trauma. *Psychol Serv.* 2013;10(2):213–222.
24. Josephson AM. Formulation and treatment: integrating religion and spirituality in clinical practice. *Child Adolesc Psychiatr Clin North Am.* 2004;13(1):71–84.
25. Caribe AC, Nunez R, Montal D, et al. Religiosity as a protective factor in suicidal behavior: a case-control study. *J Nerv Ment Dis.* 2012;200(10):863–867.
26. Firdous N. Khushoo in Salah. *The Ideal Muslimah.* November 9, 2017. Available from http://www.theidealmuslimah.com/2013/04/08/khushoo-in-salah/; accessed November 13, 2017.
27. American Psychiatric Association. *Diagnostic and Statistical Manual of Mental Disorders* (5th ed.). Arlington, VA: American Psychiatric Publishing, 2013.
28. U.S. English. Available from https://usefoundation.org/; accessed November 12, 2017.

29. Rumbaut G, Massey D. Immigration and language diversity in the United States. *Daedalus.* 2013;142:141–154.

30. U.S. Census Bureau. The nation's older population is still growing, Census Bureau reports. Available from https://www.census.gov/newsroom/press-releases/2017/cb17–100.html; published June 22, 2017; accessed November 14, 2017.

31. The Joint Commission. Overcoming the challenges of providing care to LEP patients. *Quick Safety,* Issue 13. May 2015. Available from http://www.jointcommission.org/assets/1/23/Quick_Safety_Issue_13_May_2015_EMBARGOED_5_27_15.pdf; accessed November 12, 2017.

32. LEP.gov. Commonly asked questions and answers regarding limited English proficient (LEP) individuals. Available from https://www.lep.gov/faqs/faqs.html#OneQ1; updated August 18, 2016; accessed November 14, 2017.

33. Hacker K, Choi YS, Trebino L, et al. Exploring the impact of language services on utilization and clinical outcomes for diabetics. *PloS One.* 2012;7(6):e38507.

34. Pochhacker, F. *Routledge Encyclopedia of Interpreting Studies.* New York: Routledge, 2015.

35. Blake C. Ethical considerations in working with culturally diverse populations: the essential role of professional interpreters. *Bull Can Psychiatric Assoc.* 2003;34:21–23.

36. Luk S. Overcoming language barriers in psychiatric practice: culturally sensitive and effective use of interpreters. *J Immigr Refug Stud.* 2008;6(4):545–566.

37. U.S. Department of Health and Human Services. Civil Rights Requirements–A. Title VI of the Civil Rights Act of 1964, 42 U.S.C. 2000d et seq. ("Title VI"). Available from https://www.hhs.gov/civil-rights/for-individuals/special-topics/needy-families/civil-rights-requirements/index.html; accessed November 12, 2017.

38. U.S. Agency for Healthcare Research and Quality. Improving patient safety systems for patients with limited English proficiency: a guide for hospitals. Available from https://www.ahrq.gov/professionals/systems/hospital/lepguide/lepguide2.html; published September 2012; accessed November 14, 2017.

13

Navigating Cultural Challenges in Patient–Clinician Dyads

JOSEPHA A. IMMANUEL, CHUN-YI JOEY CHEUNG, AND NHI-HA T. TRINH ■

The content of one's lived experience influences the instinct to search for similarities and differences when interacting with others. People often make trait inferences—level of competence, trustworthiness, likeability, attractiveness—about people they interact with at both a superficial and deeper level.[1] This instinct to make cognitive and emotional appraisals of others is no different in the psychiatric encounter. The framework of such an encounter calls for information gathering and synthesis to make treatment recommendations. The patient–clinician relationship lies at the core of this framework and drives the interaction. Historically, this relationship has been hailed as a unique component of the clinical encounter that affects patient outcome, treatment adherence, and patient satisfaction with treatment.[2] Given that the themes discussed in this chapter emerge in a dynamic process, the first part of the chapter aims to summarize the cultural and academic background regarding patient–clinician matching and to highlight some challenges that may arise in this process. The second part of this chapter aims to explore the process of navigating cultural dilemmas through three in-depth case vignettes.

The Centers for Disease Control and Prevention reported that approximately 25% of all U.S. adults have a mental illness and that nearly 50% of U.S. adults will develop at least one mental illness during their lifetime.[3] Unfortunately, most of these people do not seek or present for psychiatric care. Those who do present for treatment do so for a variety of reasons; some come of their volition, others at the behest of someone else who is impacted by the patient's symptoms, and still others seek court-mandated or involuntary treatment. Regardless of the reason, certain questions that patients often attempt to answer about the clinician throughout the encounter are, "Does this person get me?"; "Will this person judge me?"; and "Can this person help me?" The verbiage might differ, but at the heart of these questions are perhaps two main concerns: "Can I trust this person?" and "Will this person understand me?" The challenge of establishing a sense of trust and understanding within the patient–clinician relationship is critical, especially for those new to psychiatric care and patients from minority groups who may have experienced injustice at the hands of health care or general society.

Trust has been highlighted as a necessary ingredient for an effective patient–clinician relationship, but it is also a complex concept that can be difficult to define succinctly. Some have defined trust as a link between the social systems and the individual,[4] while others, such as Hall and colleagues,[5] divide trust into several dimensions: fidelity, competence, honesty, confidentiality, and global trust. Halbert and colleagues[6] went further to describe trust in the clinical setting as "a multidimensional construct that includes perceptions of the clinician's technical ability, interpersonal skills, and the extent to which the patient perceives that his or her welfare is placed above other considerations." Empathic understanding—the idea that a patient perceives that his or her feelings are both understood and accepted—is often considered to be a part of trust.[7] The concepts of trust and understanding, though related, can still be separate. A patient can believe a clinician is trustworthy, but can simultaneously feel that he or she is not being understood. Both qualities require nurturing in a therapeutic alliance.

Trust and empathic understanding are key when establishing a therapeutic relationship, as anxiety is often present in the initial clinical encounter, especially for those new to psychiatric care. Some seek to reduce this anxiety by requesting that their clinician have certain characteristics (e.g., specific race, sexual orientation, gender, age). The comfort in familiarity and the desire to seek commonality, especially in a new interaction, has underpinnings in social psychology. Since race and gender are visible characteristics, both patients and clinicians have used concordance in these features as a barometer to gauge a "good clinical fit." The assumption is that in a patient–clinician dyad with "good fit," there is an increased likelihood of an easier navigation of the relationship, and of readily established rapport.

Physical appearance, which includes gender presentation and ethnocultural characteristics, may contribute to assumptions that patients make about the clinician's background. Pairing clinicians and patients from seemingly similar cultural backgrounds has been a proposed way to establish rapport. Historically, there has been a tendency to equate culture with race and ethnicity, but in reality, culture—including cultural meanings, traditions, values, and practices—constitutes a variety of factors, including gender, class, religion, region of origin, and ethnicity. Studies have suggested that a shared background or commonality not only fosters the development of trust and mutual understanding within the patient–clinician relationship, but also positively affects patient satisfaction and outcome.[2,4,8] It has been postulated that cultural concordance fosters a shared worldview and problem definition and thus reduces or eliminates cultural barriers that would otherwise impede rapport-building and culturally sensitive assessments. Chang and colleagues[9] conducted a stratified matched-pair design in cross-racial therapy in hopes of isolating factors that predicted patient satisfaction and rapport building. Using a communication style, specifically a passive style, that shied away from "deep questioning regarding the patient's experience," proposing "textbook" recommendations that were "not tailored to the patient's specific life context and history," and minimizing the patient's experience of discrimination or oppression, were all found to be contributors to poor patient satisfaction and an unsuccessful therapeutic alliance.

Interpersonal similarities are hypothesized to influence not only the content, but also the perception of the interaction. Patients, especially those from minority groups, sometimes intentionally seek someone who appears similar to them, presuming that such a similarity will decrease the risk of discrimination and judgment. Their concerns are not unfounded, as there have been historical occurrences of systemic mistreatment of various groups by the medical community. The "Tuskegee Study of Untreated Syphilis in the Negro Male" is a classic example of the medical community's unethical behavior toward a specific minority group based on racism. In this study, conducted from 1932 to 1972, over 400 African American men with syphilis were not given informed consent and were left untreated, even when the cure for syphilis, penicillin, became available.[10] The Tuskegee study reduced the African American community's trust in the medical community and negatively affected their help-seeking behaviors. Another example illustrating the systemic mistreatment of a group occurred between 1950 and 1952, where approximately 1,000 pregnant women received diethylstilbestrol.[11] Not only was this study conducted without informed consent, but it took about 20 years to recognize the full extent of various ailments the offspring of these women developed. Recent studies comparing the level of trust in medical providers between Caucasians and African Americans continue to show that African Americans have lower levels of trust in their medical providers; long-term effects of this mistrust can influence treatment adherence and the quality of the patient–clinician relationship.[5,12]

Although researchers have generally found a decreasing trend in the incidents of blatant forms of discrimination as described above, hidden forms of discrimination, such as microaggressions, still exist.[13] *Microaggressions*, as first defined by Dr. Chester Pierce,[14] are "subtle, stunning, often automatic, and non-verbal exchanges which are 'put downs.'" Microaggressions apply not only to race, but also to gender, sexuality, religion, and cultural values, among other characteristics. The taxonomy of microaggressions includes *microinsults*, defined as indirect, often unconscious communications that put down an individual's group; *microinvalidations,* defined as "communications that negate or deny the thoughts, feelings, or experiences of a person based on their race, gender, sexuality"; and *microassaults*, which are "explicit and intentional denigration of an individual."[15,16] Because microaggressions are common human interactions, we can also expect them to occur in the clinical encounter.

Patients are not the only party considering the effects of ethnocultural, gender, sexuality, and religious concordance in the clinician–patient dyad. The experiences of both patient and clinician—which have shaped both parties' cognitive, social, cultural, and emotional worlds—undergo a dynamic and bidirectional interplay that is inescapable in the clinical encounter. The growing literature on the clinical impact of patient–clinician cultural matching has speculated that racial matching, for example, has a strong relationship to clinical outcomes.[9] Pierce and colleagues suggest that patients seeing a clinician with a dissimilar race or gender were likely to have a higher rate of attrition and to attend fewer sessions as compared to those with racial- and gender-concordant clinicians.[14] Wintersteen and colleagues[17] discovered that although their subjects assigned little importance to racial matching after the first two sessions, there was a higher treatment retention rate in the racial-concordant groups. However, meta-analytic studies have shown that racial matching alone is not directly associated with symptom improvement and is not necessary to establish an effective therapeutic alliance.[8,18,19] Rather, the clinician's cultural humility, level of attunement, and self-awareness of biases all influence the interaction between clinician and patient.

With this in mind, it is important to note that cultural matching may be helpful, but only to an extent. Relying solely on ethnocultural, gender, and sexuality concordance in the patient–clinician dyad can result in transference and countertransference reactions that can inhibit clinical gains. Overgeneralization, for example, is an inter-ethnocultural reaction that can blind us to the reality that people who share a sociocultural attribute (e.g., race, gender, sexuality, religion) might not automatically share the same opinions, understanding, or worldview. Clinically, overgeneralization can result in bidirectional trait projection and stifle therapeutic progress. Clinicians might assume they "know" the patient so well that they "fill in the blanks" without fully listening to the patient. Conversely, patients might imagine their clinician understands them so well that they do not need to provide a comprehensive narrative. Subsequently, when the clinician does not show a synchronized understanding as the patient in such a dyad, there can be an even greater sense of disconnection. Hook and colleagues[13] point out that in racially concordant dyads, patients reported that microaggressions in the encounter had more impact, as compared to racially dissimilar pairings, again strengthening the consensus bias theory: people expect others within their group to share similar perspectives.[19]

WORKSHOP

Both culturally similar and dissimilar dyads can be challenging and require psychological processing and interpersonal negotiations, but can ultimately be therapeutic. Given the current political and social climate emphasizing group divisions, there is a greater potential for the appearance of cultural mismatch between clinician and patient, even between dyads who might at first glance share similar cultural identities or backgrounds. In addition, it can feel easy to talk in the abstract about what one might do in a given scenario, but it is another matter entirely to work through the discomfort of clinical impasses in real time.

With these themes in mind, as part of the MGH/McLean Sociocultural curriculum, a two-hour advanced workshop for PGY-3s was developed to bring these topics alive, with the goal of examining these potential impasses in depth in an experiential manner. In some ways, this workshop is a "capstone" in the curriculum and pushes residents to synthesize their experiences of self-examination in PGY-1, and of knowledge and attitudes of cultural constructs and cultural humility in PGY-2 and PGY-3. In designing a curriculum, educators can decide whether to include such a workshop based not only on logistical constraints such as time and faculty availability, but also whether they feel residents have the necessary orientation and skills to engage in such a workshop. More information regarding curriculum development is provided in Chapter 14 in this textbook.

As a means of exploring clinical dilemmas, the workshop leaders use adaptations of their own clinical cases adapted from real-life scenarios. Initially, leaders begin by setting a frame for safety and exploration. Establishing a safe space in which trainees and faculty can explore these dilemmas is of utmost importance. The leaders emphasize that these clinical dilemmas have no "one right answer"; rather, the purpose of the workshop is to prompt residents to imagine what they might do in similar situations and to promote discussion. The ultimate goal is for residents to feel better prepared should they be confronted with similar "sticky" situations. The leaders brainstorm with residents regarding a few clinical cases from either the leaders' or the residents' practices. A group agreement is reached regarding which two to three cases will be explored. Resident volunteers are solicited to act as the clinician, while the group leader assumes the role of the simulated patient. After a role play of 5 to 10 minutes, group discussion follows for 15 to 20 minutes. Common themes discussed include clinician overidentification with the patient (like Cases 1 and 2) and ensuing therapeutic impasses and challenges of self-disclosure on the part of the clinician.

Below are three case examples to illustrate the cultural negotiations that can occur in clinical encounters, in each case followed by thoughts for discussion. The identities of the patients and clinicians have been disguised to preserve anonymity. When reading through these cases, we encourage readers to reflect on the merits and challenges encompassed in the patient–clinician dynamic on their personal clinical experiences.

CASE 1: OVERIDENTIFICATION BASED ON RACIAL MATCHING

Case Vignette

You are a clinician in a community clinic and receive a message from the practice manager asking if you will accept a new patient described as "A 30-year-old African American female, new to psychiatric care, requesting to be seen by a Black woman, saying that she would feel more comfortable because a female Black clinician would understand 'my struggle'." You accept the case but sense that the notification from the clinic manager was a formality, as you are the only female Black clinician in the clinic. Besides, this is not the first time you have been paired with a patient based on race, gender, or both.

When you call the patient from the waiting room, she says, "It's so good to see you." As you direct her to sit, she states in the same familiar tone, "I'm Grace . . . I'm so glad it's you." You ask her if she's met you before, to which she responds, "No, but I thought they would give me another white lady like last time." She appears relieved. She explains that she had an initial evaluation with another clinician, but left that appointment feeling "like she didn't get me" and searched for another clinician. The familiarity in Grace's first statement feels welcoming for you. While you have a positive reaction to Grace's initial comments, it does cross your mind that there is an unspoken pressure to give her an experience different from her previous clinician. Although Grace does not explicitly state that she did not feel understood because of the racial discordance with her previous clinician, it seems implied. You have a brief pang of worry, which is not unfounded, as you recall that throughout high school, you were called an "Oreo"—a term used to describe someone who is "black on the outside but white on the inside," leaving you feeling separate from your black peers. You often wondered if you were "black enough" because of this experience. You brush that worry away and proceed with the appointment.

As the intake progresses, Grace describes a history of stagnancy in her life. She explains, "I've been working hard all my life but I feel that life is so hard . . . I feel like I have to work twice as hard just to be on the same level as everybody else," then ends the statement with, "You know what I mean, right?" You smile and say, "I know exactly what you mean," to which Grace responds, "I knew you would, 'cuz you seem like you would keep it real." The remainder of this session includes Grace disclosing spoken and unspoken pressures from her Ghanaian parents to be wealthy and married, neither of which she has attained. She was born in the United States and voices a pervasive conflict managing Ghanaian and American culture. She again says, "You know what I mean, right?" You reflexively respond "yeah," despite not knowing much about Ghanaian culture, except for limited knowledge about similarities between Ghanaian and Nigerian cuisine. She discloses that based on your last name, she deduced that your family is from Africa. You again respond "yes" and reveal that you were born in Nigeria and have lived in the United States for 20 years. She proceeds to tell you that she has several Nigerian friends who are "just the best."

You redirect her to discuss her concerns. She describes the constant fear that any deviation from perfection at work could lead to immediate termination. She remarks, "You get it, right? As a professional, you know how hard it is for us to make it." You nod because you have had similar worries and ideas throughout your career. She too nods and smiles. You end the session feeling confident that you can help Grace. She states: "I've got a really good feeling about you . . . like you're really going to help me feel better." She leaves your office assuring you that she will return for her follow-up.

The next five sessions begin in a similar manner: Grace complimenting you on your attire, your compassion, your level of competence such that she feels that she doesn't have to "talk a lot" because "you really seem to care and get me." She describes a pattern of "feeling so happy in here" but as soon as she leaves your office, "I feel sad again." You notice that she often offers to change her work schedule rather than miss a session. You applaud her for being motivated and treatment adherent.

You have supervision but typically discuss the more difficult cases; considering Grace as one of the "easy" cases, you did not discuss her case in supervision. You have three more sessions and you notice a change in your reaction to Grace—you feel physically drained throughout the appointment. There is a new awareness of monotony and redundancy in your dynamic with her—she compliments you, you reciprocate with affirmations, she talks about her difficulties and frustration, you agree with her, and the appointment ends. You identify feeling stuck, despite your simultaneous belief that you understand Grace and she is a "really good patient." You discuss your observations with your supervisor, who speculates that you may be overidentifying with Grace because of your similar backgrounds. You disagree, as you have past success with other patients whose backgrounds were just as similar, but out of respect consider the possible validity of your supervisor's comment.

The next session is different. You repeatedly remind yourself that you should be curious about whatever Grace presents. She informs you about an African American colleague whom she assumed would "have my back" but didn't. She once again says, "I bet you've dealt with this in your work." Your instinct to once again agree resurfaces, but you decide to ask more questions. You respond, "I might have some ideas about this experience but I want to make sure I fully understand, so can you tell me more?" She is visibly upset as evidenced by her irritable tone, audible breaths, and frowning. You ask how she is feeling, to which she responds, "Fine." You point out the incongruence in her affect and stated mood, and she responds, "You know how it is . . . can't be the angry Black woman in the office." She describes a pattern of both her parents and past boyfriends "not having my back," once again ending with, "You know." You quietly gather your thoughts. In an irritable tone, she says, "I'm sorry, you probably don't know what it's like to be me. You're a doctor and everyone is probably proud of you." You choose to ask her what it would mean if you did feel the same way that she was feeling. She immediately retorts, "But you don't" in an irritable tone, her eye contact averted. She then intones, "You must be one of those who gets to the top and forgets where they came from and all the lil' folks they left." As you begin to speak, she interrupts, stating that the session is almost over, so she'd like to schedule a follow-up time. You discuss the case with your supervisor, who encourages you to explore this session further, specifically what it means to Grace if or when you don't "get it."

For the first time, Grace misses an appointment, but she does reschedule. She smiles as she walks into your office with a plate of cookies, apologetically saying, "I was really stressed out, and it just came out like that last time." She appears uncomfortable when you state you'd like to discuss the previous session. You wonder out loud if there were times that you assumed an understanding of what she intended to convey and did not fully "get it." She appears perplexed and responds in an irritable tone, "I don't get it. I thought you liked being my doctor." You attempt to placate the situation by giving an example of how assumptions can lead to inaccurate conclusions. She proceeds to state, "What wrong assumptions do you have about me? I thought that both of us being Black independent women that you could help me move forward . . . I guess not." She sighs, turns her body and legs toward the door, and averts eye contact. She does not return for subsequent appointments.

Discussion

Spontaneous projective identifications, where patients assign qualities and values to the clinician based on their own ethnocultural values and background experiences, occur throughout the clinical encounter. The initial reaction from this patient when she meets the Black female clinician is a sense of relief, as this pairing not only means that her request was acknowledged, but implicitly provides the space for her to feel understood, not judged or dismissed. Grace imagines that the clinician has the ability to empathize with her difficulties navigating her conflicts. Race is not explicitly stated as a reason Grace did not follow up with her previous clinician, but it is implied. On the one hand, the clinician's awareness of the patient's hidden intent in her request introduces an unspoken but loaded challenge for the clinician to "get" the patient better than her previous clinician. On the other hand, the clinician's own experience of being labeled an "Oreo" creates an ambivalent countertransference reaction, one where Grace could also reject the clinician as she did her previous therapist.

Often when a patient makes a specific request like this, there is a perception of an unconscious defense and resistance to underlying conflict. In this case, there appears to be a conflict of both hope and despair. There is a powerful hope that her pairing with the clinician—who looks like her, shares assumed similarities, and is perceived as successful—will help her resolve and perhaps undo her supposed missteps. This palpable transference reaction of hope sets the stage for the assumed strong therapeutic alliance. Grace's initial transference reaction of hope weaves into her other reaction of overcompliance and idealization. The statements of praise and the nods of affirmation nurture this reaction. The shared identification between Grace and the clinician is initially comforting for both parties, as there is often safety in the familiar. However, with subsequent appointments, we begin to see how the overidentification between both parties inadvertently creates and encourages therapeutic blindness and a faulty sense of omniscience. In the absence of a self-reflective attitude early on in this case, the clinician unconsciously substitutes her experiences for those of the patient and likely misses vital information. The clinician inadvertently "fills in the blanks," thus contributing to the stagnancy in therapeutic progress. This omniscient countertransference, coupled with the patient's transference reaction of idealization of a clinician who both "keeps it real" and "really cares and gets me," ultimately compromises the therapeutic alliance. When the clinician reveals a semblance of not being "all-knowing," there is an immediate disruption in their dyad, catalyzing the conversion of Grace's initial hope to despair, anger, and mistrust.

The clinician's acknowledgment of the overidentification dynamic's contribution to hindering therapeutic progress creates the possibility of both therapeutic chaos and reparation. Shared experiences and ethnocultural similarities can help create the framework for an initial therapeutic alliance and therapeutic progress, but relying solely on these similarities can be detrimental to the ultimate success of the treatment.

CASE 2: OVERIDENTIFICATION BASED ON SIMILAR DEMOGRAPHICS IMPEDES ALLIANCE-BUILDING

Case Vignette

A colleague refers you, a straight Caucasian male clinician in your 40s, a patient named Dr. C, with a history of treatment-resistant depression. At the first interview, upon taking the social and cultural history, you realize numerous demographic similarities. The patient is a straight Asian American man in his 40s who grew up in the same metropolitan area. You find out that you both went to the same Ivy League college within 5 years of each other, have served on the same community service organizations, and both have young children around the same age. The patient is also in the mental health profession as a PhD-level clinician. You learn that at the core of the patient's presentation is a sense of shame that his career did not take off in the trajectory he had hoped due to his psychiatric illness, and, coupled with a recent divorce, he feels his life "is in shambles." Additional stressors, including financial instability and a sense of social isolation, compound his low mood and despair.

Dr. C feels embarrassed about being a patient while other members of his cohort are all thriving in academic careers and do not seem to be struggling with their mental health. He describes being embarrassed about asking for money from his mother, a retired law professor, and the discomfort he feels at family gatherings, where his younger sister is an accomplished prize-winning poet with "the perfect life." He describes a family wedding he went to recently, and how his mother remarked that his teenage niece and nephew "are so well-behaved" while looking askance at his own children, who appeared to be wrestling in the corner. The patient laments: "This just reinforces to me how I am such a failure, in my professional life, in my personal life . . . everything I do gets fouled up."

During the initial visit, he has a hard time making eye contact with you in the room. He chokes up while describing his story and parenthetically remarks, "I am so embarrassed to be talking about this." He remarks on your numerous diplomas "showcasing your impressive pedigree" hanging in your office, and you observe him lingering on the college diploma of your shared alma mater.

Over the next few sessions, it becomes quite difficult for you to develop a therapeutic alliance. The patient perseverates on the shortcomings in his life. He repeatedly says, "It's so embarrassing to tell you all that I've f'ed up in my life." Thematically, the patient comes back to this at his follow-up appointments and talks about "just giving up." When you probe for suicidality, however, the patient bristles and yells back, "Just because I am telling you this doesn't mean I'm going to do it! I know what you're doing here; I'm in the business, too!"

After about three or four sessions, the patient pages you after work in crisis. Without a place to speak privately during dinnertime, you retreat to your home office to answer the call. While the patient is explaining his dilemma, a yell from one of your children is heard in the background. The patient stops midsentence and asks directly, "Do you have kids?" Awkwardly, you reply a simple "yes," and a quiet pause follows on the phone. The patient breaks the silence, saying, "I'm just a bother to you and your family," and hangs up.

During the subsequent session, the patient begins to debunk your suggestions and repeatedly injects comments about the superb skill of his prior clinician, a more senior academician. The patient says to you condescendingly, "Dr. S always had ideas, and you never have any. I feel like you are too young and overwhelmed by me. I don't know what we should be doing here." You feel stuck in your clinical judgment and unconfident in your ability to help the patient. You suggest restarting a medication that was helpful but caused difficult side effects. In hearing this, the patient becomes livid and storms out of the office.

After the above encounter, you talk with the patient's prior clinician to understand the treatment course. She describes how the patient, when doing well, is relatively high-functioning, but struggles immensely when he is not. She suggests the termination with her may be a source of distress, as the patient had a difficult termination with a prior clinician as well.

With this knowledge, you seek consultation from your peer supervision group; your colleagues also have strong reactions to this patient. One is concerned that this patient is still seeing his own patients; another is hyperfocused on the types of medications and trials, hoping to help you "find the right medication." However, hoping to seek advice on how to normalize some of the alliance difficulties, you reach out to a senior clinician in your group for consultation. The senior clinician suggests you have been too passive and should be more direct with treatment suggestions with this patient. You explain you are seeking consultation because you did strongly suggest a medication (which the patient vehemently refused) and receive no further advice from your colleague. You turn to the director of your clinic to discuss the case. She perceptively notes that alliance-building (not medication choice) is the challenge, and agrees to see the patient. Although the director returns with a laundry list of medications to consider, the patient appears disgruntled and the few trials of medications (with the lengthy insurance prior authorizations) that followed are not successful. You feel caught in a cycle of disgruntled phone visits, brief medication trials (and discontinuations), and frustrated phone calls from the patient that "nothing is working."

After a year of working together, breakthrough seems to happen during a phone call between sessions. The patient comments to you, "Everyone just wants to leave me." You reply off the cuff, "It sounds like you have written off our relationship as well." There is a pause on the phone. You notice that over the next few months, the patient appears relatively more relaxed and less frustrated with your recommendations.

Discussion

In the first case, the patient found initial concordance with the clinician based on gender and ethnoracial identity, while the second case presents an example where overidentification occurs based on demographic characteristics (socioeconomic status, profession, geography, community affiliation, education) that are not immediately observable. Although the teaching in psychotherapy has traditionally focused on maintaining a neutral therapeutic stance, clearly there are aspects of our own identities as clinicians that we cannot necessarily keep at bay. Our race, ethnicity, and gender are all aspects of our cultural identity that can often be readily visible to patients. Similarly, there are other subtle clues available to the patient, including socioeconomic status (especially as pertaining to educational achievement), or marital status, as suggested by the presence or absence of a wedding ring. Other aspects of cultural identity, including sexual identity, political or community affiliation, spiritual or religious orientation, or family background, may not be as accessible at first glance, but assumptions, inferences, or fantasies about these may impact both the transference reaction of the patient and the clinician's countertransference reaction.

As clinicians, we often assume that having a background similar to our patients will help us better understand them. In this case, there is a common geographical background, educational background, profession, and stage of life. Like the cultural background of race and ethnicity, these are all cultural communities to which both patient and clinician belong, and for which there are norms of behavior and success. However, for the patient, seeing a clinician who may mirror his cultural experience feels quite shameful. Noticing the similarities between their lives, this form of overidentification brings up feelings of failure and regret for the patient, who wonders why his life did not turn out to be as "successful" as the clinician's life.

Depending on the size of the community, these feelings may differ in degree. While in the first case, similarities ultimately impeded the therapeutic process due to unspoken assumptions and perceived connectedness, the impasse in this case initially emerged from the unshakable overlapping identities between the clinician and the patient. Communities based on gender and ethnocultural communities are relatively large, but then split off into smaller subgroups depending on various details (e.g., nationalities, values). In this case, the clinician and patient belong to a relatively small community of practicing Ivy League–educated mental health clinicians in the same geographical area with similar family backgrounds. With this clear set of mirroring identities, the therapeutic alliance is initially stuck, as the patient feels trapped by seeing a clinician in his same social circle.

Given the similarities in professional training, there is an interesting power differential present in this dynamic between clinician and patient. There is an inherent power dynamic built into the therapeutic relationship, with the clinician adopting a position of authority as opposed to the patient who has come to seek help. As a trained clinician himself, however, the patient has an in-depth understanding of his treatment options and "insider information" about the techniques used to build therapeutic rapport. Possibly to prove himself to be just as capable as his clinician, the patient becomes defensive and lashes back at the clinician by asserting his own knowledge and undermining the clinician's. It is possible that because the patient overidentifies with the clinician while simultaneously self-loathing, he also has difficulty trusting the clinician just as he has difficulty trusting himself. Undermining the clinician by bringing his previous clinician into the conversation works to affirm this belief. Like the first case, the clinician is given a loaded challenge to be better than the patient's previous clinician.

For the clinician, mixed feelings may arise from seeing a patient from such a similar background unable to move forward with his life given his illness. On one hand, the clinician could feel, "Maybe this could've been me," engendering more empathy. On the other hand, the clinician could feel impatient with the patient and expect the patient to have more agency given the patient's similar intellectual and educational background. The clinician must remember, however, that the very nature of mental health disorders can impede cognitive function, as well as judgment and insight.

Alliance-building is more than shared identities; it comes from an established trust between the clinician and the patient. In this case, trust came eventually with time, despite the challenges of working with him.

CASE 3: WHEN TO DISCLOSE?

Case Vignette

You are a clinician in a group practice. You have an appointment with a 5-year-old girl named Chloe who presents with both parents, Linda and Scott, at her school's request for "behavioral issues." She is her parents' only child. As they walk into your office, Chloe asks for her tablet and headphones, and her mom immediately obliges. Linda and her husband, Scott, both express their displeasure that the school made the referral but state they brought Chloe to appease the school. Scott expresses his displeasure that the school's staff "couldn't handle a little tantrum here and there."

Based on the documentation you received from the school, you sense that Chloe's parents are minimizing Chloe's behavior. Linda states, "Well, Chloe is bossy, but she's not a bad child," while Scott describes Chloe as a "child who knows what she wants. She is a very advanced child . . . too advanced for her age." You begin to speak when Scott interrupts you and asks you if you have children of your own. You feel a tightness rise from your abdomen and rest at the base of your neck. You can sense that you are frowning as you stare at him in silence. A series of thoughts swirl in your mind—What is he implying by his question? How should I answer this question? How can I get out of answering this question? What does it mean if I tell him that I don't have kids? You decide not to respond to his direct question for fear that you might lose credibility. All you say is, "I am well trained in child psychiatry and how to manage difficulties that may come up, and right now, it seems that Chloe is having some difficulties in school."

Your response seems to do the trick as it shifts his attention from you, back to the school's staff.

You offer supportive statements about the frustration both parents might be experiencing as they decide how to manage the reports about Chloe. Both parents nod in agreement. Linda proceeds to say, "I know that I might spoil her sometimes, but you don't know what we went through to have her." As you begin to explore mom's state- ment, Chloe takes off the headphones and states in an irritable tone that she's hungry and would like to leave. Scott begins to stand but you redirect him that you'd like to discuss recommendations in the time left. You start off stating that Chloe appears to be outgoing and intelligent but sometimes might need "just a little bit of help in some areas." Both parents seem amenable and agree to make a follow-up appointment. You sense some ambivalence and don't believe they'll return to the clinic, but you make the appointment. Your next available appointment is in 2 weeks. You notice that the tight- ness at the base of your neck resolves as they walk out.

Linda comes to the next appointment stating that Scott will remain in the waiting room with Chloe. She wants to speak to you separately. Linda explains that after reading several blogposts and speaking to friends who have worked with clinicians, they decided to give behavioral therapy a chance. She begins to tell you that she has been more ob- servant of Chloe's interactions with her peers during play dates and does see a "bossy" side to Chloe, but adds, "She does play really well with the other kids. It's just sometimes she wants to do what she wants to do." She becomes tearful, stating, "I know part of this, I guess, is my fault, but she's my miracle baby, so I give her everything she wants."

You ask Linda to elaborate and she responds that after she married her husband, they tried for years to have a child without success. She begins to cry and says, "I haven't told anyone this, not even Scott . . . but I had an abortion in my 20s and all those nega- tive pregnancy tests were a reminder of my punishment for what I did . . . Having Chloe was a miracle for me. I thought I lost my chance to have kids after the abortion." With her eye contact averted, she remarks, "My parents would disown me if they ever found out." She explains, still with her eye contact directed towards the floor, "I was raised in a good Catholic home so. . . I actually don't know why I just told you all of that, but I guess it's important just so you get how important Chloe is to me."

You nod in agreement and thank her for sharing that information with you. She sighs and laughs nervously as she dries her tears. You say nothing. She apologizes for crying, to which you respond, "There's no reason for an apology. Crying is a normal reaction to a painful situation." She states, while laughing nervously, "Well, you probably think I'm crazy, though," to which you begin to respond stating, "No . . ." but she interrupts and says, "I'm going to guess you're Jewish or Catholic because of how your last name is spelled. It's just like in the Old Testament." She asks if you are Catholic or Jewish and you are taken aback by her statement. In your training, you were taught to be careful about self-disclosure. You recall your countertransference reaction when her husband, Scott, asked if you had children of your own, and how you skirted the question. You suspect lingering pain and shame in her narrative and wonder if self-disclosure would be helpful in this case, but also wonder if it is necessary.

She chuckles, shakes her head, then says, "You're probably trying to think of some- thing to say to make me feel better because I know it's a sin." She is silent so you ask if she'd like to share what she's thinking. She responds, "Nothing . . . it's just that I've had conversations about abortion with so many people . . . and people always want to be politically correct so they say the right things, but in their hearts, they still judge, so . . ."

She shrugs. You validate her skepticism about your response and highlight that not all stereotypes are true. You give an example of how assumptions can be inaccurate, which seems to resonate with her; she smiles, nods, and responds "You're right, you're right." She lets out an audible breath and says, "I guess I've just had experiences where it felt that people weren't sincere, so it's hard for me to trust what people tell me about this be-cause I guess I've not really dealt with how I feel about it. I've just kept it in." She thanks you for listening.

Her demeanor shifts—her eye contact is no longer averted; she sits upright and smiles. She apologizes, stating, "Sorry, I just turned this into my own therapy session even though we're here to help Chloe." She asks for your recommendations of how they both can help their daughter. You further explore their dynamic and parenting style with Chloe. You discuss typical developmentally appropriate defenses, the psychoso-cial dilemmas Chloe is attempting to resolve, and ways to help her manage difficult emotions that she might struggle to manage. Linda smiles, places her hand on her cheek, and asks, "How do you know all this stuff about children? Did you learn all of this from your own children? They must be so happy to have you as a mom."

You feel confused because you don't have children. You feel shame as both your parents have repeatedly asked you why you are not married or have children. Your mom often reminds you of your "biological clock." That tightness from the first ses-sion when her husband, Scott, asked a similar question returns and remains in your abdomen.

You choose to disclose that as part of your training, you observed and interacted with children in different age groups, and personally you have a 5-year-old niece. You are about to conclude your statement emphasizing that all these experiences make you a competent child clinician when Linda interrupts you and states, "That's probably why you understand this so much." She goes further to say, "You must have so much fun with your niece with playing dress-up. It's such a fun age!" You invite Scott and Chloe into the room, and Linda explains what was discussed during the session. She reports that she'll have a more in-depth conversation with Scott before their next session.

They all present to the next several sessions. They are engaged and treatment ad-herent. Both parents are pleased with the progress Chloe has made both at home and school. Linda, and sometimes Scott, occasionally ask about your 5-year-old niece. Chloe also suggests some games she plays at home that you can play with your niece when you babysit. After eight sessions, both Scott and Linda feel comfortable with the behavioral changes and plan to continue on their own.

Discussion

In the above case, we see several shifts in the dynamic between all parties. At the beginning of the interaction, we see both the clinician and the parents negotiating how to define and assign meaning to the reports from school about the identified patient, Chloe. During this negotiation, the patient's father asks about the clinician's life outside of the role of being a clinician. One can postulate that the question was asked to identify a shared lived experience of parenting as a way of facilitating con-nection and shared understanding. The question of having children of her own has a different meaning for the clinician, including a countertransference reaction of shame, ambivalence, and disconnection. The clinician considers the implications of his question and decides to maintain a stance of authority and limit self-disclosure, so she redirects his focus without answering the question. We see that by the end of the intake, there is no sense of connection. In fact, it appears both parties are going through the polite routine of arranging a follow-up appointment, with neither party expecting to honor this arrangement.

In the subsequent session, Linda's revelation about her abortion introduces a shared experience of shame—from the clinician's experience when Linda's husband asks her the question about having children, and Linda's shame about her abortion years ago—that allows for a deeper alliance. The clinician's ability to acknowledge and validate Linda's concerns allows for trust and a display of empathic understanding in that relationship. The shift in the dyad between clinician and mother allows for further understanding of the patient. It is important to always note that although the child is the identified patient, without an alliance with the parents, the patient–clinician relationship and treatment will be handicapped. As the session progresses, the same question asked in the intake is presented again, and is more directed and layered. The clinician has a different reaction to this question given her increased comfort with Linda. There is still a fear of the implication, but we see that a small familial self-disclosure from the clinician promotes a sense of connection and trust rather than undermining the clinician's position. Linda then includes both her husband and child in the positive treatment dynamic.

Table 13.1 Factors to Consider Regarding Clinician Self-Disclosure

When Direct Disclosure May Be Beneficial	When Withholding Disclosure May Be Beneficial
Patient feels comfortable asking the clinician directly about his or her identities as the therapeutic alliance is just developing	Patient's fantasies or assumptions about the clinician produces material for further exploration
Patient identifies resolving conflicting feelings about his or her own identity as a treatment goal, and the clinician shares said identity	Patient is particularly defensive against exploring questions of his or her own identities
Patient expresses continued indirect inquiries on the clinician's identities	Patient expresses particularly violent views against the clinician's identities
The clinic openly advertises as a safe space for all communities and identities	Clinician has unresolved feelings about his or her own identities
Not disclosing would undermine the therapeutic alliance	Patient already has knowledge on the clinician's identities but is inquiring in an uncomfortable, indirect manner
Patient's misunderstanding of the clinician's identity can further reinforce the patient's self-hatred or damage trust	

Adapted from Levounis, P., Drescher, J., & Barber, M. E. (2012). *The LGBT Casebook*. Washington, DC: American Psychiatric Publishing.

The desire to find a similarity in interactions is instinctive, even when the similarity is not obvious from superficial physical features such as race, clothing, body habitus, and so forth. A sense of a shared experience can provide a gateway for connection, but there must be openness to vulnerability on the part of both the clinician and the patient and family, as in this case. There is no universal rule guiding whether disclosure is necessary or beneficial to the therapeutic process; some may argue that withholding personal information may hinder trust-building, while others argue that too much honest disclosure can represent a boundary crossing or violation with serious transference and countertransference effects.[21] However, people are generally curious about the lives of others, and a clinician's thoughtful self-disclosure can be powerful for the patient. Disclosure, however, should occur after the clinician has had a thorough understanding of the patient's intention and what the patient's response might be to the disclosure (Table 13.1).

Patients exercise their own intuition when interacting with the clinician and are often trying to interpret verbal and nonverbal cues to better understand the person with whom they are sharing their intimate lives. It is important to note

---

Box 13.1

What Do You Do Now?

1. At the end of your third appointment, your patient comments that she's so glad you speak "American," unlike the other clinicians in your practice, who "talk funny." How do you respond?
2. You are of Jewish decent and notice that your new admission is a patient who has a tattoo of a swastika. You feel angry as soon as you see this tattoo and also when the patient comments on your Jewish surname. How will you handle the situation?
3. Your patient is complaining about how stressful it is to raise children and asks if you have children and a spouse, followed by saying that only someone who is married and has children could possibly understand what a parent is going through. What do you say?
4. It is election season. Your patient has strong ideas about politics and does not hesitate to voice them in depth at each session. At the start of the session, your patient asks you who you are going to vote for this election season. How do you respond?
5. The parents of one of your young adult patients are very involved in their treatment. They are also in the medical profession. They sent you a request to connect with them on LinkedIn. At the next session, they mention your profile and the request to connect. How do you respond?
6. Despite having top-level privacy settings on your Facebook profile, one of your patients discovers that you are active in the same local political organization as they are. Your patient brings this up and says it is not a big deal but they thought you should know. Now what? Would it be different if this was a weekly therapy case versus a straightforward, stable medication management case?

that disclosures happen at every point of therapy and can be the result of indirect cues. While it is impossible for a clinician to exist completely out of the public domain, ultimately clinicians are responsible to ensure that what they are disclosing to their patients would allow them to maintain professionalism with all patients.

CONCLUSION

In this chapter, we have examined challenges of bridging perceived cultural similarities and differences in the clinical encounter, and how navigating these challenges can influence the therapeutic outcome. Using three case vignettes, we have illustrated the potential effects of overidentification on therapeutic progress, background concordance on rapport-building, and self-disclosure on therapeutic outcome. The three cases discussed above and additional cases in Box 13.1 can be used as examples of the types of cases that can be used for these role-play exercises, although our experience has been that the most stimulating discussion comes from trainee cases that may be "burning" in their minds. No matter what the level of the clinician (from trainee to seasoned clinician), contemplating these challenges is of utmost importance and brings together the art and science of the therapeutic process.

REFERENCES

1. Willis, J., & Todorov, A. (2006). First impressions: Making up your mind after a 100-ms exposure to a face. *Psychological Science, 17*(7), 592–598.
2. Patel, S. R., Bakken, S., & Ruland, C. (2008). Recent advances in shared decision making for mental health. *Current Opinion in Psychiatry, 21*(6), 606–612.
3. Fact Sheet | MIS | CDC. (n.d.). Retrieved April 5, 2018, from https://www.cdc.gov/mentalhealthsurveillance/fact_sheet.html
4. Meyer, S., Ward, P., Coveney, J., & Rogers, W. (2008). Trust in the health system: An analysis and extension of the social theories of Giddens and Luhmann. *Health Sociology Review, 17*(2), 177–186.
5. Hall, M. A., Zheng, B., Dugan, E., et al. (2002). Measuring patients' trust in their primary care providers. *Medical Care Research and Review, 59*(3), 293–318.
6. Halbert, C. H., Armstrong, K., Gandy, O. H., & Shaker, L. (2006). Racial differences in trust in health care providers. *Archives of Internal Medicine, 166*(8), 896–901.
7. Kim, S. S., Kaplowitz, S., & Johnston, M. V. (2004). The effects of clinician empathy on patient satisfaction and compliance. *Evaluation & the Health Professions, 27*(3), 237–251.
8. Cooper, L. A., Roter, D. L., Johnson, R. L., et al. (2003). Patient-centered communication, ratings of care, and concordance of patient and clinician race. *Annals of Internal Medicine, 139*(11), 907–915.
9. Chang, D. F., & Berk, A. (2009). Making cross-racial therapy work: A phenomenological study of patients' experiences of cross-racial therapy. *Journal of Counseling Psychology, 56*(4), 521–536.
10. Tuskegee Study—Timeline—CDC—NCHHSTP. (2017, August 30). Retrieved April 5, 2018, from https://www.cdc.gov/tuskegee/timeline.htm

11. Capron, A. M. (1989). Human experimentation. In R. M. Veatch (Ed.), *Medical Ethics* (125–172). Boston: Jones & Bartlett.

12. Musa, D., Schulz, R., Harris, R., et al. (2009). Trust in the health care system and the use of preventive health services by older black and white adults. *American Journal of Public Health*, *99*(7), 1293–1299.

13. Hook, J. N., Farrell, J. E., Davis, D. E., et al. (2016). Cultural humility and racial microaggressions in counseling. *Journal of Counseling Psychology*, *63*(3), 269–277.

14. Pierce, C. M. (1974). Psychiatric problems of the black minority. In G. Caplan (Ed.), *American Handbook of Psychiatry*. New York: Basic Books.

15. Sue, D. W., Capodilupo, C. M., Torino, G. C., et al. (2007). Racial microaggressions in everyday life: Implications for clinical practice. *The American Psychologist*, *62*(4), 271–286.

16. Sue, D. W. (2010). *Microaggressions in Everyday Life: Race, Gender, and Sexual Orientation*. Hoboken, NJ: John Wiley & Sons.

17. Wintersteen, M. B., Mensinger, J. L., & Diamond, G. S. (2005). Do gender and racial differences between patient and therapist affect therapeutic alliance and treatment retention in adolescents? *Professional Psychology: Research and Practice*, *36*(4), 400–408.

18. Shin, S., Chow, C., Camacho-Gonsalves, T., et al. (2005). A meta-analytic review of racial-ethnic matching for African American and Caucasian American patients and clinicians. *Journal of Counseling Psychology*, *52*(1), 45–56.

19. Cabral, R. R., & Smith, T. B. (2011). Racial/ethnic matching of patients and therapists in mental health services: A meta-analytic review of preferences, perceptions, and outcomes. *Journal of Counseling Psychology*, *58*(4), 537–554.

20. Kimball, R. A., Weller, S. C., & Batchelder, W. H. (2009). Culture as consensus: A theory of culture and informant accuracy. *American Anthropologist*, *88*(2), 313–338.

21. Magee, M., & Miller, D. C. (2013). *Lesbian Lives: Psychoanalytic Narratives Old and New*. London: Routledge.

22. Levounis, P., Drescher, J., & Barber, M. E. (2012). *The LGBT Casebook*. Washington, DC: American Psychiatric Publishing.

14

Teaching Sociocultural Psychiatry Throughout the Lifespan

PRIYA SEHGAL, MAYA NAUPHAL, AND JUSTIN A. CHEN ∎

CASE

You are a 40-year-old faculty member with a teaching appointment at an academic medical center that trains 12 psychiatry residents per year. In response to resident feedback, you want to create a curriculum in cultural psychiatry.

One of the constant themes from the residents is that they feel they do not get enough exposure to sociocultural issues in psychiatry, which they point out are increasingly important to understand given ongoing discussions of class, race, and religion that dominate the national political discourse and that arise in their clinical work. They describe clinical impasses with patients with whom they feel they cannot relate due to cultural, religious, and other psychosocial differences. While you empathize with their dilemma, you feel overwhelmed when considering how to design and implement a curriculum on topics that may be sensitive, vague, and hard to teach compared to the "bread and butter" topics of psychopharmacology and psychotherapy. You are wary of coming across as "tokenist" or stereotypic in your approach. Compounding this problem, you realize that you received very little teaching on sociocultural psychiatry during your own training.

INTRODUCTION

The U.S. population continues to become increasingly diverse. Census data indicate that ethnic minorities make up about 30% of the population, and demographic trends anticipate that by 2050, racial and ethnic minority populations will account for 90% of the increase in the U.S. population. By 2020, the U.S. Census Bureau reports that over 50% of youth under the age of 18 will be a part of an minority or ethnic group.[1]

The increase in racial, ethnic, and linguistic diversity in the United States offers opportunities for the synthesis of new ideas and the potential for a more accepting society. Unfortunately, there are historical, persistent, and often growing health disparities among racial and ethnic minority groups in the United States. According to the 1999 supplement to "Mental Health: A Report of the Surgeon General," there are significant disparities in mental health services among minorities, who have historically had less access to mental health services than whites, are less likely to receive mental health care, and often receive lower-quality care.[2] The 2003 Institute of Medicine (IOM) report "Unequal Treatment: Confronting Racial and Ethnic Disparities in Healthcare" emphasized the extent of racial and ethnic disparities in medical treatment and disease burden.[3] Racial and ethnic minorities continue to be disproportionately affected by cardiovascular disease, diabetes, HIV/AIDS, cancer, and tuberculosis compared to nonminority patients. Health care providers and organizations are thus faced with addressing the cultural needs and potentially growing health disparities of an increasingly diverse patient population.

Regulatory bodies and health care institutions have responded to this increasing diversity and associated health disparities by mandating efforts to improve cultural competency in health care organizations and in medical education. In 2000, the Office of Minority Health of the U.S. Department of Health and Human Services published the first National Standards on Culturally and Linguistically Appropriate Services for health care organizations to help mitigate health disparities. Among those 14 standards was a recommendation to "Educate and train governance, leadership, and workforce in culturally and linguistically appropriate policies and practices on an ongoing basis."[4]

The need to train medical personnel is not limited to practicing physicians, but also expands to a need to train medical students, residents, and fellows. In their 2003 report, the IOM called for medical education programs to "integrate cross-cultural education into the training of all current and future health professionals."[5] The Liaison Committee for Graduate Medical Education and the Accreditation Council on Graduate Medical Education (ACGME), which are the accrediting bodies for allopathic medical schools and residency and fellowship training programs in the United States, both recognize the need to be sensitive to diversity and have incorporated this tenet into medical education and postgraduate training standards.[6,7]

In psychiatry, the intersection of mental health and diverse societies has been a topic of interest for many years, but only in the last few decades has there been a greater effort to formally integrate culture into professional practice guidelines, clinical assessment, training milestones, and curricula. The American Psychiatric Association (APA) does not publish specific guidelines regarding cultural competence or awareness for practitioners. However, the APA guidelines for Psychiatric Assessment of Adults offer sample questions regarding obtaining sociocultural history (e.g., What are the patient's cultural, religious, and spiritual beliefs, and how have these developed or changed over time?).[8] In 1994, the APA published an Outline for Cultural Formulation (OCF) in the fourth edition of the *Diagnostic and Statistical Manual of Mental Disorders* (DSM-IV). In the most recent edition of the DSM (DSM-5), the outline of the cultural formulation became more operationalized with the creation of the Cultural Formulation Interview (CFI). The CFI comprises 16 questions that should be asked in any patient assessment.

The American Academy of Child and Adolescent Psychiatry has created a Practice Parameter on Cultural Competence in Child and Adolescent Psychiatric Practice that outlines 13 principles for providing clinical care; it addresses health disparities and is culturally sensitive, patient-centered, unbiased, strengths-based, and systems-focused, with a developmental approach.[9]

In addition to professional guidelines and formal assessment tools in culture, psychiatry residencies have incorporated standards for cultural competence in formal evaluations for trainees. The ACGME's Psychiatry Milestones identify the importance of trainees' developing an ability to reflect on their own cultural backgrounds, including how their backgrounds may affect patient interactions and care.[12] Training curricula on a range of special topics, including health disparities; lesbian, gay, bisexual, transgendered, questioning, and allied (LGBTQA) persons; women; Native Americans; Hispanics; Asian Americans; and African Americans, have been published. In particular, the American Association of Directors of Psychiatric Residency Training has published two model curricula on cultural psychiatry from New York University (NYU) and the University of California at Davis.[13,14]

These efforts are a welcome contribution and start to address mental health disparities among racial/ethnic minority groups and the increasingly diverse U.S. population. Nonetheless, much more work remains to be done in order to develop a workforce that is better equipped to address the impact of culture on clinical care and to propagate sociocultural education in medical training and lifelong learning.

This chapter describes the evolution of sociocultural medical education from teaching cultural competence to cultural humility, with its associated opportunities and challenges. Then, using a case-based approach, the chapter will propose general principles that can help psychiatric faculty design and teach sociocultural curricula for psychiatry trainees in diverse settings.

TERMS AND DEFINITIONS

It is helpful to first define the following key terms often found in the literature and used in discussions about cultural education and its goals:

- *Culture:* According to the Office of Minority Health of the U.S. Department of Health and Human Services, culture refers to integrated patterns of human behavior that include the language, thoughts, communications, actions, customs, beliefs, values, and institutions of racial, ethnic, religious, or social groups. Betancourt and colleagues (2013) summarize culture as "an integrated pattern of learned beliefs and behaviors that can be shared among groups and include thoughts, styles of communicating, ways of interacting, views of roles and relationships, values, practices, and customs."[15]
- *Cultural Competence:* "Congruent behaviors, attitudes, and policies that come together in a system, agency, or profession that enables that system, agency, or profession to work effectively in cross-cultural situations."[16]
- *Cultural Humility:* Refers to the health care provider's commitment, active engagement in a lifelong practice of self-evaluation and self-critique within the context of the patient–provider relationship through patient-oriented interviewing and care.[17]

CULTURAL COMPETENCE EDUCATION: INTENTION, DESIGN, AND FLAWS

In the 1990s, cultural competence programs were originally designed to address barriers to care for immigrants, refugees, and those on the sociocultural margin, with the hope of reducing the "cultural gap" between patients and providers.[5] In medical education, teaching cultural competence often focused on teaching about specific cultural groups and their beliefs and illness interpretations.

Cross-cultural education programs have traditionally focused on providing knowledge, attitudes, values, beliefs, and behaviors about specific cultural groups.[15] Dogra (2003) refers to this cultural education as "cultural expertise"—an emphasis on factual information embedded within the biomedical framework.[18] The definition of culture can then be oversimplified as a fixed process that guides behavior in a linear fashion and risks reinforcing stereotypes rather than decreasing cross-cultural misunderstanding.[5] According to Muntinga and colleagues (2016), culture in medical education has been narrowly defined as "ethnicity, nationality, language, and migrant status."[19] Individuals often conflate the terms "ethnicity" and "culture," suggesting that they are equivalent, but they are not: Persons who share an ethnic background may share particular cultural beliefs and behaviors, but a shared ethnic background does not necessarily or invariably predict shared cultural traits.[5] Thus, cultural competence education does not highlight how heterogeneous cultural norms can be, or that many individuals identify with multiple cultural groups/definitions, and these cultures do not always coherently fit together.[5]

For example, the anthropologist Janelle Taylor offers a critique of Anne Fadiman's novel *The Spirit Catches You and You Fall Down*, about the often conflicting interactions between a Hmong refugee family and the health care system in California. She writes that although the book provides one example of how a Hmong family navigates the health system, it presents a static, simplistic notion about Hmong culture. Thus, those who did not act according to "Hmong culture" were viewed as being "American or not being Hmong," an impression that minimizes the heterogeneity in belief systems among those in the same community.[20]

This example highlights that individuals who share the same "culture" (understood as ethnic or immigrant background) might share many beliefs and behaviors, but may also differ based on the fact that they belong to myriad other social identities that significantly shape their unique cultural identity. Other categories that contribute to social identities include gender, race, social class, ethnicity, and religion/spirituality; individual experiences of these roles are contextualized by systems of oppression and privilege. Individuals do not ascribe to only one social identity. However, cultural competence education can oversimplify identity as having a single role (race or ethnicity), which inherently minimizes the interaction of multiple identities.

Intersectionality, a critical strand of diversity theory, aims to analyze human experience beyond single categories of difference.[19] Several authors have suggested that intersectionality can provide a more complex and dynamic framework for diversity teaching in medical education. By analyzing how intersections of multiple sociocultural group memberships influence identity and health, learners can increase their understanding of patients' unique needs and experiences.[19]

MOVING FROM CULTURAL COMPETENCE TO CULTURAL HUMILITY

> *Any understanding of a particular cultural context is always incompletely true, always somewhat out of date and partial.*[5]

The limitations of cultural competence, including oversimplification of cultural norms, the potential for perpetuating stereotypes, a rigid notion of culture and its fluidity, and lack of provider self-awareness on diversity, have contributed to a shift from knowledge-based cultural competence education to promoting cultural humility in medical education. Often the problem is not a lack of knowledge, but rather the need for a change in practitioners' self-awareness and a change in their attitudes toward diverse patients.[17]

The Office of Minority Health of the U.S. Department of Health and Human Services distinguishes cultural humility from cultural competence based on the dynamic and contextual relationship between patient and provider. Cultural competence is defined as "having the capacity to function effectively within the realm of cultural beliefs, behaviors, and needs presented by the consumer and their communities."[16] In contrast, cultural humility "incorporates a health provider's commitment and active engagement in a lifelong practice of self-evaluation and self-critique within the context of the patient–provider (or health professional) relationship through patient-oriented interviewing and care."[17] Cultural humility is not an achieved destination, but rather a lifelong endeavor that requires sustained dedication to active engagement with patients, communities, colleagues and themselves.[17]

TEACHING CULTURAL HUMILITY

Cross-cultural training in medical education historically has comprised three conceptual approaches: knowledge, skills, and attitudes. Teaching cultural humility involves learning beyond the "facts" and emphasizes enhancing awareness and attitudes, while still teaching skills and learning relevant content. Cultural humility emphasizes communication skills, particularly learning how to communicate with patients and how to act on the information obtained and formulated. Learning to communicate better with patients and understanding their perspectives of illness are essential to providing good patient care for all patients, regardless of their cultural background.[5] Improving communication skills, however, requires cultivating a "critical consciousness" to reflect on one's norms, values, and positions, with their associated contexts, and understanding how systematic social structures determine and sustain differences in health outcomes.[19]

Providers can increase their self-awareness by reflecting on their own cultural and social identities, personal histories, biases, and assumptions to understand how their backgrounds may impact a clinical encounter.[21] Betancourt writes that first- and second-year medical students should engage in a process of reflection that explores the impact of racism, sexism, and classism on the provider's and patient's culture, and how these may influence clinical outcomes.[15]

Teaching cultural humility in medical education offers opportunities to mitigate health disparities and to deliver quality health care to an increasingly diverse patient population. Despite these opportunities, teaching culture is a challenging topic given its tremendous scope and complexity, and the heterogeneity among individuals who share a similar cultural background. In the face of these challenges, faculty may find themselves wanting to incorporate cultural humility into the psychiatric curriculum, but struggle with the actual implementation.

GUIDING PRINCIPLES FOR IMPLEMENTING A SOCIOCULTURAL PSYCHIATRY CURRICULUM

Designing a sociocultural psychiatric curriculum can be overwhelming because the definition of culture is so broad. Additionally, due to the heterogeneity, contradictions, and complexity in human behavior, teaching about particular subgroups' cultural realities can be reductive and may risk stereotyping. Thus, determining what and how to teach in cultural psychiatry is challenging. In collaboration with the Group for the Advancement of Psychiatry's Cultural Committee, Hansen completed 20 interviews with culture and psychiatry instructors in residency programs across the United States assessing nationwide best practices with regard to teaching culture[13] and recommended these strategies:

- Course content should reflect the local and specific needs of the patient populations served.
- Cultural self-awareness on the part of residents, including awareness of the professional culture of biomedicine, is important in improving communication in the clinical encounter.
- Residents should be involved in developing curricula on culture, as they may have more experience in sociocultural theory than attendings.
- Engagement with community-based organizations as part of the training provides residents with a broader set of culturally sensitive approaches to working with patients.
- Curricular processes and outcomes should be evaluated regularly to continue to develop the curricula over time.

The modalities of teaching cultural humility and addressing issues of bias and discrimination in the clinical encounter should not be viewed as an entirely separate entity from the rest of the field of medical education. Malcolm Knowles' seven principles of adult learning continue to apply to teaching cultural psychiatry:

1. Establish an effective learning climate, where learners feel safe and comfortable expressing themselves.
2. Involve learners in mutual planning of relevant methods and curricular content.
3. Involve learners in diagnosing their own needs—this will help to trigger internal motivation.
4. Encourage learners to formulate their own learning objectives—this gives them more control of their learning.
5. Encourage learners to identify resources and devise strategies for using the resources to achieve their objectives.

6. Support learners in carrying out their learning plans.
7. Involve learners in evaluating their own learning to help develop their skills of critical reflection.[23]

When designing and implementing a sociocultural psychiatric curriculum, these guiding principles can help frame the attitudes, skills, and knowledge that we are trying to teach.

Creating a Holding Environment

The opening case raises questions about the type of curriculum the faculty member is hoping to create. Is the curriculum designed for a longitudinal program integrated into the entire duration of a training program? Or is it limited to a series of individual classes for a particular group of trainees? When designing a curriculum, it is also important to embed and/or consider one's method of teaching, a primary vehicle for bringing meaning, relevance, and utility to the material.

Regardless of the scope of the curriculum, creating a "safe space" or a "holding environment" is the essential first step for effectively discussing matters of culture and diversity.[23] A safe space cultivates rapport, safety, and trust. A "holding environment" mirrors the atmosphere that one hopes to create in a clinical encounter. The instructor can create this by using therapeutic techniques such as recognizing and welcoming different meanings, validating varying voices, tolerating uncertainty, encouraging narrative co-construction, engaging in countertransference issues, and encouraging clinicians to recognize the limitations of their knowledge.[23] One way to encourage vulnerability and courageous discussion regarding issues of diversity is for the course instructors to introduce how they became interested in the topic of cultural psychiatry, and what it means for them professionally and personally.

Shifting Attitudes

The tripartite model in curriculum design has often been categorized as knowledge, skills, and attitudes. Teaching cultural humility emphasizes gaining awareness while continuing to teach skills and relevant content. It does not mean that one teaches just one of the three areas without the others. Cultural humility emphasizes communication skills, which requires an awareness to reflect on one's values and belief systems. As noted above, the literature suggests that providers can increase their self-awareness by reflecting on their background and how it could affect a clinical encounter.[21]

For general psychiatry training programs, the University of California Davis School of Medicine published *A Four-Year Model Curriculum on Culture, Gender, LGBT, Religion and Spirituality for General Psychiatry Training Programs*.[14] It outlines various objectives in each of the three categories (awareness, knowledge, and skills) at each level of training, from PGY-1 to PGY-4. For instance, one of the objectives in the first year of adult psychiatry training is to understand one's own cultural identity. In small groups, first-year psychiatry trainees are asked to answer the following questions in a Cultural Identity Awareness Exercise:

1. What is your cultural identity?
2. What was your first experience with feeling different?
3. What is your ethnic background?
4. What has it meant to belong to your ethnic group?
5. How has it felt to belong to your ethnic group?
6. What do you like about your ethnic identity?
7. What do you dislike?
8. What are your feelings about being white or a person of color?
9. How do you think others feel?

The questions ask residents to reflect on topics ranging from cultural identity to ethnicity and race. The first question broadly asks residents about their cultural identity, asking them to define what cultural identity means. Depending on the discussion, the instructor can question the participants about how they define cultural identity, highlighting potential narrow definitions of culture. The subsequent questions, particularly the ones regarding experiences of feeling different, aspects of one's ethnicity one dislikes, and feelings about one's race, have the potential to evoke discomfort, shame, and possibly pain—underscoring the need to create a safe or a holding environment so that residents feel comfortable expressing these narratives. However, helping residents tolerate their own discomfort and vulnerability may help them better empathize with patients' cultural experiences.

Using an auto-ethnography or Kliman's Social Matrix Wheel can help residents generate greater awareness about their own values and beliefs. An auto-ethnography is a qualitative research method in which the author engages in a personal reflection to connect his or her autobiographical narrative to a broader cultural, political, and social meanings. The Social Matrix Wheel (Figure 14.1) can help trainees identify the diversity of privilege and how one's privilege and power can change depending on one's context. The matrix features 33 domains of social identity or group membership that intersect with seven concentric circles indicating degree of privilege (centrality) or marginalization (outer circles). Participants plot their sense of marginalization in each of these domains along one of the seven circles, with the center indicating the greatest centrality (privilege) and each outer circle representing larger degree of marginalization.[24]

Developing Skills

Becoming aware of one's own values and beliefs related to the impact of cultural factors on clinical care is a vital component of developing one's self-reflective capacity. However, physicians early in training want to develop skills in understanding cultural explanatory models of illness, stress, coping, help-seeking behavior, and the impact of culture on issues of transference and countertransference in the clinical encounter. Incorporating the CFI in the curriculum can help residents practice culturally aware interview techniques that can be applied to all patients. The conceptualization and operationalization of cultural factors in psychiatric treatment in DSM-5 is explored more fully in Chapter 3. Here we will summarize the main areas that are relevant to educators seeking to incorporate sociocultural psychiatry topics into a curriculum.

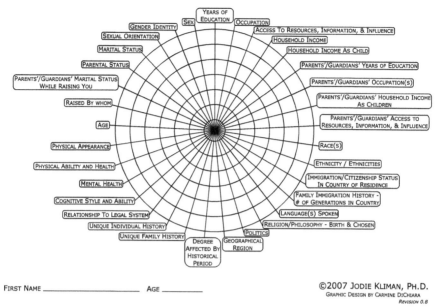

Figure 14.1 Intersecting Domains of Privilege and Marginalization: Locating Oneself in a Social Matrix.
Reproduced with permission from Kliman J. Intersections of social privilege and marginalization: a visual teaching tool. In: *Expanding Our Social Justice Practices: Advances in Theory and Training*. AFTA Monograph Series: A Publication of the American Family Therapy Academy. 2010;6:39–48.

In the early 1990s, the OCF was incorporated into DSM-IV, thereby recognized the importance of culture in clinical practice. However, the OCF was not an operationalized set of questions. Nearly two decades later, the CFI has been developed into a 16-question interview with 12 supplemental modules. Among the topics addressed in the 16 questions are the cultural definition of the problem; cultural perceptions of cause, context, and support (subsections: stressors and support and role of cultural identity); cultural factors affecting self-coping and past help-seeking (subsections: self-coping, past help-seeking, and barriers); and cultural factors affecting current help-seeking (subsections: preferences and clinician–patient relationship).

The CFI is a helpful set of interview questions to enhance cultured meanings in a clinical encounter, but it is not a structured diagnostic interview. Interviewers can ask questions from the 12 supplemental modules to obtain a more comprehensive cultural assessment. The first eight supplementary modules inquire in greater depth about the domains of the core CFI (i.e., explanatory model, level of functioning, social network, psychosocial stressors, spirituality, cultural identity, coping and help-seeking, and the patient–physician relationship). The next three modules focus on specific populations (children and adolescents, older adults, and immigrants and refugees). The last module further explores the cultural experiences of caregivers to assess how caregiving affects social support in the patient's immediate environment.[26]

TEACHING THE CFI

The Cultural Consultation Service (CCS) at McGill's Division of Social and Cultural Psychiatry can offer a framework in teaching the CFI.[25] The CCS model provides specialized consultation when "care as usual" is not sufficient, and difficulties with intervention may be related to social and cultural issues. In the CCS, child psychiatry trainees and allied professionals are involved in a two-part model. First, the trainee participates in a family interview with a supervisor and possibly an interpreter and/ or cultural broker (a person who has comprehensive knowledge of the family's cultural background), observing how the supervisor introduces cultural dimensions into the interview. Second, the trainee participates in a multidisciplinary setting to share the formulation and refine how to present the information obtained to the primary clinical service requesting the consultation.

Most training programs in the United States do not have a cultural consultation service, but in a structured teaching setting, residents could role-play interviewing patients using the CFI, paying attention to how the "interviewer" introduces or makes transitions in the CFI. The role-play can also help the trainee practice obtaining relevant cultural information that can be incorporated into not only a cultural clinical formulatioh, but also a bio-psycho-social formulation.

Teaching Content

Knowing what content to teach in a cultural psychiatric curriculum can be daunting given the breadth and scope of cultural topics, such as race, ethnicity, spirituality, religion, gender, gender identity, sexuality, bias, and discrimination. As indicated in the NYU model curriculum, the content should reflect the local needs and problems of the community that providers are serving. Thus, course directors of a cultural psychiatry curriculum should obtain local or national epidemiological data about demographic changes, disease prevalence, culture-bound syndromes, and strategies for improving the care of diverse populations within a health system.

Both the NYU and UC Davis model curricula incorporate epidemiological and health disparities data. Based on Knowles' adult learning theory principles, engaging trainees in designing course content and assessing their learning goals can help instructors tailor content to the learners' needs. Residents are self-directed learners and can be co-teachers; many have had a great deal of exposure to these topics in their own educations and life experiences, and some may have had formal training in anthropology, sociology, and psychology. Residents may be very helpful when designing the content for a cultural psychiatric course.

Alternative Ways of Teaching

Teaching about the implications of culture on clinical encounters does not have to be limited to the formal teaching curricula. Given the current sociopolitical environment, communities are faced with increased division and a questioning of our collective identity that may impact clinical encounters. Creating forums for providers to gather and share their reflections on the impact of current events on the physician–patient relationship promotes greater self-reflection and a space for providers to process how their personal identity may interface with clinical interactions. Analyzing editorials written by physicians who have encountered clinical situations where they have faced discrimination or have had their personal identity and integrity questioned can help spark this discussion.[27,28]

Voluntary and open forums offer an invitation for reflection but may serve a self-selected audience. Organizing community visits and tours of neighborhoods, schools, local markets, parks, and playgrounds for all trainees in the cultural psychiatric course can provide trainees with a small window into the lives of their patients. Although the formal course curricula can set the stage for generating awareness, building skills, and learning content, creating training partnerships with community health centers can expand residents' direct experience with local cross-cultural issues. Many racial/ethnic minority patients obtain health care from community health centers, which have often found innovative ways to serve their patients with limited resources, including embedding bilingual/bicultural social workers as both therapists and cultural brokers in the clinical encounter.[29] Residency programs can thus make rotations at community health centers mandatory as part of the cultural psychiatric clinical curriculum.

In addition to creating a formal didactic curriculum in cultural psychiatry, there are alternative ways to bring attention to the role of culture in psychiatric encounters. For instance, a program can offer monthly case conferences dedicated to discussions regarding special topics such as race, ethnicity, asylum cases, refugees, sexuality, gender, and religion/spirituality. Programs can also incorporate cultural grand rounds where invited speakers can present on current matters related to cultural psychiatry, sociology, and anthropology.

REVISITING THE CASE

The faculty member in this case faces a common challenge about how to best incorporate complex sociocultural teaching into an already saturated psychiatric curriculum. Although there is no "one size fits all" approach to curricular design, the following steps provide a sample approach.

The faculty member could gather residents' feedback regarding the need for sociocultural psychiatry teaching in the formal curriculum and present it to members of the residency administration responsible for training and education. Depending on availability, the faculty member could petition for a longitudinal series spanning multiple years of psychiatric residency training. Following the example of our authors' institutions (JAC and PS) as well as Hansen's recommendations, a curricular "content team" or working group could be assembled consisting of interested faculty and a selected number of residents with a passion for this topic. This content team would meet and discuss the background, needs, and preferences of trainees at their institution to help guide the content, breadth, and depth of the curriculum.

Following Betancourt's recommendation, didactics during the earliest years of training could focus on a process of reflection that explores residents' cultural identities and influences, for example using the Cultural Identity Awareness Exercise described in the UC Davis model curriculum or Kliman's Social Matrix Wheel. This conversation will likely begin to touch on potentially sensitive topics such as privilege, racism, and identity; therefore faculty should endeavor to create a safe, holding, and nonjudgmental environment that encourages vulnerability and personal disclosure, and that specifically attempts to avoid shaming any particular set of beliefs. Such activities could be supplemented by discussions of topical lay press articles relating to cultural or personal identity characteristics that could impact the clinical encounter, as well as a discussion regarding differences between the cultures of internal medicine, psychiatry, neurology, and other hospital-based disciplines to which learners are being exposed daily. Residents should be encouraged to bring their own experiences and cases to these sessions.

We have found that learners in the PGY-2 stage of training, struggling to consolidate their identities as psychiatrists rather than general medical professionals, are often eager to learn discrete skills and knowledge as it relates to their chosen field. Therefore, this year of sociocultural didactics may focus more on content knowledge, with topics including local, national, or global psychiatric epidemiology, health disparities, culture-bound syndromes, and teaching the DSM-5 CFI.

By the time residents have reached their PGY-3 and PGY-4 years, they have a more sophisticated understanding of the dilemmas and limits of the practicing psychiatrist. Thus, more advanced topics can be introduced at this point, including the role of religion and spirituality in clinical care, ambiguous concepts of what is considered normal and abnormal in psychiatry as they relate to deeply personal topics such as sexuality, patient–provider matching, and clinical impasses. Many of the other chapters in this textbook offer examples of fruitful topics for discussion during this year of training, for example discussing the ethical, personal, and professional dilemmas that might arise when a patient's family requests a doctor of a different race (see Chapter 12).

Box 14.1 outlines a general format and guideline to creating a formal sociocultural psychiatric curriculum. Of course, sociocultural education does not have to be limited to a course. In line with Hansen's recommendation to include residents' experiences, at the institution of one of the authors (PS), an annual retreat for trainees from the departments of psychiatry, child psychiatry, social work, and psychology is held to discuss how their personal cultural experiences and identities influence clinical encounters and professional development. The retreat was developed by trainees with faculty and institutional support. Unlike in a formal course, the retreat offers an opportunity for trainees from multiple disciplines, at different levels in training, to convene and to share the complex intersection of personal identities with those of a trainee, a clinician, and a citizen in a larger sociopolitical context. The faculty member could assess, through a survey or with a "content team," trainees' interest in developing a retreat and, depending on the level of support from the trainees, approach the residency program for financial support.

Although trainees are exposed to sociocultural psychiatric education, faculty may not receive similar training, which can lead to inconsistency and a lack of cultural humility in clinical practice, potentially leaving residents feeling that their newly gained sociocultural knowledge has been invalidated. Thus, the faculty member could also consider creating a series of continuing education workshops featuring aspects from the PGY-1 through PGY-4 sociocultural curriculum for teaching faculty. Finally, the faculty member leader must endeavor to practice and embody the tenets of cultural humility in his or her attitude and approach to teaching, knowing

Box 14.1

APPROACH TO DESIGNING SOCIOCULTURAL PSYCHIATRIC CURRICULUM

1. Create a working group with interested trainees and faculty.
2. Work with the training program's educational committee to determine the length of the course: Is this a longitudinal course or a course in a particular training year? If time is not available for an actual course, consider a case conference, journal club or grand rounds on cultural psychiatry.
3. Assess trainees' areas of interests in sociocultural psychiatry through an internal program survey.
4. Assess the cultural needs of the patient population served in the local community through an internal hospital system survey or informal focus groups.
5. Create a list of topics based on the input of trainees and the community that the health care system serves.
6. Determine the course objectives for domains of awareness, knowledge, and skills.
7. Plan instruction, thinking about how to make the learning relevant to trainees and to create active learning.
8. Create an evaluation form assessing how well objectives were met and ways the course could be improved.

that the process of learning and teaching sociocultural issues is indeed a lifelong endeavor.

CONCLUSION

The U.S. psychiatric workforce must enhance medical training and education in order to meet the increasingly diverse cultural needs of patients and providers. Medical education is moving away from cultural competence to teaching cultural humility, a lifelong inquiry into understanding one's own relationship to people from different backgrounds. While this is an admirable goal, it is also more complicated than prior approaches emphasizing teaching discrete facts. Promoting greater reflection requires faculty leaders to alter the psychiatric curriculum to provide more opportunities for trainees to critically appraise themselves in relation to clinical encounters and a larger sociopolitical context. Nonetheless, an emphasis on cultural awareness does not mean that we can neglect to teach specific skills and content related to culture, diversity, and health disparities; these elements must continue to be present within the curriculum. Curriculum design should involve trainees and should reflect the needs of the local community. Faculty should view their role as leaders who can advocate for making space within the overall curriculum to deepen the conversation about diversity, with the ultimate goal of better serving our increasingly diverse patient populations.

REFERENCES

1. It's official: the U.S. is becoming a minority-majority nation. *US News & World Report*. Retrieved from https://www.usnews.com/news/articles/2015/07/06/its-official-the-us-is-becoming-a-minority-majority-nation; accessed November 12, 2017.

2. U.S. Department of Health and Human Services, Public Health Service, Office of the Surgeon General. *Mental Health: A Report of the Surgeon General*. 1999. Retrieved from https://profiles.nlm.nih.gov/ps/retrieve/ResourceMetadata/NNBBHS

3. Shaya FT, Gbarayor CM. The case for cultural competence in health professions education. *Am J Pharm Educ*. 2006;70(6):124.

4. National Standards for Culturally and Linguistically Appropriate Services (CLAS) in Health and Health Care. Think Cultural Health. Retrieved from https://www.thinkculturalhealth.hhs.gov/; accessed November 12, 2017.

5. Gregg J, Saha S. Losing culture on the way to competence: the use and misuse of culture in medical education. *Acad Med*. 2006;81(6):542–547.

6. Liaison Committee on Medical Education. Full text of LCME Accreditation Standards. Retrieved from http://www.lcme.org/stnd-text.htm#educationalprogram

7. Swing SR. The ACGME outcome project: retrospective and prospective. *Med Teach*. 2007;29(7):648–654.

8. American Psychiatric Association. *The American Psychiatric Association Practice Guidelines for the Psychiatric Evaluation of Adults*, 3rd ed. Washington, DC: American Psychiatric Publishing; 2015.

9. Pumariega AJ, Rothe E, Mian A, et al. Practice parameter for cultural competence in child and adolescent psychiatric practice. *J Am Acad Child Adolesc Psychiatry*. 2013;52(10):1101–1115.

10. American Psychiatric Association. Outline for Cultural Formulation. In: *Diagnostic and Statistical Manual of Mental Disorders*, 4th ed. Washington, DC: American Psychiatric Association; 1994.

11. Lewis-Fernández R, Aggarwal NK, Hinton L, et al. *DSM-5 Handbook on the Cultural Formulation Interview*. Arlington, VA: American Psychiatric Publishing Inc.; 2015.

12. Accreditation Council for Graduate Medical Education. The Psychiatry Milestone Project. July 2015. Retrieved from https://www.acgme.org/Portals/0/PDFs/Milestones/PsychiatryMilestones.pdf

13. Levin Z, Caligor E. Culture and psychiatry: a course for third-year psychiatry residents. NYU Medical Center Psychiatry Residency Training Program, Cultural Psychiatry Model Curriculum Nomination. 2010. Retrieved from https://nyculturalcompetence.org/; accessed May 25, 2018.

14. Lim R. A four-year model curriculum on culture, gender, LGBT, religion, and spirituality for general psychiatry residency training programs in the United States. University of California at Davis. Retrieved from http://www.academia.edu/765843/A_Four-Year_Model_Curriculum_on_Culture_Gender_LGBT_Religion_and_Spirituality_for_General_Psychiatry_Residency_Training_Programs_in_the_United_States; accessed November 12, 2017.

15. Betancourt JR. Cross-cultural medical education: conceptual approaches and frameworks for evaluation. *Acad Med*. 2003;78(6):560–569.

16. Cross TL, Bazron BJ, Dennis KW, Isaacs MR. *Towards a Culturally Competent System of Care: A Monograph on Effective Services for Minority Children Who Are Severely*

Emotionally Disturbed. Washington, DC: CASSP Technical Assistance Center, Georgetown University Child Development Center; 1989.

17. Tervalon M, Murray-García J. Cultural humility versus cultural competence: a critical distinction in defining physician training outcomes in multicultural education. *J Health Care Poor Underserved*. 1998;9(2):117–125.

18. Dogra N. Cultural expertise or cultural sensibility? A comparison of two ideal type models to teach cultural diversity. *Int J Med*. 2003;5(4):223–231.

19. Muntinga ME, Krajenbrink VQE, Peerdeman SM, et al. Toward diversity-responsive medical education: taking an intersectionality-based approach to a curriculum evaluation. *Adv Health Sci Educ*. 2016;21(3):541–559.

20. Taylor JS. The story catches you and you fall down: tragedy, ethnography, and "cultural competence." *Med Anthropol Q*. 2003;17(2):159–181.

21. Kirmayer LJ. Rethinking cultural competence. *Transcult Psychiatry*. 2012;49(2): 149–164.

22. Kaufman DM. Applying educational theory in practice. *BMJ*. 2003;326(7382):213–216.

23. Willen SS, Carpenter-Song E. Cultural competence in action: "lifting the hood" on four case studies in medical education. *Culture Med Psychiatry*. 2013;37(2):241–252.

24. Kliman J. Intersections of social privilege and marginalization: a visual teaching tool. In: *Expanding Our Social Justice Practices: Advances in Theory and Training*. AFTA Monograph Series: A Publication of the American Family Therapy Academy. 2010;6:39–48.

25. Rousseau C, Guzder J. Teaching cultural formulation. *J Am Acad Child Adolesc Psychiatry*. 2015;54(8):611–612.

26. Lewis-Fernández R, Aggarwal NK, Hinton L, et al. Supplementary Modules. In: *DSM-5 Handbook on the Cultural Formulation Interview*. Arlington, VA: American Psychiatric Publishing Inc.; 2015.

27. https://www.statnews.com/2017/10/18/patient-prejudice-wounds-doctors/

28. http://www.wbur.org/commonhealth/2016/01/08/hospital-bigotry-opinion

29. Lokko HN, Chen JA, Parekh RI, Stern TA. Racial and ethnic diversity in the US psychiatric workforce: a perspective and recommendations. *Acad Psychiatry*. 2016;40(6):898–904.

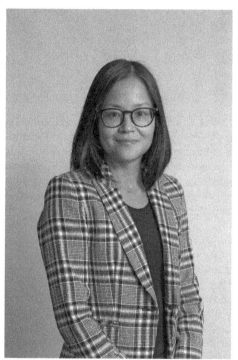

Nhi-Ha T. Trinh, MD, MPH, serves as Director for the MGH Department of Psychiatry Center for Diversity as well as the Director of Multicultural Studies and the Director of Clinical Services at the MGH Depression Clinical and Research Program. As Assistant Professor of Psychiatry at Harvard Medical School and Associate Director, HMS Holmes Society, she is committed to medical student and psychiatry resident education and mentorship. Her academic work focuses on sociocultural issues in psychiatry, and she shares her passion for this topic as course Co-Director of the MGH/ McLean Residency Sociocultural Curriculum. Dr. Trinh earned her medical degree at the University of California, San Francisco and her Master of Public Health at the University of California at Berkeley, specializing in epidemiology. She completed residency training in Adult Psychiatry at the Mass General/McLean Adult Psychiatry Training Program and a fellowship in Geriatric Psychiatry at McLean Hospital.

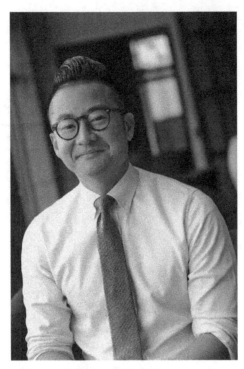

Justin A. Chen, MD, MPH, is Medical Director of Ambulatory Psychiatry and Co-Director of Primary Care Psychiatry at Massachusetts General Hospital. His interests include cross-cultural psychiatry, stigma, racial/ethnic disparities in mental health service utilization, and medical education. He is dedicated to teaching and mentorship, serving as Associate Director of Medical Student Education in Psychiatry at Harvard Medical School, as a Training Mentor and Co-Director of the longitudinal Sociocultural Psychiatry curriculum for MGH/McLean psychiatry residents, and as an Assistant Professor at Harvard Medical School. As Executive Director and Co-Founder of the MGH Center for Cross-Cultural Student Emotional Wellness, a nonprofit consortium of clinicians, educators and researchers, he delivers talks and trainings for families, clinicians, and educators throughout the United States on promoting the emotional health and psychological resilience of diverse student populations. Dr. Chen received his undergraduate and medical degrees from Yale University. He completed his residency in adult psychiatry at MGH/McLean followed by a Master of Public Health degree in Clinical Effectiveness at the Harvard-T.H. Chan School of Public Health and a Dupont-Warren Research Fellowship focused on improving engagement of depressed Chinese immigrants into mental health care at South Cove Community Health Center.

Page numbers followed by t, f *or* b *refer to tables, figures, and boxes on respective pages.*